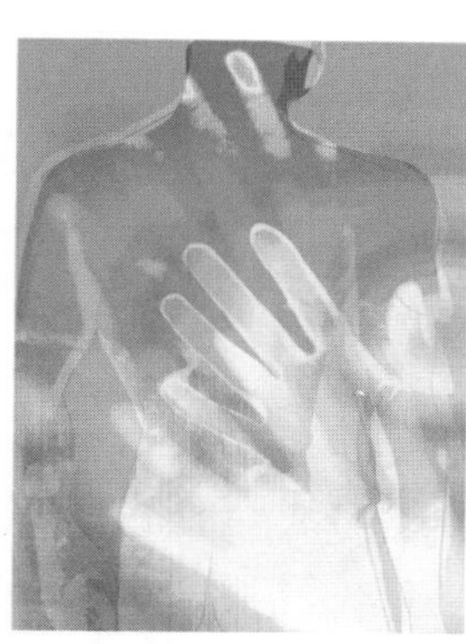

lifestyle medicine

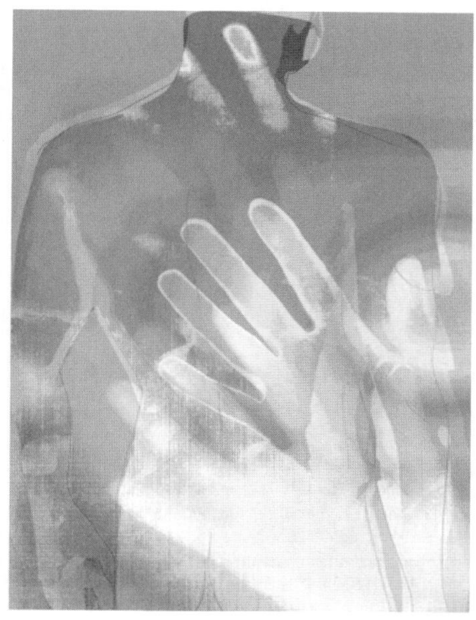

lifestyle medicine

GARRY EGGER, ANDREW BINNS AND STEPHAN ROSSNER

The McGraw·Hill Companies

Sydney New York San Francisco Auckland
Bangkok Bogotá Caracas Hong Kong
Kuala Lumpur Lisbon London Madrid
Mexico City Milan New Delhi San Juan
Seoul Singapore Taipei Toronto

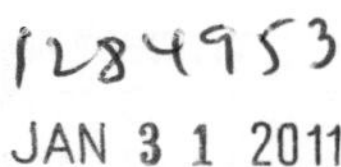

The McGraw-Hill Companies

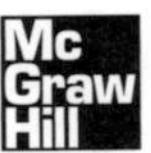

Notice

Medicine is an ever-changing science. As new research and clinical experience broaden our knowledge, changes in treatment and drug therapy are required. The editors and the publisher of this work have checked with sources believed to be reliable in their efforts to provide information that is complete and generally in accord with the standards accepted at the time of publication. However, in view of the possibility of human error or changes in medical sciences, neither the editors, nor the publisher, nor any other party who has been involved in the preparation or publication of this work warrants that the information contained herein is in every respect accurate or complete. Readers are encouraged to confirm the information contained herein with other sources. For example, and in particular, readers are advised to check the product information sheet included in the package of each drug they plan to administer to be certain that the information contained in this book is accurate and that changes have not been made in the recommended dose or in the contraindications for administration. This recommendation is of particular importance in connection with new or infrequently used drugs.

First published 2008

National Library of Australia Cataloguing-in-Publication Data

Egger, Garry.
Lifestyle medicine.

Includes index.
ISBN 9780070138179 (pbk.).

1. Medicine, Preventive. 2. Health promotion. 3. Health behaviour. I. Binns, Andrew, (Andrew Frederick). II. Rossner, Stephan. III. Title.

613

Published in Australia by

McGraw-Hill Australia Pty Ltd
Level 2, 82 Waterloo Road, North Ryde NSW 2113

Publisher **Nicole Meehan**
Associate Editor **Hollie Zondanos**
Managing Editor **Kathryn Fairfax**
Manager, Rights and Permissions **Philip Millard**
Production Editor **Nicole McKenzie**
Copy Editor **Kathy Kramar**
Cover design **Patricia McCallum**
Internal design **Natalie Bowra**
Illustrator **Alan Laver**
Typesetter **Aptara Inc., New Delhi, India**
Proofreader **Terry Townsend**
Indexer **Mary Coe**
Cartoonist **Suzanne Plater**
Printed in **China on 80 gsm woodfree by 1010 Printing International Ltd**

To Leigh and Tyler

The only commandment is to do your best with what you were given, while not hurting anyone.

brief contents

contents

about the authors

Professor Garry Egger MPH PhD MAPs is the Director of the Centre for Health Promotion and Research in Sydney and Adjunct Professor in Lifestyle Medicine at Southern Cross University in Lismore. He has worked in clinical and public health since 1972 and has been a consultant to the World Health Organization, industry, and several government organisations, as well as being involved in medical and allied health education. He is the author of twenty-five books, over a hundred scientific articles, and numerous popular press articles and has made numerous media appearances.

Dr Andrew Binns AM BSc MBBS DRCOG DA FACRRM is a general practitioner in Lismore in rural NSW. He has a special interest in lifestyle medicine and its relevance to primary care. He is Adjunct Professor with the Division of Health and Applied Sciences, Lismore Campus, Southern Cross University. He is also medical editor of GP *Speak*, a bi-monthly magazine for the Northern Rivers General Practice Network.

Professor Stephan Rossner MD PhD is Professor of Health Behavior Research at the Karolinska Institute in Stockholm and Director of the Obesity Unit at the Karolinska University Hospital. He has worked with international obesity-related matters for more than twenty years and served as the Secretary, Vice-President, and President of the International Association for the Study of Obesity (IASO). He has published more than 500 scientific articles on nutrition and lifestyle-related matters, written more than twenty books for the lay press, appeared repeatedly in media, and promoted health as a stand-up comedian in 'science theatre'.

about the co-authors

Dr Mike Climstein PhD FASMF FACSM FAAESS DE is a clinical exercise physiologist, Director of Chronic Disease Rehabilitation at Freshwater Rehabilitation (one of Australia's largest community rehabilitation programs), and Director of Diabetes Rehabilitation at the Vale Medical Clinic. Mike is Adjunct Clinical Associate Professor with the Faculty of Health Sciences, Australian Catholic University (NSW). He is also on the editorial board for the *Australian Journal of Science and Medicine in Sport* and a columnist for 'Research Reviews' in the *Australian Fitness Network* magazine.

Dr Maximilian de Courten MD MPH (Univ Basel, Switzerland) is Associate Professor of Clinical Epidemiology with Monash University in Melbourne. His medical education started in Switzerland where he undertook clinical research in the area of hypertension and insulin resistance. In the U.S. he worked at the National Institutes of Health on diabetes. His international experience was enhanced through positions at the World Health Organization as a scientist at HQ and a Medical Officer, Chronic Disease Control, for the South Pacific.

Rosanne Coutts BHM ExSci (Hons) AEp Sp MAAESS is an accredited exercise physiologist and sports scientist. She is a member of the Australian Psychological Society and lectures at Southern Cross University in sport and exercise psychology. Her interests include the support of a lifestyle approach to the enhancement of health and wellbeing. She also coordinates the Exercise Physiology Clinic within the School of Health and Human Sciences at Southern Cross University.

Professor Rob Donovan PhD (Psychology) is Professor of Behavioural Research at the Centre for Behavioural Research in Cancer Control in the Division of Health Sciences at Curtin University and Professor of Social Marketing and Director of the Social Marketing Research Unit in the Curtin Business School. Current interests include regulation of the marketing of 'sin' products, mental health promotion, racism, violence against women, Indigenous issues, and doping in sport.

Dr David Colqhoun MBBS FRACP is a consultant cardiologist at the Wesley Medical Centre in Brisbane and Associate Professor of Medicine at the University of Queensland. He is also actively involved in research in national and international trials and is currently the coordinator of the SCOUT trial for Australia. His areas of interest are lipids and dietary management in metabolic disease and the role of psychological factors in coronary heart disease.

Dr Bernadette Drummond BDS MS PhD FRACDS is a specialist in and Associate Professor of Paediatric Dentistry in the Faculty of Dentistry at the University of Otago in Dunedin. She is an active clinician, teacher, and researcher with a particular interest in understanding and preventing dental problems in young people.

Dr Michael Gillman MBBS FRACGP is the Director of the Brisbane Health Institute for Men. He has worked in the area of men's health for over fifteen years and sits on several national advisory boards concerned with male sexual health. He has given presentations extensively throughout Australia and internationally to medical and community groups, has a regular state-wide radio talkback segment, and is actively involved in clinical work and clinical research.

Dr Julian Henwood BSc PhD is a medical writer and Managing Director of PharmaView, a medical education agency based in Sydney. He trained as a pharmacologist in the U.K. and has spent twenty years researching and writing about drugs. He has written for independent international publications aimed at specialists (e.g. the journal Drugs) or at general practitioners (e.g. the monthly magazine Medical Progress), as well as on numerous publications supported by the pharmaceutical industry.

Dr Neil King BSc PhD is Senior Lecturer at Queensland University of Technology in Brisbane. He is an expert on the relationships between physical activity, appetite control, and energy balance. He has published extensively on physical activity, diet, and obesity.

Dr John Litt MBBS Dip RACOG MSc (Epid) FRACGP FAFPHM PhD is an academic general practitioner and public health physician at Flinders University in Adelaide. He is also the Deputy Chair of the Royal Australian College of General Practitioners National Quality Committee. He has been involved in prevention research and teaching for fifteen years and was a key contributor to the RACGP monograph Guidelines for prevention in general practice. He has been involved in running lifestyle intervention workshops for many years.

Dr Joanna McMillan Price BSc (Hons) PhD is a nutrition scientist and fitness leader, based in Sydney. She is a popular media spokesperson, appearing regularly on the Today show, a health writer for Life etc magazine, and an author of several nutrition books. Her PhD looked at the role of the glycaemic index and protein intake in weight loss, body composition, and cardiovascular disease risk.

Barbara O'Toole RN BBus (Econ) Intensive Care Certificate Cert IV Assessment and Workplace Training has worked as an independent consultant/contractor to general practice for the past six years both at practice and Division levels. She has a special interest in diabetes and is currently completing a Graduate Certificate in Diabetes Education and Management. For the past eighteen months she has been directly involved in the provision of chronic disease management (CDM) services to practices as well as being engaged in educating doctors and nursing staff on the effective implementation of EPC and CDM programs in general practice.

Dr Hugh F. Molloy MRCS (Eng) LRCP (Lond) DObst RCOG (Lond) DDM (Syd) FACD is a retired Sydney dermatologist. He began his medical career as a GP in the U.K., before becoming a surgeon at sea. He then moved to Australia where he trained and practiced in dermatology. In the 1980s, he spent time in Oxford investigating the effects of overheating, especially at night in bed using doonas (douvets). He has a particular interest in the effects of the local environment on skin and general body functions.

Suzanne Pearson BBiolSc (Hons) MNutrDiet is a practicing dietitian and postgraduate student, based at the University of Sydney and studying weight control practices.

Dr Robert Reznik MBBS MPH MSc MD FAFPHM FRANZCP is a consultant psychiatrist in private practice in Sydney. He also works as a consultant psychiatrist for a rural area of NSW, is part of the chronic pain management team at the Prince of Wales Private Hospital, and is a Senior Forensic Psychiatrist for Justice Health within NSW Correctional Services. He was previously the Director of Community Medicine at Royal Prince Alfred Hospital and part of the WHO Collaborative Centre for Early Intervention for Alcohol Abuse at Royal Prince Alfred Hospital and had a major interest in the effects of cardiovascular disease in the community.

Dr Caroline West Warne MBBS specialises in healthy lifestyle medicine. Her areas of interest include preventative health, weight management, smoking cessation, mental wellbeing, and sleep medicine. She combines her clinical work in a busy Sydney city medical practice with her role in the media. She is a well-known print and television health journalist and her credits include presenting for the television shows *Beyond Tomorrow, Beyond 2000,* and *Good Medicine.*

Dr Kevin Wolfenden PHD MHA has over thirty years practice and policy experience in mental health and population health. He has worked as a senior clinical psychologist and been a mental health consultant to the Australian Government. As a population health practitioner, his specialist area has been injury prevention. He has held senior population health positions in Australia and been a long-term international consultant.

preface

With more than 120 years of combined experience, ranging from clinical practice and research to epidemiology and public health intervention, we have become increasingly frustrated with the inability of established primary care to deal adequately with modern disease conditions. Far from creating the health utopia described glowingly in the popular press, advances in health care have been limited and confusing. Decreases in deaths from heart disease, for example, seem set to be reversed by the march of obesity and its associated metabolic disorders, for which the most pessimistic of us can see no solution, save a major economic slowdown, energy crisis or world event.

In The Rise and Fall of Modern Medicine, author James Le Fanu states that medical advances have been vastly exaggerated (by the public), as well as confused by the changing nature of modern disease. It is true that we have managed to delay mortality, but it may be argued that this has come with increases in many diseases that diminish life's exuberance. Diabetes, heart disease, cancers, fatty liver, sleep apnoea, sexual dysfunction and many other conditions are problems related not to micro-organisms that can be managed through the magic bullets of pharmacopoeia, but to the lifestyles we now lead in environments designed to improve life's quality—although perhaps only through the blinkered eyes of economic rationalists rather than those of the concerned health practitioner. Ironically, the material advances achieved over the past century, which suggest to the populace that simplistic, effort-free technological fixes will solve all our health woes, in fact advance the need for greater patient involvement in their own health, suggesting a revolution in primary care.

Lifestyle medicine—contrary to the belief of one GP attending one of our workshops who thought it was about 'how to incorporate golf into my practice'—is aimed at correcting this situation. We hope that through this book we have at least made a start in doing so. It is certain that there will be much more to come.

Garry Egger
Andrew Binns
Stephan Rossner

CHAPTER 1

Introduction to lifestyle medicine

GARRY EGGER, ANDREW BINNS, STEPHAN ROSSNER

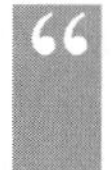

Life is a sexually transmitted disease with 100% mortality and inevitable intermittent morbidity.

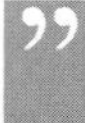

R.D. LAING

What is lifestyle medicine?

The rise in obesity worldwide has focused attention on lifestyle as a prominent cause of disease in modern times. However, obesity is just one manifestation, albeit an obvious one, of a range of health problems that have arisen from the environment and behaviours associated with our modern way of living. Inactivity, poor and over-nutrition, smoking, drug and alcohol abuse, inappropriate medication, stress, sexual behaviour, inadequate sleep, risk taking, and environmental exposure (sun, chemical, the built environment) are significant modern causes of disease that call for a modified approach to health management. 'Lifestyle medicine' is a relatively new and different approach to doing this.

While there is not yet a universally accepted definition, we define lifestyle medicine as 'the application of environmental, behavioural, medical and motivational principles to the management of lifestyle-related health problems in a clinical setting'. It involves the therapeutic use of lifestyle interventions in the management of disease at all levels.

This book summarises aspects of lifestyle medicine, examining the causes, measurement and management of a range of modern health problems with predominantly lifestyle-based aetiologies. The need for such an approach stems from economic advancement, which has changed the environments in which humans live (both 'macro' and 'micro') and, in doing so, the lifestyles and behaviours associated with those environments. Up to 70% of all visits to a doctor are now thought to have a predominantly lifestyle-based cause (AIHW, 2006), hence the need for a new approach to dealing with the problem. As we will see, an appropriate response leads to a convergence of a range of diverse issues confronting humankind in the third millennium, from personal and population health to pollution, climate change, social equity, population stabilisation and globalisation. We concentrate largely on the contribution that can be made directly by the clinician at the personal level and conclude in Chapter 22 with a discussion of personal carbon trading schemes and economic reform as a potential encompassing 'distal' approach to health and the environment.

The scope of lifestyle medicine

The practice of lifestyle medicine extends from that of *primary* prevention (preventing a disease from developing by modifying the behavioural or environmental cause) to *secondary* prevention (modifying risk factors to avert the disease) to *tertiary* prevention (rehabilitation from a disease state and prevention of recurrence). For example, helping prevent a person become overweight by implementing lifestyle changes is *primary* prevention; helping an overweight person with pre-diabetes avoid diabetic complications is *secondary* prevention; and advising a morbidly obese patient with poor diabetic control to undergo bariatric surgery to avoid the need for insulin is *tertiary* prevention.

Although it is a clinical discipline, lifestyle medicine forms a bridge with health promotion, where health promotion is defined as 'the combination of educational and environmental supports for actions and conditions of living conducive to health' (Green and Kreuter, 1991).

In contrast to population and environmental interventions, lifestyle medicine focuses on individuals (and, in some cases, small groups), where interventions are typically administered in a primary care setting. Just as in any specialised area, there is a body of knowledge and skills that needs to be mastered to become involved in lifestyle medicine. However, the involvement of different disciplines ensures a greater availability of these skills within a practising team.

Historical background

Around 500 BC, the Greek philosopher and founder of modern medicine, Hippocrates, first hinted at the notion of lifestyle medicine by suggesting that in order to keep well one should simply 'avoid too much food, too little toil'. For the ensuring two and a half millennia, humans had little difficulty conforming to Hippocrates' lifestyle recommendations. Indeed, the problem was getting *enough* food and having to toil *too much* in order to survive the trials and tribulations of human evolution. Their problem was more the acute ravages of infection.

A change came with the industrial revolution of the late nineteenth century. Machines began to replace people, thus making physical effort in the gathering of food less necessary, as well as increasing the availability (and density) of energy in such food. Leisure time was more at a premium, population and work stresses increased, access to ingestible and mind-altering substances increased, and social and community structures changed.

As a result, the Hippocratic prescription now needs to be expanded. To the above, we could add: 'and don't smoke, don't eat too much fat (or eat or drink too much in general), don't drink too much (or too little) alcohol (while having a couple of alcohol free days a week), try not to get anxious or depressed, get just the right amount of stress, don't do too many drugs (of all kinds), don't have unsafe sex, eat breakfast, keep regularly active, sleep well and for long enough, do some stretching and strength work every other day, wear sunscreen, use a moisturiser, avoid airconditioning where possible, keep the skin well hydrated, chew gum, floss regularly, and, remember, moderation in all things—including moderation'!

Lifestyle medicine includes these preventive tactics. It can combine changes in behaviour or the environment with medical management and, at another level, does this in the absence of conventional medical intervention.

Lifestyle medicine in the context of chronic and acute disease

Acute diseases are those that usually have a short prodrome and cause debilitating symptoms but in an otherwise healthy person resolve completely and relatively quickly, without sequelae. These are usually caused by infectious agents and include diseases such as rubella, measles and influenza. Chronic diseases are usually those with a long prodrome and which require ongoing management over an extended period—sometimes a lifetime.

In earlier times, the acute, infectious diseases often resulted in death because there was no treatment for the secondary complications of illnesses, such as pneumonia or rheumatic fever. People who developed more serious illnesses—such as insulin dependent diabetes, tuberculosis or typhoid—usually died from the disease itself.

With improved living standards and health care, people with illnesses that once would have caused death are now able to live with their disease into later life. Crohn's disease, ulcerative colitis, multiple sclerosis, ischaemic heart disease and diabetes are all examples of diseases that could previously have been fatal but which are now manageable. HIV and hepatitis B and C are more recent examples. At the other extreme, some chronic diseases (e.g. cystic fibrosis, haemochromatosis, polycystic kidneys) have a significant genetic component and could not be classified as lifestyle based. Consequently, the boundary between chronic and acute diseases and the scope of lifestyle medicine is much less discrete than it may have been in the past (Figure 1.1).

Differences between traditional/conventional and lifestyle medicine

Lifestyle medicine differs from traditional/conventional medicine (hereafter called 'conventional') in that it is aimed at modifying the behavioural and lifestyle bases of disease, rather than simply treating the disease. As such, it requires the 'patient' to be an active partner in the process, rather than a passive recipient of medical care. In

FIGURE 1.1 The place of lifestyle medicine

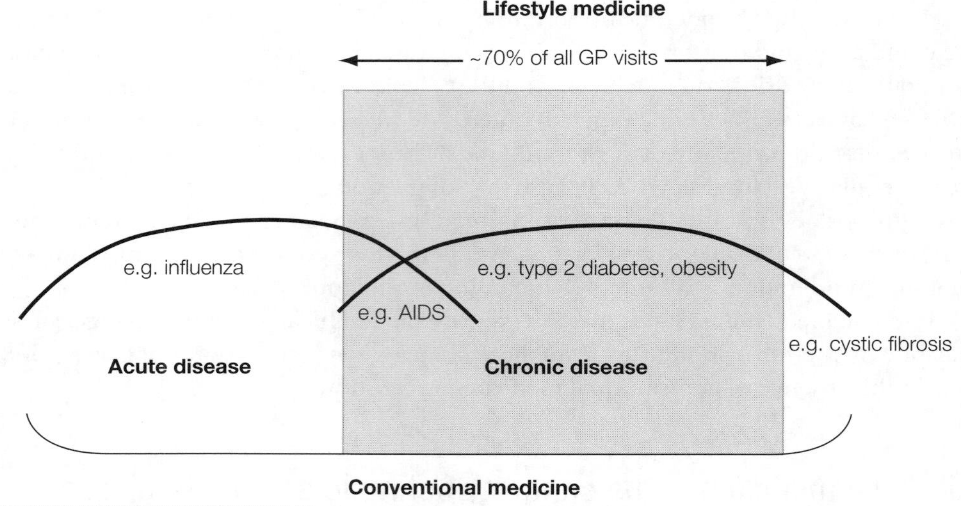

fact, the term 'patient' is really no longer appropriate in this setting; unfortunately, no fully acceptable alternative term has presented itself.

It differs from non-medical clinical practice in that it may include medication (e.g. for smoking cessation or hunger control) and even surgery where this is appropriate (e.g. for weight control), and it differs from purely behavioural approaches in that it examines environmental aetiologies as well as individual behaviours. Some of the other main differences between the two approaches are shown in Table 1.1.

TABLE 1.1 Differences between traditional/conventional and lifestyle medicine approaches in primary care

Traditional/conventional medicine	Lifestyle medicine
treats individual risk factors	treats lifestyle causes
patient is a passive recipient of care	patient is an active partner in care
patient is not required to make big changes	patient is required to make big changes
treatment is often short term	treatment is always long term
responsibility is on the clinician	responsibility is on the patient
medication is often the 'end' treatment	medication may be needed but the emphasis is on lifestyle change
emphasises diagnosis and prescription	emphasises motivation and compliance
goal is disease management	goal is primary/secondary/tertiary prevention
less consideration of environment	more consideration of environment
side effects are balanced by the benefit	side effects that impact on lifestyle require greater attention
involves other medical specialties	involves allied health professionals
doctor generally operates independently on a one-to-one basis	doctor is part of a team of health professionals

The links that justify lifestyle medicine

It is not drawing too long a bow to suggest that the aspects of lifestyle covered in this book are closely linked. Poor sleep, for example, can lead to fatigue; fatigue to inactivity; inactivity to poor nutrition or over-eating; and all these can exacerbate obesity and depression, leading to the metabolic syndrome, type 2 diabetes, sex and mood problems, and possibly heart disease. In reverse, poor nutrition, inactivity, and smoking or alcohol abuse may result in injury, poor sleeping habits or disease proneness that can make the process cyclical. Medication can help manage this but may also, if misused, have side effects such as weight gain and sexual dysfunction. Antidepressant medication can cause weight gain, which may cause greater psychological disturbance than the original depression. All of this—the predisposing factors, cause, the disease and the treatment—are part of lifestyle medicine.

Exercise and nutrition are the 'penicillin' of lifestyle medicine; hence, the early chapters are devoted to these, albeit modestly, as both topics are covered in much greater detail in other individual texts. Psychology is the 'surgery' by which homeostasis is restored in lifestyle-based diseases; hence, psychological processes litter the text. Together with other more specific treatment approaches, these make up the bulk of lifestyle medicine.

Who is best qualified to practice lifestyle medicine?

In our view, there is currently no single discipline equipped to practice lifestyle medicine alone. Medical practitioners have the training to diagnose and treat disease but little time to supervise and motivate patients through complex lifestyle change. Nurses are equipped for ongoing management and care of patients, but they often lack specific knowledge about nutrition, exercise and behaviour change (the emerging breed of practice nurses may be able to fill this gap).

Dietitians can advise on the basis of existing nutritional knowledge but the ground is constantly changing under their feet and they often have a minimal background in exercise or behaviour change. Exercise physiologists are knowledgeable about the physical activity requirements for specific problems but have less complete knowledge of nutrition and psychology. Psychologists and complementary medicine practitioners bring their own advantages but lack the prescribing ability and often the physiological background of the doctor and other mainstream disciplines.

University courses are now being tailored to try to fill this gap. Courses are being offered in the combination of nutrition, exercise and psychology (i.e. metabolic health). Many medical degrees now also include a related non-medical discipline as a prerequisite and are increasingly emphasising the role of prevention, as well as treatment, and an understanding of psychology and behaviour. However, it is unlikely in the near future that any one professional will be able to assume the mantle of the fully fledged lifestyle medicine 'expert'. As a result, the practice is likely to be carried out by a team of health professionals with the doctor, very often a general practitioner (GP), as the coordinator of the team.

Yes, I believe in prevention. So can you give me a pill that will prevent me from having to exercise, eat less, and stop smoking and drinking?

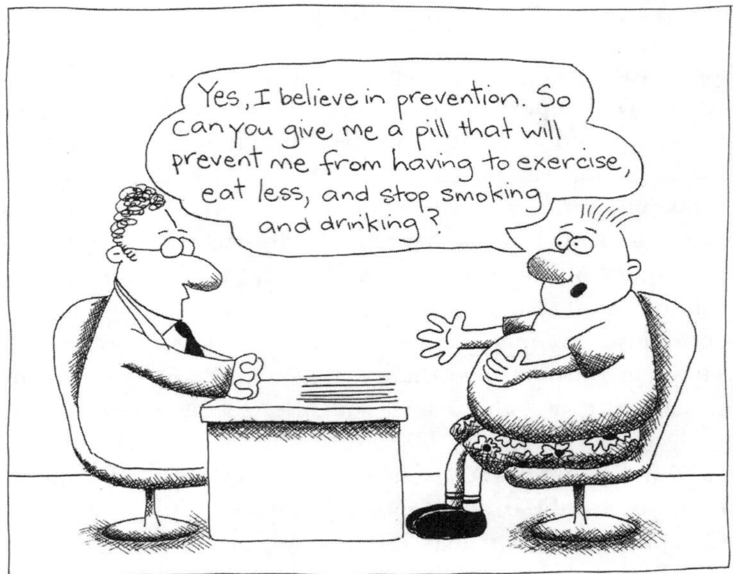

The evidence base

Where possible, we use evidence-based information to make recommendations for lifestyle-based prescriptions. However, as lifestyle medicine is a developing area, there is still much to be learned and much that is difficult to objectify. This becomes particularly apparent when discussing exercise prescription for various ailments (Chapter 7) or learning positive psychology to combat mood disorders (Chapter 14). Although specific prescriptions for different lifestyle-based ailments are now emerging, there has only recently been an appreciation of the general importance of lifestyle in what have often otherwise been thought of as medical issues. Hence, evidence-based prescription is not yet available in several areas. Where this is the case, we have attempted to compensate by providing recommendations based on the available data and the careful reasoning of our experienced contributors.

Other publications cover the more theoretical rationales for lifestyle medicine, its evidence base, and specific areas of lifestyle medicine such as sports medicine, women's health, and pulmonary and paediatric medicine (e.g. Knight, 2004; Rippe, 1999), so these are not dealt with in detail here. We have also not covered each area of lifestyle medicine exhaustively, given that most have extensive literatures of their own elsewhere. The idea is to synthesise these topics into one unified concept.

Frameworks for lifestyle medicine

The recent interest in lifestyle medicine has generated a number of frameworks to assist clinicians in dealing with lifestyle-based disease. The SNAP (smoking, nutrition, alcohol, physical activity) framework in Australia was initially developed to draw attention to the need for dealing with these lifestyle factors in the medical environment (RACGP, 2004). The Australian Government initiative *Lifescripts* represents an extension of this and provides extensive accompanying resource materials

(DoHA, 2005). Both SNAP and *Lifescripts* have been developed on an evidence base and trialled.

Because lifestyle medicine is in its early stages, it is still a work in progress, influenced by its developing status, the norms and aspirations of the population and ongoing feedback. This book represents an attempt to capture the best in an embryonic field, accepting that this is only a beginning in a developing process. We have adopted and adapted existing initiatives to suit changing conditions. The five As of *Lifescripts* (ask, assess, advise, assist, arrange), for example, have been reduced to three As (assess, assist, arrange) for easier recall, and are provided at the end of each chapter, and practical applications have been summarised for medical practitioners and practice nurses.

Developing and using care plans and other aids

The advent of the Enhanced Primary Care (EPC) scheme under the Australian Government's Medicare system has improved the viability of lifestyle medicine in the primary care system. The scheme first requires a GP to perform a GP Management Plan (GPMP), which is essentially a strategy to manage chronic disease. A Team Care Arrangement (TCA) is then completed, outlining the roles of two additional accredited allied health professionals working in conjunction with the GP. These may be dietitians, exercise physiologists, psychologists, physiotherapists, Aboriginal health workers, chiropractors, etc. (other professions are occasionally being added). Allied health workers report back to the GP, and a coordinated team approach to chronic care is thus established. This is a different way of practising for GPs used to conventional, reactive, one-on-one consultations and to treating health problems as they present (or at least to slowing down the progression of the disease process), rather than taking a proactive approach and preventing disease in the first place. The EPC system has facilitated the development of the lifestyle medicine approach to modern health care (RACGP, 2006).

In the following chapters, we look at various areas of lifestyle medicine that are particularly applicable to the primary care setting. The approach is based around practicality, with sufficient theoretical background given to validate the process. Current procedures involving the EPC system are discussed in the Appendix at the end of the book. Because it is in its early days, however, this system is constantly changing. We have done our best here to signal the aspects of the system that are likely to remain constant over time.

What can be done in a standard consultation

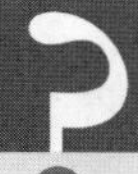

Ask what aspects of the patient's lifestyle she or he thinks could be improved.

On the basis of the above, enquire in more depth about the areas identified.

Suggest/refer to an allied health specialist in this area or make another appointment to discuss these in more detail.

If appropriate, carry out some basic measurements (e.g. waist circumference, weight, bio-impedance).

Provide written material on the lifestyle areas identified.

Summary

Lifestyle medicine represents a different approach to dealing with the significant proportion of patients with ailments caused predominantly by lifestyle and now presenting to healthcare practitioners. Managing these problems changes the emphasis from conventional treatment to one where the patient needs to be more involved in his or her care, and this requires considerable knowledge about motivation and motivational skills on the part of the clinician. New developments in health funding involving allied health professionals as part of a healthcare team now make this not only financially feasible but necessary for dealing with the changes in disease aetiology associated with our modern way of life.

references

REFERENCES

AIHW (Australian Institute of Health and Welfare) (2006) *Australia's health 2006: the tenth biennial report of the Australian Institute of Health and Welfare,* Canberra: AIHW. cat no. Aus 73.

——AIHW (2006) *Chronic disease and associated risk factors,* Canberra: AIHW. cat no. Aus PHE 81.

DoHA (Department of Health and Ageing) (2005) *Lifescripts.* Practice and Resource Kits. Canberra: DoHA. Available from www.health.gov.au/internet/wcms/publishing.nsf/Content/health-pubhlth-strateg-lifescripts-index.htm.

Bodheimer T. (2006) Primary care—will it survive? *NEJM* 355(9): 861–64.

Goodyear-Smith F, Arroll B, Sullivan S et al. (2004) Lifestyle screening: development of an acceptable multi-item general practice tool. *N Z Med J* 117(1205): U1146.

Greene LW, Kreuter MW. (1991) *Health promotion planning: an educational and environmental Approach.* Palo Alto, Ca: Mayfield Publishing Co.

Knight JA. (2004) *A crisis call for new preventive medicine: emerging effects of lifestyle on morbidity and mortality.* New Jersey: World Scientific Publishing Co.

RACGP (Royal Australian College of General Practitioners) (2004) *SNAP (smoking, nutrition, alcohol, physical activity): a population health guide to behavioural risk factors in general practice framework.* South Melbourne: RACGP. Available from www.racgp.org.au/Content/NavigationMenu/ClinicalResources/RACGPGuidelines/SNAPapopulationhealthguidetobehaviouralriskfactorsingeneralpractice/SNAPguide2004.pdf.

Rippe J. (ed) (1999) *Lifestyle medicine.* NY: Blackwell Publishing.

PROFESSIONAL RESOURCES: A LIFESTYLE SCREENING QUESTIONNAIRE

Patient instructions: For each question, give a score from 1 to 5 based on the following scale: 0 = Don't do, 1 = Never do, 2 = Rarely do, 3 = Sometimes do, 4 = Often do, 5 = Very often do.

And tick the column that best answers the question *Would you like help with this?* (Yes, No, Later)

	SCORE	YES	NO	LATER
Do you ever feel the need to cut down on your smoking?				
Do you ever feel the need to cut down on your alcohol intake?				
Do you ever feel the need to cut down on other drug use?				
During the past month, have you often been bothered by feeling down, depressed or hopeless?				
During the past month, have you often been bothered by having little interest or pleasure in doing things?				
Have you been worrying a lot about everyday problems?				
Do you spend most days being physically inactive?				
Are you concerned about your current weight?				
Are you unhappy with the quality of your sleep?				
Do you eat less than about three serves of fruit and vegetables each day?				
Do you suffer side effects from any medications you take?				
Do you have concerns about the state of your skin/hair?				
Are you concerned in any way about your sexual performance?				
Do your teeth/gums cause you any problems?				
Do you regularly drink large amounts of soft drink or fruit juice?				

Source: Adapted from Goodyear-Smith et al., 2004

CHAPTER 2

The epidemiology of chronic disease

MAXIMILIAN DE COURTEN, GARRY EGGER

> *For if medicine is really to accomplish its great task, it must intervene in political and social life. It must point out the hindrances that impede the normal social functioning of vital processes, and effect their removal.*
>
> RUDOLF LUDWIG KARL VIRCHOW, 1849
> (QUOTED IN P. FARMER *PATHOLOGIES OF POWER,* 2004)

A (very) short history of disease

About five million years ago, a variation of a common ape began to walk out of the jungles of Central Africa. Not much is known about this antecedent of *Homo sapiens,* but we can speculate on a couple of things. First, it is highly unlikely that these creatures were obese. Although having the genetic capacity for storing fat (something which evolved in the early mammals as a means of getting through the inevitable lean times), the prospects of achieving this were almost certainly limited by a harsh environment and competition for scarce resources. Second, they were exposed to all manner of diseases, most of which were likely to be acute and contagious and for which protection would evolve through the development of disease-fighting antibodies. In the ensuing millennia, life would revolve around getting enough to eat, not being eaten or killed in warfare, and battling the countless co-evolving disease micro-organisms, some of which still plague humanity today.

How are these things connected? Until the late twentieth century this was not clear. Humans had progressively survived the 'four horses of the apocalypse' to increase exponentially as a result of developments in disease prevention. Changes in public health and hygiene around the time of the industrial revolution of the late nineteenth century and the development of medical marvels, such as vaccination and antibiotics, resulted in a massive blow to infectious diseases. In the euphoria of the 1960s, it appeared that the battle against disease had been all but won. Few would have predicted that the (apparent) demise of infectious diseases would be accompanied by a rise in diseases largely caused by the factors underlying this decrease in infections, namely, industrial development, 'modernisation' and economic growth (Lucretius may have been an exception when he wrote in 50 BC, 'In primitive times, lack of food gave languishing bodies to death; now, on the other hand, it is abundance that buries them.' Trans. Latham, 1994).

The emergence of chronic diseases began with the industrial revolution, which, for the first time, allowed machines to carry out much of the work otherwise done by humans. The increased production of food not only made what was once a relatively scarce resource into a common commodity, but also increased the energy density, or fattening capacity of food. The technological revolution of the late twentieth century then hastened the process. With greater access to mass-produced food pleasing to our primitive taste and obtainable with ever decreasing effort, humans began to fulfil their genetic potential to store excessive fat. In fact, an epidemic of fatness of national and international scope began in the 1980s and, by the turn of the millennium, it involved at least half of the adult population and one-quarter of adolescents in industrialised countries. Because obesity has been shown to have a causal link to many diseases, this significantly changed the pattern of disease from those caused by an outside agent (e.g. bacterium, virus) to those primarily caused by the way we live. This has not been helped by a return of acute and infectious problems, such as SARS, AIDS and bird flu, which are also related to the way we live (e.g. overcrowding, over-population, international travel, sexual behaviour) but are less relevant to the discussion here, which we will confine to non-infectious, lifestyle-related chronic disease problems.

Lifestyle-related causes of disease

Epidemiologists have traditionally used mortality (death rates) from a particular disease as an indication of the severity of that disease. With chronic diseases, however, mortality tells only a part of the story. Morbidity (sickness statistics) are also limited in this respect. However, there is a new measure called 'disability adjusted life years' (DALYs). DALYs for a disease are the sum of the years of life lost due to premature mortality and the years lost due to disability in a given population (WHO, 2007). The DALY is a health gap measure that extends the concept of potential years of life lost due to premature death to include equivalent years of healthy life lost to states of less than full health (broadly termed disability). One DALY represents the loss of one year of equivalent full health.

Table 2.1 shows the highest causes of DALYs in Australia in early 2000 (AIHW, 2006a). (The main lifestyle factors and DALYs associated with disease for males and females in Australia are shown in Table 2.2.) The plusses in the right hand side of Table 2.1 indicate the degree to which each of these has a lifestyle-based aetiology. As can be seen, heart disease holds the number one ranking in DALYs (as it does with mortality). Stroke and chronic obstructive pulmonary disease (COPD) come second

TABLE 2.1 The fifteen leading causes of disability affected life years (DALYs) in Australia, 2000

Disease	% of total DALYs	Lifestyle cause or component?
1. ischaemic heart disease	12.4	+++
2. stroke	5.4	+++
3. COPD	3.7	++
4. depression	3.7 (4.9 if suicide included)	++
5. lung cancer	3.6	+++
6. dementia	3.5	++
7. diabetes	3.0 (4.9 if CHD included)	+++
8. colorectal cancer	2.7	++
9. asthma	2.6	++
10. osteoarthritis	2.2	++
11. suicide/injury	2.2	++
12. traffic accidents	2.2	+++
13. breast cancer	2.2	++
14. hearing loss	1.9	+
15. alcohol dependence	1.8	++

Source: AIHW, 2006a

TABLE 2.2 Proportion of disease burden (attributable DALYs as a proportion of total DALYs) attributed to selected determinants of health (%)

Risk factor	Males (%)	Females (%)	Total (%)
overweight	8.8	8.3	8.6
tobacco smoking	9.5	6.5	7.9
high blood pressure	7.5	7.0	7.3
physical inactivity	6.5	6.8	6.7
high cholesterol	6.5	5.7	6.1
alcohol harm	5.3	2.2	3.8
alcohol benefit	−1.6	−2.1	−1.8
occupational exposure	2.6	1.3	2.0
illicit drugs	2.6	1.2	1.9
lack of fruit and vegetables	1.9	1.0	1.4
intimate partner violence	n.a.	2.1	1.0
child sexual abuse	0.3	1.3	0.8
unsafe sex	0.1	0.6	0.5

Source: AIHW, 2006

and third, respectively. The increase in diabetes and pre-diabetes of around 1% per year also makes this one of the most rapidly growing problems in the modern world. Overall, it can be seen that a large burden of modern disease is currently being imposed by potentially preventable lifestyle causes.

Table 2.2 holds a few surprises. Although smoking is still one of the main preventable causes of disease, this has now been overtaken by overweight as the major preventable cause of DALYs and is rapidly being caught by inactivity. This can probably be attributed to the significant successes achieved in Australia through systematic anti-tobacco campaigns since the 1970s. Inactivity is increasing consequentially as widespread technology (e.g. cars, TV, computers) further reduces the need for physical activity both at work and at play. It is also of note that the much-publicised benefit from drinking alcohol (in moderation) is, on a population level, more than cancelled out by the harm caused by drinking.

Four main causes—excess weight, poor diet, physical inactivity and smoking—account for most of the mortality and morbidity of the major diseases of modern society, such as heart disease, stroke, colorectal cancer, depression, kidney disease, diabetes, osteoarthritis and osteoporosis.

Assessing risk factors

Risk factors are characteristics that are associated with an increased risk of developing a particular disease or condition. They can be demographic, behavioural, biomedical, genetic, environmental, social, or other factors, and they can act independently or in combination. Such a broad definition includes biomedical concepts of risk and behaviours considered as 'risky' based on social values and cultural norms. A risk factor can therefore be understood as something lying within the realm of personal responsibility (something the individual can control) or something that either cannot be altered at all (e.g. genetic factors) or is very intangible and therefore hard to address (e.g. cultural traditions). To identify risk factors, then, does not necessarily lead to their swift reduction.

Biomedical risk factors are derived from body measurements, such as overweight, high blood pressure and high blood cholesterol. Because they are 'within the body', biomedical risk factors carry comparatively direct and specific risks for health.

Biomedical risk factors are often (but to varying degrees) a result of *behavioural factors* that are in turn influenced by *socioeconomic factors* and other even more distal determinants. Health behaviours such as eating healthy foods and being active tend to interact with each other and to influence a variety of biomedical factors (e.g. body weight, blood levels of glucose, cholesterol). Both physical activity and diet, for example, can affect body weight, blood pressure and blood cholesterol. Each health behaviour can exert this influence alone but act with greater effect when combined with other behaviours. Behavioural and biomedical risk factors tend to amplify each other's effects when they occur together; for example, smoking tobacco and high blood pressure escalate the risk for stroke.

Assessing risk factors for disease is at the core of preventive clinical medicine. Risk factors in individuals can be measured by interview (e.g. questionnaires) physically (i.e. anthropometry), or biochemically (i.e. based on blood samples). Some of the common biomedical risk factor measures used are shown in Table 2.3 (the clinical relevance of some of these is discussed at the end of each of the relevant chapters dealing with their lifestyle-related links). Risk factor questionnaires are discussed in each chapter to follow.

While many of the risk factor measures have been around for some time, new measures and markers are continually being assessed. Some of these extend existing measures, such as the inclusion of an ApoB/ApoA ratio, which further refines the risk of abnormal lipid levels for heart disease (Yusuf et al., 2004). Others, such as C-reactive

TABLE 2.3 Common biomedical risk factor markers for lifestyle-related diseases

Physical measures	Biochemical measures
blood pressure fitness: • step test • submaximal test • stress test weight/body fat/fat distribution: • BMI (weight in kg/height in metres^2) • body fat (%) • waist circumference (WC) • waist-to-hip ratio (WHR)	standard measures: • fasting lipids (TC, TG, HDL, LDL) • fasting plasma glucose (FPG) • HbA_{1c} • uric acid • liver function tests other measures: • glucose tolerance test • homocysteine • ApoB/ApoA ratio • C-reactive protein

protein (CRP) and homocysteine, take us into different areas of risk measurement (CRP reflecting chronic subclinical inflammation and homocysteine folic acid metabolism), the meanings of which are often unclear (Hankey et al., 2004). Still others increase the predictive potential of individual measures by combining more than one measure (Wang et al., 2006); the combination of a high triglyceride and large waist circumference, for example, has been shown to be a reliable proxy measure of insulin resistance (Esmaillzadeh et al., 2006) and may be the first indication of insulin resistance.

However, as was recently pointed out, identification of new risk factors for specific diseases is an enduring theme in medical research (Ware, 2006). This type of research often increases our understanding of the causes of diseases better than it actually translates into practice for treatment or prevention. Research done by Wang and colleagues is a good example: adding ten novel biomedical risk factors for predicting the risk of cardiovascular events to the classic risk factors, such as blood pressure, cigarette smoking and total cholesterol, resulted in only very small increases in the ability to classify risk (Wang et al., 2006). There is a real potential for contemporary medical risk factor research to get caught in Pareto's trap where 20% of the risk factors explain 80% of the disease but researchers try hard to chase the remaining 20% of disease with ever increasing effort (Rose, 1991), even though there is already sufficient grounds to act. One should not underestimate the power of the classic risk factors at hand (abnormal lipids, smoking, hypertension, diabetes, abdominal obesity, psychosocial factors, inactivity, lack of consumption of fruits and vegetables, and alcohol), which accounted for more than 80% of the risk of myocardial infarction in a worldwide study (Yusuf at al., 2004). Such findings suggest that approaches to prevention can be based on similar principles worldwide and have the potential to prevent most premature cases of cardiovascular disease.

Beyond single risk factors

Narrow attention on single risk factors and their association with disease led to clinical recommendations focused primarily on managing these individual risk factors, particularly raised blood pressure and cholesterol. Typically, separate guidelines were then developed for each risk factor and treatment was recommended when that factor was above a specified level. Only in the past decade have we witnessed a remarkable change from these recommendations based on relative risk to those based on absolute or total risk. According to Rose (1991), 'All policy decisions should be based on absolute measures of risk; relative risk is strictly for researchers only.' This should also apply to risk management in lifestyle medicine.

The newer clinical guidelines recommend that priority for treatment be given to patients with a high absolute risk of disease or death, defined as the probability of developing a particular end-point over a specified period, instead of undue emphasis being placed on an individual risk factor. New and simple clinical tools for assessing absolute risk were developed and are being constantly refined and made available over the internet (for example, from the New Zealand Guidelines Group at www.nzgg.org.nz or the National Heart Foundation, Australia, at www.heartfoundation.com.au).

Clinical trial evidence clearly shows that the absolute benefits of treatment are directly proportional to the risk level before treatment. The absolute risk of a person's future cardiovascular disease is therefore strongly influenced by the combination of risk factors already present, particularly history of cardiovascular disease, age, gender, diabetes, smoking, blood pressure and blood lipid concentrations. For example, a fifty-year-old, non-smoking woman with a blood pressure of 180/105 mm Hg, a total cholesterol of 7.0 mmol/L, and a high density lipoprotein (HDL) cholesterol of 1.0 mmol/L has about a 7.5% chance of suffering a major cardiovascular event in the next five years, if you calculate her risk using the National Heart Foundation of New Zealand's *Estimating CVD risk and treatment benefit* (available from www.clinicalevidence.com/ceweb/resources/women_no_diabetes.jsp#cvdChart). However, a sixty-year-old male smoker with a blood pressure of 160/95 mm Hg, a lower total blood cholesterol values (6.6 mmol/L), and slightly higher HDL value of 1.1 mmol/L has about a 27.5% risk.

With antihypertensive or lipid lowering drugs both these patients could reduce their risk of cardiovascular disease (CVD) by up to a quarter over the next five years. The woman's absolute risk over the five years could fall from about 7.5% to 5.6% and the man's from about 27.5% to 20%. In other words, about fifty such women would require five years of treatment to prevent one cardiovascular event but only fifteen such men. What is even more striking is the contribution of smoking to the high cardiovascular risk of our male example: if he gave up smoking, his five-year CVD risk would rapidly drop from the 27.5% to about 17.5%, a greater reduction than he could experience by adhering for five years to drug treatment of his high blood pressure or elevated lipids. This illustrates the importance of selecting lifestyle-related disease management based on the (evidence-based) impact any intervention could have (Tonkin et al., 2003).

Beyond risk factors altogether

Risk factor assessment and monitoring leading to corrective therapy and prescription of medication is often at the centre of clinical management but it is merely the start of diagnosis in lifestyle medicine. The task of the modern clinician is not only to recognise the importance of the immediate causes or markers of disease probability, but also to address associated factors (e.g. mechanical and other problems such as joint problems associated with obesity, impaired vision with diabetes). Because these can often cause vicious cycles, they can hinder a lifestyle change being effectively undertaken or sustained by the patient (Swinburn and Egger, 2004). After all, a key characteristic of lifestyle-related diseases is that they are caused not by a single factor but by several factors. Consequently, merely correcting one risk factor (such as lowering blood glucose levels with medication) will often not suffice to cure the problem that caused blood sugars to rise in the first place (e.g. poor diet, inactivity).

Looking beyond immediate causes of disease

While Tables 2.1 and 2.2 give a general picture of causality, this needs to be expanded. As can be seen in Figure 2.1, there is a hierarchy of causality in modern diseases which needs to be discussed in any considered analysis. In the first place, there are the measurable risk factors discussed above. These are a result of more proximal causes such as smoking, obesity or alcohol use, which are often not considered further. However, these proximal causes in turn have more medial and, ultimately, distal causes that present the true basis of disease.

FIGURE 2.1 A hierarchy of chronic disease causes

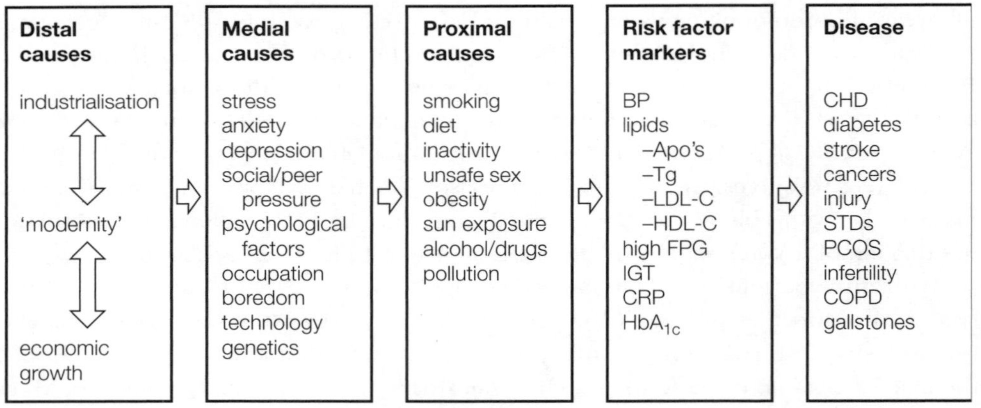

Tracking disease causes back like this helps to explain why a disease like type 2 diabetes is closely associated with affluence, industrialisation and 'modernity', and hence is a consequence or fault of modern society. At face value, diabetes appears to be caused by inactivity and poor nutrition, and so could be regarded as the fault of the individual (Chakravarthy and Booth, 2004). And while a clinician could be expected to have little effect on the more distal causes, these need to be recognised in a comprehensive public health approach and any sophisticated epidemiological analysis. Each level in this causal hierarchy and its measures and implications for the clinician are discussed below.

Proximal causes

Immediately recognised causes of disease usually represent the reach of medical investigation into disease causality at the practice level, beyond measuring and monitoring the biomedical risk factors. Smoking, drinking habits, inactivity, obesity, drug use, unsafe sex and poor diet are often pinpointed as the primary aetiologies the treating physician will focus on. However, as argued below, they are *at least* only secondary causes. Proximal causes are often seen as the end-point of the causality chain when in fact they are not. This may be a consequence of the busy time schedules GPs face: rarely is there enough time to explore and address the underlying psychosocial experiences that resulted in disturbed body perception and eating patterns which in turn caused obesity. For example. 'Eat healthier and move more' is often the only advice dispensed—well meant but hardly appropriate.

Another glaring example is the failure to realise and act upon the significance of psychological factors such as stress and depression in the aetiology of heart disease. The results of the recent Interheart study (Yusuf et al., 2004, which involved more than 11 000 cases of myocardial infarction in fifty-two countries and various ethnic groups) have now objectively indicated the need to extend the epidemiological analysis to include 'causes of causes'—and stress in particular.

Medial causes

Medial causes lead to the more obvious proximal causes of disease. Tobacco smoking, for example, is prevalent because of peer pressure, social stress, anxiety, and other psychological factors. Regular smoking is not a behaviour that occurs without a precipitating drive. Similarly, obesity is undoubtedly influenced by factors such as social pressures to eat, binge eating due to depression or anxiety, and genetic influences, among other things.

The value in identifying medial causes as driving forces behind the proximal causes of disease is that any success in positively influencing these may lead to profound and long-lasting changes of a greater significance than treating the biomedical or proximal risk factor alone would produce. For example, mediating a bad relationship (be it at home or at work) can change eating and drinking habits and reinvigorate physical activity; the resulting joy in life in turn reduces overweight, blood pressure and blood sugar probably more sustainably than a combination drug could have achieved. It is this potential widespread impact medial causes have on lifestyle-related diseases that makes recognising and influencing them so important. And, unlike with distal causes, the clinician has the potential to influence them—in fact, it is the hallmark of a good family doctor to address medial causes while accompanying patients through their life.

What can be done in a standard consultation

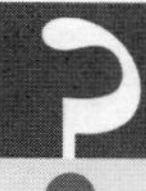

Discuss the lifestyle basis of much modern illness.

Explain the concept of a hierarchy of risk factors.

Measure anthropometric risk factors that can be done on the spot (e.g. weight, waist circumference, bio-impedance).

Refer for appropriate tests of further biomedical risk factors (see text).

Distal causes

It is hard to escape the conclusion that many modern diseases have deep-seated environmental and economic grounds beneath their more apparent causes (Marmot, 2006). In the words of one writer, 'We have dallied too long at the banquet of natural resources, only to discover that the only way out is past the cashier . . . the general consensus seems to be that with the aid of a little fast technological tap dancing most of us may make our escape without paying the full price. Not only would this involve a drastic and immediate reduction in the daily rate at which we gobble up the world's energy resources and dump our wastes, but we would have to sacrifice two of western civilisation's most sacred cows—Growth and Progress—to do it' (Morrison, 2003).

Growth economics has served humanity well over the past century, but there is little doubt that exponential development—of both population growth and resource use—cannot continue unabated (Egger, 1978). The debate on global warming suggests that carbon emissions are the problem, yet, seen more 'distally', carbon emissions are influenced by population size, industrialisation and the economic growth imperative (see Chapter 22). On the one hand, growth economics has led to prosperity and the defeat of many health scourges; on the other, it is responsible for some of the world's most prominent current problems, including obesity and its associated diseases.

The answers to these problems are unlikely to be simple, because they go to the heart of how we (currently) live. Sceptics argue that a failure to act now may lead to the irreversible depletion of resources such as oil and clean water and bring on a major world conflict or economic crisis. The influence of technology on health can be seen in the rate at which cars, computers and effort-saving machines have reduced the need for humans to be physically active. These are macro-environmental issues which the clinician may not be able to influence but which need to be recognised and which call for a fundamental shift in thinking. Nevertheless, clinicians may be able to influence micro-environmental issues, particularly around the house or neighbourhood.

Pervasive and occasional causes

A final striking feature of causality in lifestyle medicine is that a small number of lifestyle choices—poor nutrition and inactivity, in particular—are pervasive or ubiquitous causes of many of the major reasons for DALYs, such as heart disease, diabetes and cancers. Because these are immediately associated with the disease, they are further categorised here as 'pervasive-proximal' causes. Other pervasive causes, such as stress, anxiety and depression, are further back in the causality chain and hence are considered 'pervasive-medial' causes. The distal causes, then, are those associated with general ill health, as discussed above.

Occasional causes are associated with less widespread disease outcome but can also be considered as either proximal, medial or distal. The damaging effects of sunlight on skin, for example, can be seen as an 'occasional-proximal' cause and the social pressures to tan would be the 'occasional-medial' cause in the chain. An illustration of this is shown in Figure 2.2.

FIGURE 2.2 Examples of pervasive and occasional causes of lifestyle-based disease

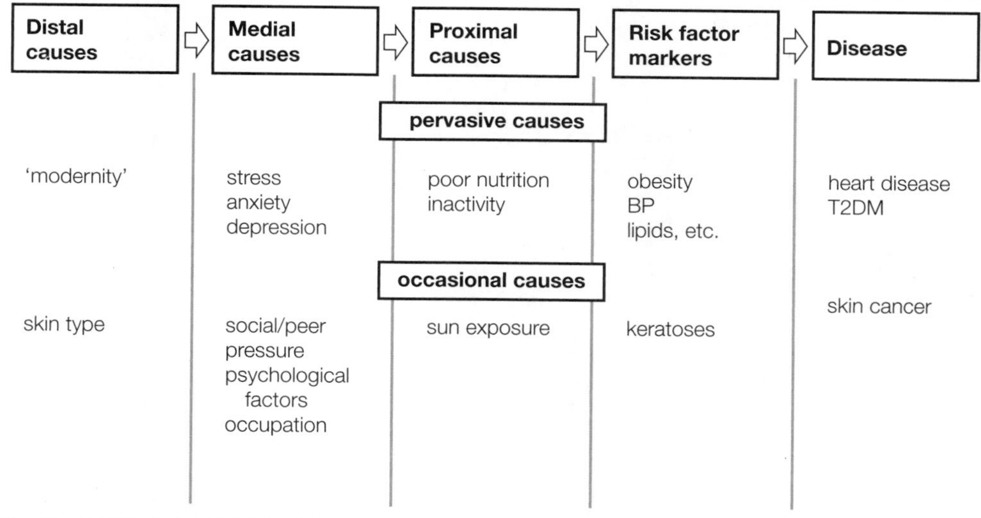

Pervasive causes and methods of correction are discussed in detail in the first half of this book. Occasional causes in problems such as sleep, skin care, sexual behaviour, and oral health are considered in the later chapters.

Expanding the concept of disease and intervention

Although we have discussed the hierarchy of disease aetiology from end-point disease to its distal causes, a lifestyle medicine perspective calls for a more integrated understanding of disease outcomes and risk factors. Often the disease itself leads to a reduction in the capacity to change the lifestyle that is causing it. Damaged joints that result from being overweight, for example, lead to reduced activity which, in turn, can increase body weight in a vicious circle (Swinburn and Egger, 2004). Consequently, increasing levels of effort and motivation are needed to make the required lifestyle changes to reduce illness.

In addition to this negative feedback between outcomes and preventive factors, there is also an incremental relationship between the motivation and effort needed to successfully implement lifestyle change, the complexity of the intervention required, and the barriers encountered along the scale of predominant disease determinants from proximal to distal causes. Figure 2.3 shows that the complexity of the intervention recommended and the amount of motivation needed or barriers experienced when managing a specific chronic disease are dependent on its predominant underlying determinant. For instance, a clinician may focus on the biomedical risk factor of an elevated LDL, which almost dictates the intervention chosen (e.g. lipid lowering drugs) and the amount of motivation needed or barriers to be overcome (e.g. obtaining the pills and taking them regularly). Looking at the other end of the spectrum, where more medial factors (psychosocial and cultural) are at the core of the lifestyle-related disease problem, much larger amounts of motivation are needed—not only by the 'patient' but also by the family and society, who are called

FIGURE 2.3 The MIB (motivation/intervention/barriers) model of disease

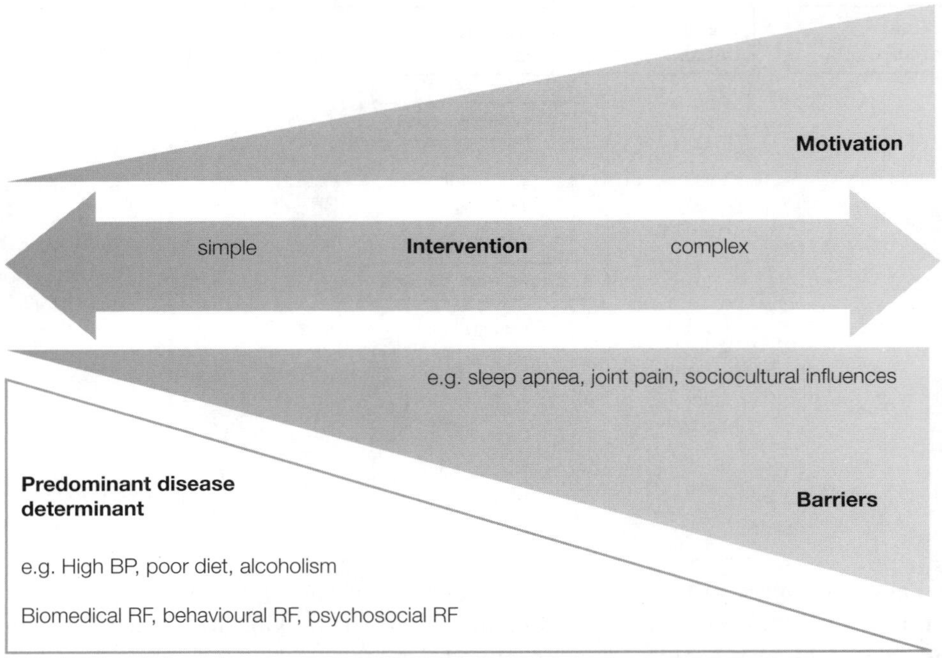

on to provide support—to counter the massive barriers our complex intervention efforts face. Such interventions are likely neither to bring easy gains nor be popular, but again if it is true that distal causes are the root of the problem then there is no easy way out.

The clinician's role in managing lifestyle-related diseases

Understanding the aetiology of disease is a significant part of primary health care. Yet in the area of chronic multifactorial diseases, our knowledge about causality is often less than in other medical areas. Research provides only probabilities, not straight causal relationships; a simple measurement of risk can give a probability estimate but is rather limited as a curative guide.

At the outset, the clinician should identify the problem and measure the obvious risks factors and assess overall risk. A practice nurse can usually undertake much of this. Immediate treatment of risks is often necessary and involves, especially at heightened risk levels, pharmaceutical management by a GP or specialist. Identification of the more distal causes and possible management of lifestyle-related disease, however, is vital for a holistic treatment of the patient. Identification may be part of a GP's diagnosis, but management is likely to take more time and may need to be left to the allied health team in collaboration with the GP. Detailed lifestyle management will require general skills in motivation (discussed in Chapter 3), as well as knowledge about the specific aspects of lifestyle associated with the measured risks.

In lifestyle medicine, motivation is crucial because a change in complex behaviour requires a greater involvement than a relatively simple action such as taking medication. However, it should be apparent that governments also need to play a part by creating conducive and supportive environments through public health measures. Highlighting this, our experience with running quit smoking programs has shown that in the absence of a non-smoking social and physical environment, those programs had little effect on smoking rates. Only when cigarette advertising was banned from the media in the 1980s and smoking became unacceptable in public places were significant inroads made into the smoking epidemic, shown by the decreases in smoking rates from about 40% during the 1950s to less than 15% today (Chapman, 1999).

practice tips

PRACTICE TIPS: MANAGING LIFESTYLE-BASED CHRONIC DISEASES

	Medical practitioner	Practice nurse
Assess	Medical and family histories, focusing on lifestyle factors. Refer for laboratory tests and treat appropriate risk factors. Distal levels of causality (e.g. stress, depression, social factors). Whether lifestyle change has been a consideration. Motivational factors.	Blood pressure, weight and waist circumference, routinely. Smoking and alcohol consumption habits, routinely. Diabetes risk with the Diabetes Risk Assessment Tick Test (see *Professional resources*, Chapter 5).
Assist	Identification of the lifestyle changes required. Risk reduction with medication where appropriate.	Understanding of the proximal causes of risk factors. By reinforcing motivational factors. Discussion of possible lifestyle changes. Negotiation of reduction of barriers to change. Development of a strategy for putting this into action.
Arrange	List of other health professionals for a care plan. Referral to a specialist where indicated.	Care plan. Contact with and coordination of other health professionals.

key points

KEY POINTS FOR CLINICAL MANAGEMENT

- While treating proximal causes of disease, do not ignore the medial and distal factors.
- Check for co-morbidities, such as depression or anxiety, with manifest disease.
- Use adequate measures for standard risk factor analysis.
- Use waist circumference in all standard consultations.
- Consider mechanical and other risks and their effects on compliance through reduced motivation.
- Be aware of the multiplicity of metabolic and mechanical risk factors of obesity and their impact on each other.

REFERENCES

AIHW (Australian Institute of Health and Welfare) (2006a) *Australia's Health 2006: the tenth biennial report of the Australian Institute of Health and Welfare*, cat no. Aus 73. Canberra: AIHW.

——. (2006b) *Chronic disease and associated risk factors,* cat no. Aus PHE 81. Canberra: AIHW.

Bray G, Bouchard C. (2004) *Handbook of obesity*. NY: Marcel Dekker.

British Cardiac Society, British Hyperlipidaemia Association, British Hypertension Society, British Diabetic Association. (2000 and 2001) Joint British recommendations on prevention of coronary heart disease in clinical practice: summary. *BMJ* 320(7236): 705–08 and 323(7316): 780.

Chakravarthy MV, Booth FW. (2004) Eating, exercise, and 'thrifty' genotypes: connecting the dots toward an evolutionary understanding of modern chronic diseases. *J Appl Physiol* 96(1): 3–10.

Chapman, S. (1999) Scare tactics cut smoking rates in Australia to all time low. *Br Med J* 318(7197): 1508.

Czernichow S, Bruckert E, Bertrais S et al. (2006) Hypertriglyceridaemic waist and 7.5 year prospective risk of cardiovascular disease in asymptomatic middle aged men. *Int J Obes* 30: 463–68.

Diabetes Australia (2002) Diabetes Risk Assessment Tick Test. Available from www.diabetesaustralia.com.au/multilingualdiabetes/English/TickTest/ticktest.htm

Egger GJ. (1978) Medical nemesis and economic health or economic nemesis and medical health: the modern dilemma. *Aust J Soc Iss* 12(4): 287–301.

Esmaillzadeh A, Mirmiran P, Azizi F. (2006) Clustering of metabolic abnormalities in adolescents with the hypertriglyceridemic waist phenotype. *Am J Clin Nutr* 83: 36–46.

Farmer P. (2004) *Pathologies of power: health, human rights, and the new war on the poor*. California Series in Public Anthropology, 4. California: University of California Press.

Hankey GJ, Eikelboom JW, Ho WK et al. (2004) Clinical usefulness of plasma homocysteine in vascular disease. *Med J Aust* 181(6): 314–18.

Latham RE (trans.). (1994) Titus Lucretius Carus, *On the nature of things,* Book V. London: Penguin Books.

Marmot M. (2006) Health in an unequal world: social circumstances, biology and disease. *Clin Med* 6(6): 559–72.

Morrison R. (2003) *Plague species*. Sydney: Reed New Holland.

National Health and Medical Research Council. (2000) *National clinical guidelines in weight control and obesity management.* Canberra: Australian Government Press.

Rose G. (1991) Environmental health: problems and prospects. *J Royal Coll Phys Lond* 25(1): 48–52.

Rosengren A, Hawken S, Ounpuu S et al. Interheart investigators. (2004) Association of psychosocial risk factors with risk of acute myocardial infarction in 11 119 cases and 1348 controls from 52 countries (the INTERHEART study): case-control study. *Lancet* 364(9438): 953–62.

Swinburn B, Egger G. (2004) The runaway weight gain train: too many accelerators, not enough brakes. *Br Med J* 329(7468): 736–739.

Tonkin AM, Lim SS, Schirmer H. (2003) Cardiovascular risk factors: when should we treat? *Med J Aust* 178(3): 101–02.

Ware JH. (2006) The limitations of risk factors as prognostic tools. *NEJM* 355(25): 2615–17.

Wang TJ, Gona P, Larson, MG et al. (2006) Multiple biomarkers for the prediction of first major cardiovascular events and death. *NEJM* 355(25): 2631–39.

Whelton PK, He J, Appel LJ et al. (2002) Primary prevention of hypertension: clinical and public health advisory from the National High Blood Pressure Education Program. *JAMA* 288(15): 1882–88.

WHO (World Health Organization). (2007) *Disability adjusted life years (DALY).* Geneva: WHO. Available from www.who.int/healthinfo/boddaly/en/index.html.

——. (2002) *The world health report 2002: reducing risks, promoting healthy life.*——. Geneva: WHO.

——. (1999) *Obesity: preventing and managing the global epidemic: report of a WHO consultation. Second edition. WHO technical report series.* Geneva: WHO.

Yusuf S, Hawken S, Ounpuu S et al. Interheart Study Investigators. (2004) Effect of potentially modifiable risk factors associated with myocardial infarction in 52 countries (the INTERHEART study): case-control study. *Lancet* 364(9438): 937–52.

professional resources

PROFESSIONAL RESOURCES: RISK FACTOR MEASURES

Patients having or suspected of having lifestyle-related chronic disease can be tested or screened with a number of readily available standard measures. The following is a list of common measures used. More specific measures are covered in the individual chapters dealing with each lifestyle-related cause or outcome.

Non-intrusive measures

- tobacco consumption—see Chapter 15.
- alcohol consumption and dependency—see Chapter 15.
- Diabetes Risk Assessment Tick Test—see Chapter 5.
- resting pulse—a non-specific indicator of possible health problems and potential lack of fitness. Tachycardia may indicate lack of fitness (see Chapter 6) or an alcohol problem (Chapter 15).
- blood pressure (BP)—approximately 50% of hypertension is lifestyle based (Whelton et al., 2002).

Blood assays

- fasting lipids
- total cholesterol—not a sensitive measure alone, except as an indicator for more detailed testing when very high.
- LDL cholesterol—regarded as the 'bad' form of cholesterol.
- HDL—the 'good' form of cholesterol.
- triglycerides (TG)—an important dyslipidaemic risk factor and often associated with a low HDL and increased girth.
- blood sugars and glucose tolerance—see Chapter 5.

Other

- thyroxine stimulating hormone (TSH)—a sensitive test for thyroid dysfunction, although much less often associated with obesity than is often thought.
- measures of body fatness—see Chapter 4.
- measures of fitness—see Chapter 6.

CHAPTER 3

Everything you wanted to know about motivation

GARRY EGGER, ROSANNE COUTTS, JOHN LITT

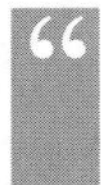

What people really need is a good listening to.

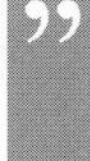

MILLER AND ROLLNICK, 2002

Introduction

The principal patient requirement in lifestyle medicine is change. However, encouraging an individual to change requires the clinician to have an inherent ability and/or a significant understanding of motivational principles. It is these principles that are at the core of lifestyle medicine and that differentiate it from conventional medicine.

Unlike a medication, which should have similar effects at different times across different individuals, motivation to act in a certain way will differ both between individuals and within the same individual at different times. A person who has little motivation to quit smoking can become extremely motivated by the death of a smoking friend or an X-ray that suggests possible cancer; for others, these things may have little impact. It is for this reason that there is no motivational pill, no single solution which suits all. It is also wrong for clinicians to think that they alone can motivate a patient to act.

The verb to motivate means 'to provide a prompt or incentive for a person to act in a certain way' (*Macquarie Dictionary*). The clinician can provide the prompt or incentive, frame an agenda for the patient, and explore the costs and benefits associated with lifestyle-related behaviour, but it is up to the patient to carry out the activity. Also, prompting on its own may generate resistance in patients especially if:

- they feel there is a judgment involved;
- the prompt cannot easily be connected to their health complaints; and
- they perceive that the doctor does not really appreciate their difficulties or has not heard their concerns.

It is important to remember that the way the communication is provided often has just as big an impact as what is said (Epstein, 2006). Strategies that demonstrate a non-judgmental approach and a sense of support help to encourage the patient to self-explore.

Addressing motivation has been shown to be effective in changing a range of behaviours including alcohol use, smoking, diet and weight loss (Burke et al., 2003), exercise and physical activity (Kirk et al., 2003; van Sluijs et al., 2004), and weight loss in diabetes (West et al., 2007). It is the basis of the process known as motivational interviewing (Miller and Rollick, 2002; Riemsma et al., 2003)

Motivational goals and strategies

Motivation is the key to lifestyle medicine. The ultimate goal of a motivator should be to move an individual from requiring *extrinsic* motivation through prompts or incentives (e.g. money, praise, support) to *intrinsic* motivation, or that which is internal and requires no outside prompting (although it may benefit from constant reinforcement). The process could be likened to switching on a motor and making sure it keeps running. To do this, it is necessary to do two things.

1. Make conscious (or create) a discrepancy between where an individual is and where he or she would like to be.

Motivation comes from desire—to have, to do, to maintain or to change. In lifestyle medicine, the desired form of motivation is one that would encourage the patient to change his or her unhealthy lifestyle behaviours. But for many people, the benefits of doing this, of moving from a current to a desired position, are often unclear or seen as too difficult to obtain. In some cases, the discrepancy is obvious (for example, the desire to feel and look better) and needs little amplification. But for others it may be more obscure, as in the experience of someone with an existential dilemma, who has abused drugs or alcohol, being sober and having a greater enjoyment of family and friends instead of avoiding them.

A useful strategy is to use a decisional balance approach. An example is provided in Chapter 15. In a nutshell, the client is asked to look at and balance the benefits and costs (likes and dislikes) associated with making a change such as quitting smoking or taking up exercise. The suggestions all need to come from the client and provide rich material to explore what is underpinning the patient's motivation. The ways of drawing this out are considered in the discussion of motivational practices below.

2. Help reduce the ambivalence about getting there.

If there is a discrepancy about where a person *is* and where he or she *wants to be,* it is because there is ambivalence about the two positions. Quitting smoking, for example, involves denying oneself a pleasure that may help relieve tension in order to get a perceived benefit of reducing the risk of a cancer that may not occur for decades.

A genuine desire to change can only be increased by reducing the barriers and/or increasing the triggers associated with this ambivalence by discussing the costs, as raised by the patient. For example, a barrier to losing weight may be the perceived pain of having to exercise or the perceived difficulty of losing weight, reinforced by many previous unsuccessful attempts. Triggers could be the desire for fresh breath from quitting smoking or the desire to reduce impotency caused by an expanded waistline. The clinician can then use this knowledge to reduce clients' ambivalence and move them towards a greater state of readiness to change.

Focusing

Within a 'helping' approach (Egan, 1998), three questions make the framework for focusing the individual. These are a starting point for encouraging new thinking and the gathering of information, so that interventions can be tailored to individuals within their current circumstances. The first question is, *What is going on?* This is where patients speak about themselves and describe aspects of their current lifestyle, often with suggestions for changes that they would like to make. The second question is, *What solutions would make sense for me?* This is where the clinician can guide and assist individuals to think about solutions that will support the changes. The third question is, *How can I make this happen?* This is about what individuals will actually do towards achieving the new goals.

Important findings by Landry and Solomon (2004) provide guidance on motivational strategy. They suggest that:

- strategies that rely on coercion do not, in the long term, encourage lasting change;
- the more reinforcing or encouraging forms of motivation will be more effective in encouraging change;
- various rewards and threats have been found to be poor motivators when trying to encourage individuals to be more active or change their eating habits;
- strategies reinforcing a more self-regulated approach (the individual organising it themselves) are more likely to foster lasting change.

An understanding of how *ready, willing* and *able* a patient is to make a change—as well as the *barriers* preventing and the *triggers* encouraging any particular change—will facilitate shifting the patient from requiring *extrinsic* motivation to being *intrinsically* motivated.

Being ready, willing and able

Miller and Rollnick (2002) use the terms 'ready, willing and able' to understand the processes inherent in a high level of motivation for change. These provide a format for discussing how to move patients closer to long-term change for a healthier lifestyle.

Being willing defines *why* a patient should change. Being able explains *how.* The only remaining question is *when.* This is where motivational instruction is probably most relevant, particularly the trans-theoretical, stages-of-change model of readiness developed by US psychologists Prochaska and Velicer (1997). The stages-of-change model proposes that individuals go through about six stages in changing any behaviour from the time that this is not even being considered to the adoption and maintenance of the new behaviour as a part of their lives. The stages of change are shown in Figure 3.1. The process is not necessarily a linear one and usually occurs in a more

FIGURE 3.1 The stages-of-change model of readiness to act

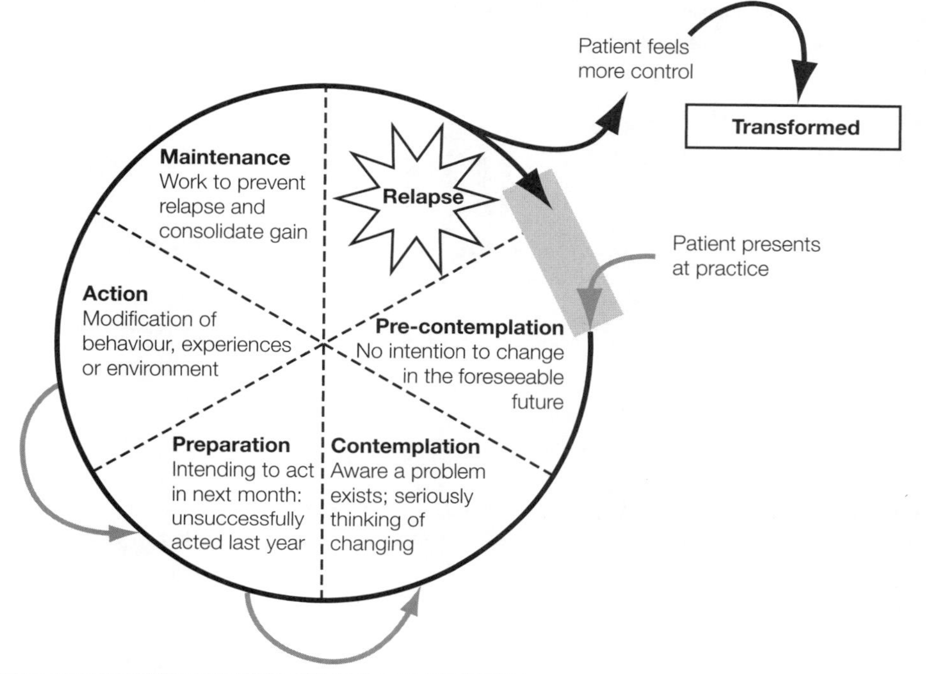

spiral form, with relapse and recovery over anything up to a two-year period until final adoption.

Interventions can be designed to encourage the individual to make forward moves from one stage to next. It is important to know which stage an individual is at because different interventions (processes of change) may work better in one stage than in another.

The first three stages—pre-contemplation, contemplation and preparation—are about thinking (cognitive processes). Action and maintenance are about actions and doing (behavioural processes). The Stages of Readiness to Change Scale allows the clinician to categorise an individual and then work on interventional approaches to assist with moving on. For example, for individuals in the contemplation stage, a discussion that may prove beneficial could be about how increasing physical activity, improving eating behaviours or reducing smoking (whichever might apply) would enhance their lifestyle. For individuals in the action stage, assisting them with further social support can encourage or facilitate a move forward into the maintenance phase.

Of the six stages seen in Figure 3.1, the first three are the main concerns of the clinician because during the stages beyond this—decision, maintenance and transformation—the impetus will come more from the patient and the main clinical requirement is for support and encouragement. A description of the first three stages and consideration of strategies for moving patients on to the next stage is shown in Table 3.1.

TABLE 3.1 Stages of change and strategies to shift

Stage	Description	Clinician's goal	Strategies to shift
Pre-contemplation (not ready)	Not considering change	Get the patient to consider the advantages of change.	Ask, 'Have you thought about…'. Check 'importance' and 'confidence'. Find where the patient 'would like to be' and work on barriers and triggers to getting there. Discuss past failures and 'reframe' these as learning experiences. Systematically explore perceived benefits and costs associated with a behaviour. **If this does not work:** Heighten awareness (but with options for reducing fear). **If this does not work:** Wait.
Contemplation (unsure)	Moving toward thinking about change	Get the patient to reduce their ambivalence about changing behaviour.	Provide information. Discuss outcomes if nothing is done. Discuss alternatives (e.g. exercise, diet). Set a manageable short-term goal around behaviour change (e.g. steps/day). Use motivational interviewing and decisional balance techniques. Provide evidence that underpins your concern by showing links with health effects of illness (but with options for reducing this). **If this does not work:** Keep reminding.
Preparation (ready)	Ready to make a change but has not yet done so	Move the patient into making a change and then maintaining this over the long term.	Discuss options. ACT—set a time and date and just 'do it'. BELONG—ask about someone (e.g. partner, club) for ongoing commitment. COMMIT—set some short and long-term goals (e.g. see weight goals in Chapter 4). **If this does not work:** Provide evidence that underpins your concern by showing links with health effects of illness.

An example of a readiness test using physical activity is included in *Professional resources* at the end of this chapter. This can be changed according to the behaviour being tested. A positive response reflects the stage of readiness to act. The individual is asked to choose one statement. For example, people who choose option three (I currently am physically active, but not on a regular basis) are in the prep ration stage. Stages of change can usually be determined early in a consultation. It is important to recognise that the stages can be quite fluid and vary considerably with time (and clinician!).

Being willing: how important is it to change?

The extent to which a person wants to change is summed up in his or her willingness to do so. Willingness to change is in turn influenced by the discrepancy between the status quo and the goal (i.e. where he or she is and where he or she wants to be), the level of ambivalence this has created, and the perceived importance of wanting to move closer to the goal. If the clinician has done the job right and reduced ambivalence by helping remove barriers and increase the triggers to action (either physically or psychologically), there should be greater willingness to move towards the goal.

Willingness can be determined by a simple question: *On a scale of one to ten (where one is not important at all and ten is extremely important), how important is it for you to [reach the goal discussed]?* If the answer score is high, the patient is willing to act and only his or her readiness and ability to do so need to be considered. If the answer is low, greater emphasis needs to be placed on increasing importance and hence reducing the ambivalence to act.

It is also worth checking what underpins the motivation or importance when the patient offers a relatively high number by asking, *What contributes to your score being an eight (say) rather than a two?* This will provide insight into what the patient believes is underpinning his or her motivation. This is useful information because you, as a facilitator, can reinforce the information and further explore it to see how robust it is. Some patients may have not thought it through and therefore will be more vulnerable to failure or lack of commitment. Others may be offering a high level of importance to please you (or get you 'off their back'). An example would be an excessive drinker who sees no problem, physical or psychological, in continuing to drink excessively. In this case, the potential problems (e.g. liver damage, family breakdown) need to be highlighted to increase the discrepancy between status quo and goal and increase willingness to do something about this.

Being able: how confident is the patient about changing?

A person can be extremely willing but lack the confidence or ability to change. This does not come just from a lack of knowledge (although in some cases it may do so) but from a lack of *self-efficacy* or feeling of one's ability to succeed in reaching a specific or general goal. Weight loss for men, for example, is often hindered by their lack of knowledge. Receipt of the correct knowledge about nutrition and exercise is often enough to increase ability to change. For many women, on the other hand, biological factors make successful weight loss more difficult and previous failures, even with the right knowledge, contribute to low self-efficacy and make success less likely.

As with importance, this can be checked with a simple question: *On a scale of one to ten (where one is not confident at all and ten is extremely confident), how confident are you that you can [reach the goal discussed]?*

Again, explore the reasons underpinning a high level of confidence to check that patients are realistic. Many smokers and those with hazardous drinking habits often report high levels of confidence to quit or cut down. This belief may represent a rationalisation of the need to change. If the score is low, ask *What would need to happen to move this score from a two to a nine?* This provides an opportunity to focus the discussion on what the barriers are that you and the patient need to overcome in order to improve motivation. For example, many younger smokers state that they will quit when there is evidence of health effects. If the clinician can show how the patient's health is already being affected, for example, by reduced pulmonary function (common in smokers over the age of 35–40 years), this may alter the motivation to change.

If the score is high for both confidence and importance, there is little for the clinician to do except discuss *when* this will happen (readiness). If the ability score is low, one of two aspects of confidence need to be targeted.

Increasing task efficacy means ensuring that there is confidence in the process to be used to affect change. Can the patient feel confident, for example, that a particular weight loss or quit smoking medication will actually work, given that so many such programs may have failed in the past? In this case it is up to the clinician to convince the patient that this time it is different and to provide specific reasons that are within the patient's control.

Increasing self-efficacy means working on the patient's confidence in being able to follow and stick with the task at hand. Typical reactions may include self-blame, catastrophising and self-doubt. In these cases, modifying thinking patterns becomes the issue and there are a variety of established ways of doing this—for example, rational emotive therapy or cognitive behaviour therapy—some of which are discussed in Chapter 11 (also see Elder et al., 1999).

Case examples

Some typical responses to both the importance and confidence questions are:

- a male alcohol abuser who scores low on the importance of giving up drinking but high on confidence to do this, if he so chooses. In this case, increasing importance by showing harmful effects, such as a damaged liver or the outcome of cirrhosis, may increase the perceived discrepancy between the status quo and goal and stimulate this to be acted on.
- a woman wanting to lose weight whose rating of importance is high but confidence low because of previous failures. The goal of the clinician here is to raise the patient's confidence about being able to make the required change, or in the process. Some ideas and questions for raising importance and confidence in a patient are show in Table 3.2.

Barriers and triggers to change

At this stage it is important to reiterate that the goal of a motivator is to shift a patient from requiring *extrinsic* motivation to being *intrinsically* motivated. Intrinsic motivation comes from the benefits achieved from change. However, in the early stages these benefits are unlikely to be felt. Hence it is important to raise extrinsic motivation by removing the barriers and increasing the triggers towards achieving this goal.

Barriers to change can be either physical or psychological (Table 3.3).

In some cases these may be obvious and easy to detect using any of the techniques discussed above. In others they may be more deep seated and require extensive probing

TABLE 3.2 Tips for enhancing importance and confidence

Enhancing importance	Why did you score a one and not a ten on this scale? What would need to happen to move you from a [low] score of x to a score of eight or nine? What would encourage you to move (that is, from your low score to an eight or nine on this scale)? How would your behaviour change if you did rate a ten on this? What are the main barriers stopping you from getting a higher score? Can you see a way to remove or reduce these barriers? What are the pros and cons of trying and not making the desired changes? Pick what seems to be important to the individual (e.g. impotence in men, efficiency in women) and concentrate on this.
Enhancing confidence	Why did you score a (for example) one and not an eight or ten on this scale? What do you think could help you score higher on this scale? What have you done in the past that has been successful? Why do you think you have failed in the past? What has made it difficult to succeed? What was the trigger for the slip up? Re-frame previous failures as 'slips' or short-term inconveniences. Stress that while the patient may have tried and failed before, this time it is a different approach and outline why. Discuss the stage approach (below) and how this involves some failures as well as successes before moving to the next stage.

TABLE 3.3 General barriers to lifestyle change (see Elder et al., 1999)

Physical	Psychological	Other
mechanical problems	stress	responsibilities
weather	social pressure	lack of time
fatigue	peer pressure	
lack of equipment	laziness	
sickness	reaction to clinician	
financial	embarrassment	

and discussion. Early sexual or physical abuse, for example, can be relatively common causes of obesity in women in order to reduce attractiveness to future potential perpetrators. This requires disclosure and management through the development of trust and rapport with a clinician. Other causes are often more subtle. For example, a male patient disclosed after several weeks of treatment for obesity that he did not want to walk in public because of a fear of looking foolish to young onlookers. Providing patients with a supportive environment and encouraging them to be candid about the various triggers will help to identify these barriers.

Some common physical barriers to becoming active and some suggested solutions for these are outlined in Table 3.4. Similar tables can be drawn up for barriers to other behaviour change.

TABLE 3.4 Typical physical barriers to being inactive

Identify the problem		What does the patient attribute the problem to? Are there any medical reasons why there is a problem (that may not be directly related to the patient's behaviour)?	
Barrier	chaffing	*Possible solutions*	wear lycra bike pants; use Vaseline™
	leg pain		change shoes; stretch; see a podiatrist
	back pain		persist; walk in water/soft sand; try another form of exercise
	joint pain		use walking poles; try weight-supportive exercise
	hypoglycaemia (in diabetes)		reduce medication accordingly; carry a carbohydrate drink

There are also motivational triggers that can help overcome these barriers and shift an individual towards being intrinsically motivated. For some, these might be financial; for others, physical (e.g. looks, healthy feeling) or impact on health; and for still others, a desire to please other people, such as a partner or children. These can assist a patient to get to the next level and be closer to being intrinsically motivated. Triggers generated by the client are more likely to be salient or important because they have some meaning or relevance to the patient. This does not preclude the clinician identifying some triggers but this should occur after the patient has exhausted the list of triggers that they can think of.

How did you get the motivation to lose so much weight?
It wasn't hard
Plater & Egger

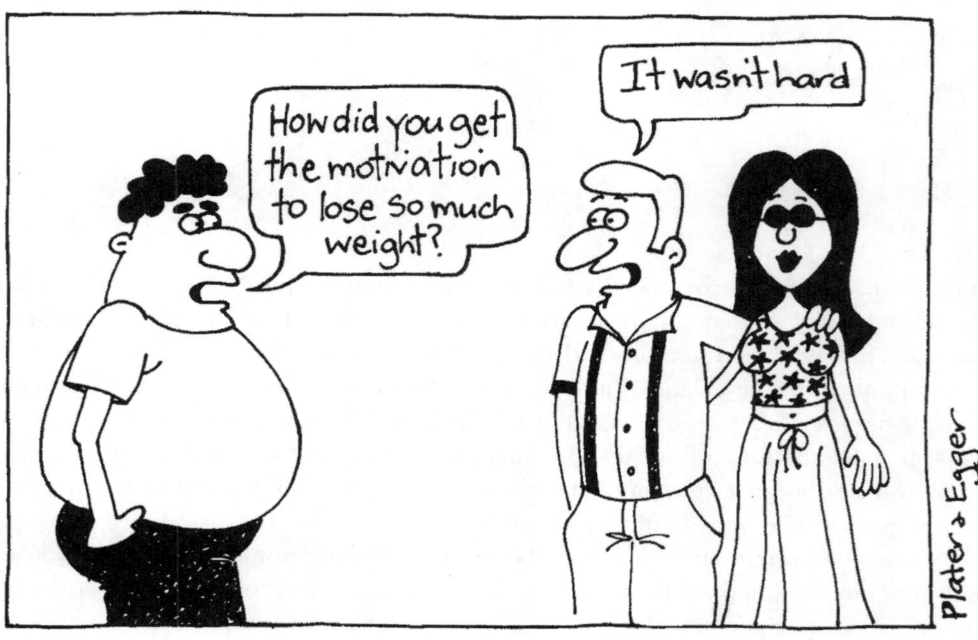

Motivation at the public health level

The above are approaches to motivation that can be used by the clinician. There are also a range of public health approaches for lifestyle change that would help support clinical initiatives. Economic incentives—such as tax rebates or legislative changes that make healthier choices the easiest choices—can add incentives to the patient environment. A lower excise/tax on low-alcohol beer, legislation mandating seat belts or allowing random breath testing, and restriction of smoking environments are good working examples. These are usually beyond the ambit of the clinician but should be encouraged as part of a wider health promotion approach to lifestyle change. For example, an approach that financially rewarded patients and clinicians for reversing early stage disease, such as type 2 diabetes, would have long-term cost saving consequences.

What can be done in a standard consultation

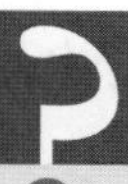

Assess the patient's readiness to change and target motivation to change.

Check willingness to change based on a ten-point scale of importance.

Check ability to change based on a ten-point scale of confidence.

Work on increasing willingness or confidence, depending on which is deficient.

Isolate and work on reducing barriers to change.

Look for and increase triggers to change.

Some motivational tactics

Set short- and long-term goals

It can take a lot of work and dedication to make substantial lifestyle changes. Accomplishments can be realised through good planning of daily, weekly and long-term personal goals. The clinician can guide a specific and measurable goal-setting exercise that captures the aims of the individual, both long and short term (Shilts et al., 2004). The goals should be accepted or internalised by the individual (Cox, 2007). An effective goal is not one that is thought about and then forgotten. Getting the patient to write goals down and monitor how they are going is most important.

Goals should be short and long term and involve processes as well as outcomes. For example, a long-term goal may be a 10 kg weight loss but a short-term goal leading to this could be a 1% decrease in waist size per week over the first 6–8 weeks. A process goal in doing this may be to walk 70 000 steps a week and cut back soft-drink consumption.

Record progress

Self-monitoring and recording of progress is one of the most effective strategies of behaviour change. This can include things such as steps measured by a pedometer, days since last drug use, or an increase in fitness. Recordings should be kept in a prominent place where they can be easily and regularly seen; they may even be kept by significant others.

Use the mate system

Where possible, involving a partner, spouse, relative or friend, or working with a group of like-minded people, can help increase adherence to a program and ensure against relapse.

Plan ahead

Planning what is going to be done in advance—for instance, on the night before—is always a good way of ensuring things are done. The busiest people in the world (e.g. politicians, businesspeople) have exercise built into their day because they have built it into their diary. Planning on the day, as a sort of second thought, increases the likelihood that things will be put off for more 'important' matters that arise.

Encourage the use of fantasy and imagination

It may not always work, but using fantasy during exercise (e.g. imagining winning the Olympic Games 10 km race) can often get the patient over the personal motivation line, if not the Olympic line.

Using imagery is associated with motivation and is a form of self-modelling. When we practice imagery, the neuromuscular patterns that are used are the same as when actually doing the activity (Smith and Collins, 2004). For example, with physical activity an individual can practice without moving a muscle. However, it must be emphasised that getting on and really doing the activity is still very important.

Imagery is helpful for gathering confidence, working through fears, exploring new skills, and generally supporting progress. Individuals who have been encouraged to use their imaginations can see themselves having increased energy, an improved appearance, or the skills to perform certain techniques, for example dancing, gardening, walking or playing a sport. Based on work by Vealey and Greenleaf (2001), a sample five-step program to enhance imagery ability is included below. This could be used to focus an individual on new tasks and goals.

1. Get comfortable in a quiet place, close your eyes, and breathe rhythmically to establish a relaxed state.
2. Visualise a coloured circle that fills the visual field initially and then sinks to a dot and disappears. Repeat the process making the circle different colours each time.
3. Select a variety of scenes and images and develop them in detail. Include scenes such as a swimming pool, a beautiful walking track or a golf course next to the ocean. Enjoy the scenes.
4. Imagine yourself in a setting of your choice doing a skill or sport that you are keenly interested in. Project yourself into the image as if you were one of the performers. Imagine yourself successfully completing the task in the scene.

5. End the session by breathing deeply, opening your eyes, and slowly adjusting to the external environment.

Find a motivational soft spot

Motivation is an intra-individual factor that varies between individuals and over time. Finding what motivates an individual at any particular time can help the clinician improve the prospects of long-term behaviour change. Avoiding disease may motivate someone to want to lose weight while increased physical attractiveness may work for someone else. Finding the motivational 'soft spot' of the moment is often the key to success.

Encourage flexibility/discourage rigidity

Rigidity in thinking is the great stumbling block to behaviour change. Perfectionism is often the cause of such rigid thinking. Flexibility allows for the odd mistake, or 'falling off the wagon', which can easily be corrected, whereas associating success with just a single, unchangeable path is a recipe for failure. Adherence is more likely when:

- people have choices;
- the intervention can be tailored to the needs of the individual;
- the process is incremental; and
- flexibility is coupled with regular review.

Intrinsic motivation: the end game

As pointed out at the start of this chapter, it is the goal of the motivator to shift the patient from needing external reward to being intrinsically motivated to maintain a lifestyle change. This is probably best seen in long-term exercisers, such as joggers, who become dedicated to their activity and need little outside prompting to carry it out, even in the presence of such negative conditions as pain, cold or lack of time. Several books have been written over the years about the stages of this process. Essentially there is a shift from a discomfort stage to one where the rewards are physical and then to one where the rewards become psychological and where there is a feeling of oneness and wellbeing when carrying out the adopted behaviour (Egger, 1981). Once the level has been achieved, the need for an outside person to motivate that individual to act becomes almost irrelevant. Anyone who has experienced this will be easier to motivate to seek that feeling again.

Knowledge is also a vital component of motivational strategy, particularly to encourage physical activity. Research by Sallis et al. (1986) found that the individuals most likely to develop a more physically active lifestyle had the following characteristics:

- confidence that they could be successful in the use of physical activity;
- knowledge about what constitutes a healthy lifestyle;
- knowledge about the importance and value of partaking in regular physical activity;
- a perception that they did have a level of self-control; and
- good attitudes about the value and importance of regular exercise.

Summary

The goal of a clinician is to move patients from requiring *extrinsic* motivation to change their unhealthy behaviours to being *intrinsically* motivated to do so, and thus not need external support. This is done by assessing the patient's *readiness, willingness* and *ability* to act, and targeting the areas of weakness that would enable them to act to reduce any ambivalence identified between where they *are* and where they *would prefer to be.* Reducing the *barriers* and increasing the *triggers* to action will assist in shifting the patient towards the desired goal.

practice tips

PRACTICE TIPS: MOTIVATING A PATIENT TO CHANGE

	Medical practitioner	**Practice nurse**
Assess	Lifestyle. Need and readiness to change. Whether it is worth putting effort into trying to bring about change at this stage. Stage of readiness to change.	Lifestyle: • the specific behaviour(s) to be changed; • how ready, willing and able the patient is to change; • importance and confidence, rated on a ten-point scale; • motivational 'soft spots'; • stage of readiness (see *Professional resources* for a test).
Assist	By providing clear, concise and non-judgmental advice to change. By providing encouragement. By Identifying potential short-and long-term goals. By using Lifescripts tools (see *References*).	By using motivational tools to encourage change. By concentrating on weaknesses in importance and confidence. By using appropriate tactics to move through stages of readiness. By helping with time planning. By using Lifescripts tools (see *References*).
Arrange	Support (e.g. family or significant others; include a motivational specialist, where appropriate). List of other health professionals for a care plan. Other resources (e.g. QUIT line).	Discussion of motivational tactics with other involved health professionals. Referral to a personal trainer, nutritionist or life coach, if appropriate. Contact with self-help groups.

key points

KEY POINTS FOR CLINICAL MANAGEMENT

- Consider motivation before giving a lifestyle-oriented prescription.
- Stress to patients that change is necessary for disease correction/prevention.
- Point out that such change will make them feel better than now.
- Make patients aware of the fact that many barriers are mere rationalisations or excuses.
- Aim for intrinsic motivation to sustain behaviour change.

REFERENCES

Burke B, Arkowitz H, Menchola M. (2003) The efficacy of motivational interviewing: a meta-analysis of controlled clinical trials. *J Consult Clin Psychol* 71: 843–61.

Cardinal BJ. (1995) The stages of exercise scale and stages of exercise behavior female adults. *J Sports Med & Phys Fit* 35: 87–92.

Cox R. (2007) *Sport psychology: Concepts and applications.* NY: McGraw–Hill.

DoHA (Department of Health and Ageing) (2005) Lifescripts. Canberra: DoHA. Available from www.health.gov.au/internet/wcms/Publishing.nsf/Content/health-pubhlth-strateg-lifescripts-index.htm

Egan, G. (1998) *The skilled helper: A problem-management approach to helping, 6th edn.* Pacific Grove: Wadsworth Publishing Company.

Egger, G. (1981) *The sport drug.* Sydney: Allen and Unwin.

Elder J, Ayala G, Harris S. (1999) Theories and intervention approaches to health-behavior change in Primary Care. *Am J Prev Med* 17: 275–84.

Epstein RM. (2006) Making communication research matter: what do patients notice, what do patients want, and what do patients need? *Patient Educ Couns* 60: 272–78.

Kirk A, Mutrie N, MacIntyre P et al. (2003) Increasing physical activity in people with type 2 diabetes. *Diab Care* 26(4): 1186–92.

Landry JB, Solomon MA. (2004) African American women's self determination across changes of change for exercise. *J Sport & Ex Psych* 11: 263–82.

Macquarie Dictionary, 3rd edn. (1997) Macquarie University: Macquarie Library Pty Ltd.

Maehr ML, McInerney DM. (2004) Motivation as personal investment. *Res Sociocult Infl Motiv & Learn* 4: 61–90.

Miller WR, Rollnick S. (2002) *Motivational interviewing: preparing people for change, 2nd edn.* New York: Guilford Press.

Morgan WP. (2000) *A simple solution to the exercise adherence problem.* Paper presented at the Annual Meeting of the American College of Sports Medicine, Indianapolis, 2000.

Prochaska J, Velicer W. (1997) The transtheoretical model of health behavior change. *Am J Health Prom* 12: 38–48.

Riemsma R, Pattenden J, Bridle C et al. (2003) Systematic review of the effectiveness of stage based interventions to promote smoking cessation. *Brit Med J* 326: 1175–81.

Sallis JF, Haskell WL, Fortman SP et al. (1986) Predictors of adoption and maintenance of physical activity in a community sample. *Prev Med* 15: 331–41.

Shilts M, Horowitz M, Townsend M. (2004) Goal setting as a strategy for dietary and physical activity behavior change: a review of the literature. *Am J Health Prom* 19: 81–93.

Smith D, Collins D. (2004) Mental practice, motor performance, and the late CNV. *J Sport & Ex Psych* 26: 412–26.

Van Sluijs E, Van Poppel M, Van Mechelen W. (2004) Stage-based lifestyle interventions in primary care are they effective? *Am J Prev Med* 26: 330–43.

Vealey RS, Greenleaf CA. (2001) Seeing is believing: understanding and using imagery in sport. In Williams JM (ed.) *Applied sport psychology: personal growth to peak performance* (pp. 247–272). Mountain View, CA: Mayfield Publishing Company.

West DS, Delillo V, Bursac Z et al. (2007) Motivational interviewing improves weight loss in women with type 2 diabetes. *Diab Care* 30(5): 1081–87.

professional resources

PROFESSIONAL RESOURCES: MEASURING MOTIVATION

The following are some simple tests to measure readiness, importance (willingness) and confidence (ability) to change a behaviour (e.g. physical activity). The type of behaviour can be changed as required (e.g. quitting smoking, reducing drinking, improving nutrition, losing weight).

Measuring readiness to change physical activity

Current physical activity status—pick the description that applies to you.

1. I am currently not physically active and do not intend to start being physically active in the next six months. (Pre-contemplation)
2. I am currently not physically active, but I am thinking about becoming physically active in the next six months. (Contemplation)
3. I am currently physically active but not on a regular basis. (Preparation)
4. I am currently physically active regularly, but I have only begun doing so within the last six months. (Action)
5. I am currently physically active regularly and have been so for longer than six months. (Maintenance)

Measuring willingness to change physical activity (importance)

How important is it for you to exercise to lose weight? (Circle the number)

1 2 3 4 5 6 7 8 9 10

NOT IMPORTANT EXTREMELY IMPORTANT

Measuring confidence in changing physical activity (ability)

How confident are you that you can exercise properly to lose weight if you try?

1 2 3 4 5 6 7 8 9 10

NOT CONFIDENT EXTREMELY CONFIDENT

CHAPTER 4

Overweight and obesity: the epidemic's underbelly

STEPHAN ROSSNER, GARRY EGGER, ANDREW BINNS

With obesity, genetics loads the gun, lifestyle pulls the trigger.

GEORGE BRAY, 2003

Introduction

In 1970 a small group of dedicated scientists met in London at the First International Congress on Obesity to discuss what was then a distinctly 'unsexy' topic. Although French endocrinologist Jean Vague had outlined the potential health problems associated with increased abdominal fat, or a 'pot belly', as far back as 1947, it had taken this long for the modern obesity epidemic to germinate. By 2006, the numbers at the Tenth International Congress of Obesity in Sydney had grown to almost 3 000, with widespread media interest in finding the answer to a problem now affecting up to 60% of people in many developed countries and an estimated 15% of the total world population (International Association for the Study of Obesity; World Health Oganization). Australian figures show that more than 67% of Australian men and 55% of women were classified as overweight or obese in 2000. This represents an average annual increase in body weight of around 1.6 g per person per day since 1980 (AIHW, 2006).

Obesity is associated with over thirty-five different diseases and a growing list of everyday ailments (discussed in Chapter 2); it is the beginning of a cascade of epidemics (Figure 4.1); and is one of the few diseases that feeds back on itself causing vicious cycles (Figure 4.2). These factors make the situation even more serious (Swinburn and Egger, 2004).

Fat distribution: not *if* you're fat but *where*

Research confirmed the early suggestion of Vague (1947) of the importance of abdominal fat. Abdominally stored fat (i.e. the android or 'apple' shape), which is most

FIGURE 4.1 The obesity cascade—some examples

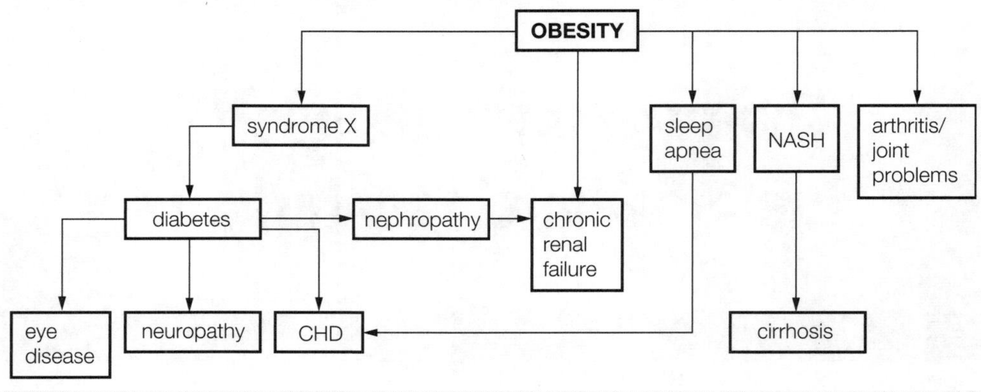

FIGURE 4.2 Vicious circles associated with obesity

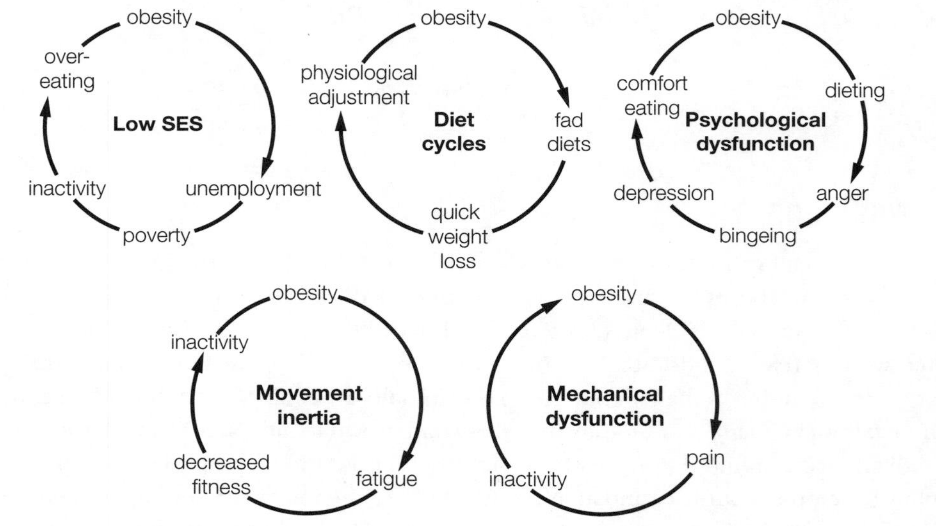

Source: Swinburn and Egger, 2004

characteristic of males and post-menopausal females, is more metabolically dangerous than gluteal stored fat (i.e. the gynoid or 'pear' shape) or fat stored around the hips and buttocks of pre-menopausal females. More recently, it has been found that internal fat, or that around the viscera of the trunk, is even more associated with metabolic risk and end-point disease than subcutaneous abdominal fat. These fat stores have implications for diagnostic measurement, as will be shown at the end of this chapter.

Perhaps naturally, the medical focus on dealing with obesity has been towards developing a pharmaceutical 'cure'; a quick fix, with little behavioural cost to the individual. Many have shown promise but none has yet yielded widespread success over the long term, and the nature of this 'disease' suggests this is unlikely to happen in the near future. As with any chronic disease, it needs to be accepted that there is unlikely to be a single, long-term solution to obesity management.

In this chapter, therefore, we concentrate on the strategies that work best for weight loss at the individual level but stress that all do so only in the context of a lifestyle change involving modification of energy intake (EI, i.e. food and drink) and/or energy expenditure (EE, i.e. exercise, metabolic rate and thermogenesis). Both EI and EE will be dealt with in detail in subsequent chapters. Here we confine ourselves to a discussion of the energy balance equation and those factors influencing energy balance. We also look at developing trends in weight control management and summarise the available strategies for dealing with the problem. This is meant to complement the *National clinical guidelines,* which provide ten steps for adults and eight steps for children (Table 4.1) and which are available from the National Health and Medical Research Council (2003) and are further discussed in Egger and Binns (2001).

TABLE 4.1 *National clinical guidelines* for weight control and obesity management

Adults	Children
1. Discuss weight and whether measurements (height, weight, BMI, WC) should be taken at this stage.	1. Assess the extent of overweight or obesity in the child or adolescent in relation to other children at the same stage of development.
2. Assess and treat co-morbidities associated with weight and determine the patient's need to lose weight.	2. Assess co-morbidities associated with weight and treat these independently where appropriate.
3. Ascertain the patient's readiness and motivation to lose weight.	3. Assess *why* energy imbalance has occurred.
4. Assess *why* energy imbalance has occurred.	4. Assess *how* energy imbalance has occurred.
5. Assess *how* energy imbalance has occurred.	5. Determine the level of clinical intervention required.
6. Determine the level of clinical intervention required.	6. Devise treatment strategy with the patient and family.
7. Devise goals and treatment strategies with the patient.	7. Devise treatment goals, including outcome indicators not related to weight.
8. Prescribe or refer for dietary and physical activity advice.	8. Review and provide regular assistance for weight management and maintenance of weight change, and change program as required.
9. Prescribe medication or refer for obesity surgery and/or conduct or refer for behaviour modification as appropriate.	
10. Review and provide regular assistance for weight management and maintenance of weight change, and change program as required.	

Source: NHMRC, 2003

Before we turn to treatments however, we need to look at the basic physics and bio-energetics of body weight.

Is a calorie really a calorie?

Traditionally, the formula for body weight has been

weight = **energy in** (from food and drink) − **energy out**
(from exercise, thermogenesis and metabolism)

This is a physics formula, with little relevance to real life. According to the equation, people eating an extra slice of toast and butter each day over the course of their lives would be approximately 170 kg heavier than if they did not eat this. This is clearly absurd. The formula, which is used widely by the public and popular media, is based on the idea that energy balance is static, rather than dynamic (as it should be in a biological organism). Egger and Swinburn (1996) have devised a more realistic formula (Figure 4.3), one that takes account of biological adaptation as well as other factors.

FIGURE 4.3 An ecological approach to obesity

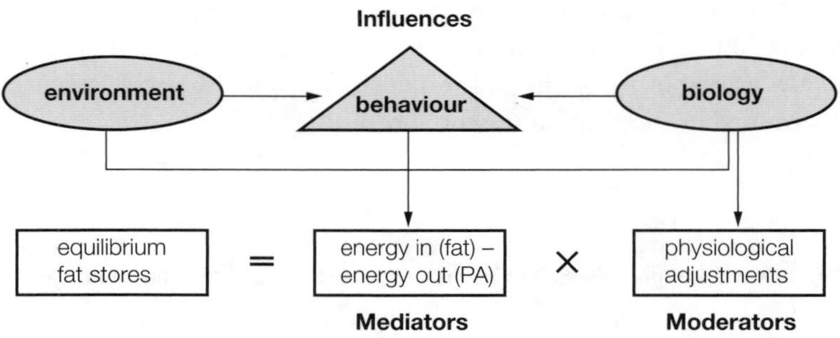

Source: Egger and Swinburn, 1996

Using this conceptual approach, it is clear that energy balance is not only influenced by a range of environmental (e.g. food availability, energy-saving devices), biological (e.g. age, gender, ethnicity) and behavioural influences (e.g. early experiences, stress, depression) but also by physiological adjustments that occur to moderate energy imbalances. In the case of the toast eater, for example, energy expenditure through heat loss, metabolism or exercise may rise to ensure that overall there is only a minor net change in body weight as a result of a small change in energy intake. These adjustments can vary between and within individuals, according to metabolic rate, effects on hunger, and other physiological factors.

Changing energy balance

Given the above proviso, it is still important to consider energy balance, within lifestyle change, as the core of weight loss instruction. This involves modifying food intake and exercise output. Although there are innumerable diets, products and programs for doing this, all effective treatments essentially involve a change in the balance of calorific volume, or the amount of calories consumed, in relation to those expended. This is relatively simply defined in both cases as being the product of three factors, as shown in Figure 4.4.

Each of these is discussed in detail in the following chapters on nutrition and exercise.

Trends in weight control management

Optimal management in weight control is unlikely to come from unlocking a lock with a single key. The appropriate analogy is more likely to be that of a barrel lock,

FIGURE 4.4 A calorific volume approach to energy balance

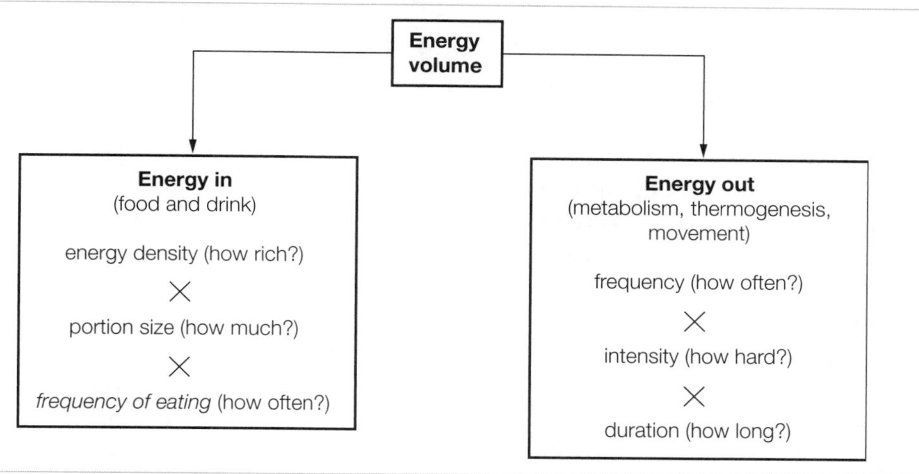

which will not open unless all locks on the barrel are lined up, as shown in Figure 4.5.

Some of these strategies are discussed in following chapters. Meanwhile, there are a number of recent developments that can help facilitate the process. Among the more recent of these are putting the emphasis on lifestyle change, matching strategies to the patient, and combining treatment strategies.

FIGURE 4.5 Unlocking the secret of lifestyle-related health

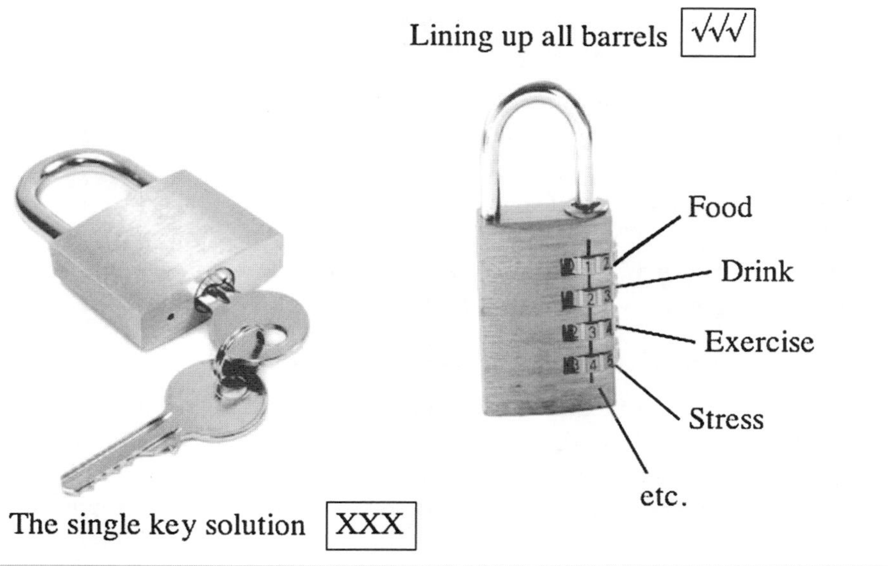

Putting the emphasis on lifestyle change

With all the 'hype' about new diets, drugs, and other weight loss treatments, it is sometimes forgotten that every treatment that works requires a lifestyle change involving the energy balance formula shown above and that such a change should be the core of weight loss management. That this is often not the case is due to the fact that, in a modern obesogenic environment, such a change is difficult to make. More detail on nutrition and physical activity is covered in the following chapters. A structured approach to this is covered in the *National clinical guidelines on weight control and obesity management* (NHMRC, 2003) and in Egger and Binns (2001).

Matching the strategies to the patient

A one-suit-fits-all approach is no longer regarded as acceptable in weight loss management. For one thing, the strategies are complementary. Furthermore, they should be used dynamically such that the strategy or strategy mix implemented at the start of a program may be totally different to that used after early losses or for long-term maintenance. The skill of the clinician is in matching the appropriate strategies (and methods within strategies) to the patient.

Recognising 'unhealthy' versus 'healthy' body fat

As discussed above, abdominal and particularly visceral fat has a close association with metabolic risk. The latter is generally correlated with the former and can usually be picked up in waist circumference measures. However, in lean individuals who are active but still have metabolic risk indicating insulin resistance, an imaging measure of visceral fat obtained from a major hospital or radiology unit is needed to assess true risk. Gluteal fat, defined by a low waist-to-hip ratio (see *Professional resources*), has been shown in several large-scale studies to have a negative association with end-point disease (Welborn and Dhaliwal, 2007). Hence, while many women may complain about the aesthetic problems of large hips, this has few adverse metabolic correlates.

Combining treatment strategies

Often in the past, only one strategy (e.g. drugs, diet) has been applied to any or all individuals. This is now considered to be less effective than combining strategies, at least in the appropriate situation. Medication and surgery, for example, can be used together with meal replacements; pre-prepared meals can be used with a nutritional education and counselling program; and exercise should always be combined with a hypocaloric diet, which can consist of meal replacements, low energy meals or a hunger suppressant drug where indicated.

Making a distinction between short- and long-term loss

It is now well recognised that short-term weight loss is relatively easy. Long-term weight loss maintenance, on the other hand, is very difficult but should be the main goal of any effective weight loss program. In the early stages, quick weight losses may be important for increasing motivation to proceed to longer-term benefits. It is much easier to do this at the outset by reducing calorific intake than by increasing exercise output. However, over the longer term, an increase in daily activity has been found to be one of the most significant factors in sustaining losses (Wing and Hill, 2001).

From diets to reduced energy eating

Because of the vagaries of physiological adjustment and the difficulty in trying to overcome psychologically a biological drive (hunger), diets (as in a structured reduction in energy intake) are unlikely to be able to be maintained over the long term. Because 'going on' a diet, usually results in 'coming off' it sooner or later, weight regain is likely. And because of physiological adjustment, this is likely to exceed that which is lost during the energy restriction phase, causing the common tick-shaped response (quick loss but over-compensated weight gain). Consequently, the modern shift is to a change in the pattern of eating, reducing (in particular) fats and other high energy-dense foods and increasing fibre and foods with low energy density.

Use of clinically supervised meal replacements

Although they have been around for some time, meal replacements in the form of powdered drinks or food bars have been generally frowned upon because they have not been nutritionally balanced and are often used over the short term only, without clinical supervision. Advances in food technology and an increase in clinical knowledge have resulted in an increase in their use under certain conditions (Egger, 2006 and below).

Practical implications of physiological adjustment

One of the most obvious implications of physiological adjustment to changes in energy balance are plateaus in weight loss. These are a source of frustration for patients and clinicians alike, many of whom often expect weight loss to occur in a perfect linear fashion. As the great Harvard nutritionist Jean Mayer once said, 'Like a wise man will reduce spending when his income is cut, the body reduces the amount of energy it expends when energy intake (food) is reduced'.

The difference between the wise person and the body is that energy use, in the form of metabolism, is dropped below that of energy intake in order to reduce the imbalance even further. In other words, a decrease of 10% in energy intake may lead to a decrease of 12–15% in energy expenditure because, like the spender without a loan, the body cannot afford to go into debt.

Plateaus occur as a result of the body's adaptation to the rate of energy intake in relation to energy expenditure. Unfortunately, nobody can say when and for how long a plateau will continue, as this is a highly individual process. It is dependant on a number of factors not yet identified but probably including the time spent being overweight, age, gender, and the actions taken to lose weight (King et al., 2006). The length of a plateau is difficult to determine because there has been little research. At this stage, and without an evidence base, there are two relevant factors. First, being on a plateau is far from a sign of failure. On the contrary, it indicates the body has adjusted to change and is re-adapting to these changes. As the average Australian is gaining 1.6 g a day, being on a plateau means a patient is winning. Second, as a plateau is a period of adjustment, it makes sense that getting off the plateau will involve change of some kind. Some possibilities are suggested in Table 4.2.

TABLE 4.2 Suggested ways of breaking through a weight loss plateau through change

General measures	Take a holiday. Go to bed earlier. Get up later. Go camping. Go bushwalking. Try a career change. Review and modify eating habits.
Changing energy intake	Change eating patterns. Try different drinks. Use meal replacements. Eat different foods. Go low carb (for a while). Monitor food intake.
Changing energy expenditure	Try different exercises. Add weights to exercise. Increase speed. Walk a different route. Walk backwards. Stand for longer. Walk instead of drive. Catch public transport.

Source: King et al., 2006

Current strategies in weight loss

A strategy is defined as a broad general approach to treatment. We have listed eleven such strategies used in the management of weight control (Table 4.3). Within these strategies there are a number of methods that are more specific ways of achieving successful weight loss. A strategy, for example, may be an exercise approach to weight loss; a method within this could be the use of resistance training. The level of evidence for these strategies is variable, so some will be treated with more detail than others. We have categorised them into strategies with a limited evidence base, those with some evidence, and those with a sound evidence base. A base of lifestyle change is assumed as a pre-requisite for success of all of the strategies listed.

Strategies with limited or no supporting evidence

(MOST) OVER-THE-COUNTER PRODUCTS

Over-the-counter (OTC) weight loss products are defined here as those ingestible substances usually (but not always) derived from herbal or natural substances for which

TABLE 4.3 Current treatment strategies for weight loss, ranked in escalating scientific strength

Treatment	Evidence	Comment
1. Herbal and other supplements; OTC products	–	May have a placebo effect with lifestyle change over the short term. No proven long-term benefits.
2. 'Alternative' treatments (e.g. hypnotherapy, acupressure)	*	May be an 'add on' to lifestyle change in some people. No proven long-term effectiveness when used alone.
3. Self-directed diets (eg. Atkins, Zone)	*	Can produce quick losses but usually not in the long-term. May help some people change lifestyle.
4. Diet-based commercial programs	*	Results not usually published. May suit females and those who respond to group/peer support.
5. Fitness programs	**	Slower, but longer-term results. Probably best for those with little weight to lose.
6. Counselling	**	Good for ingrained habits and irrational or counterproductive thoughts involving eating/inactivity.
7. Prescribed medication	**	Good adjunct to lifestyle change in select cases. Sometimes useful to develop early motivation.
8. Pre-prepared meals	**	Can be combined with and assist other techniques. Good for singles, the time poor and non-cooks.
9. Meal replacements	***	Inexpensive, balanced way of reducing food input. Needs ongoing clinical support.
10. Surgery	***	Often a last resort for the morbidly obese or those with major risks. Expensive but effective.
11. Lifestyle change	***	Should be the basis of all other treatments. Needs motivation and a level of discipline

– no evidence; * limited evidence; ** some good evidence; *** good evidence

weight loss properties are claimed. American figures show that as many as 7% of the general population and up to 28% of young, obese women regularly use OTC substances for weight loss (Allison et al., 2001). Several reviews agree that, despite their widespread use, there is no convincing evidence of efficacy for the vast majority of OTC products (Allison et al., 2001; Egger and Thorburn, 2005; Pittler and Ernst, 2004), the exception being xenical (Orlistat) which was initially a prescription-only medication in Australia before becoming available OTC and with which 4–5% of users have been able to maintain weight loss for 2–4 years (Richelson et al., 2007). Apart from this, the category should not necessarily be dismissed totally and some OTC products may benefit from further research (for a full discussion, see Egger and Thorburn, 2005). Nevertheless, a review of five meta-analyses and twenty-five additional trials, covering twelve main herbal supplements, concluded that none of the currently available substances can be recommended for weight loss (Pittler and Ernst, 2004).

ALTERNATIVE NON-INGESTIBLE TREATMENTS

'Alternative' approaches to weight loss include topical treatments such as creams or soaps, body wrapping, aromatherapy, acupuncture/acupressure, electrical stimulation, hypnosis, passive exercise devices, and yoga and other eastern meditation techniques (Egger and Thorburn, 2005). Minor weight loss benefits have been reported with treatments such as hypnosis, which could have adjunct benefits (even as a placebo) to other lifestyle change interventions. Other treatments such as body wrapping and passive exercise devices have no reliable supporting evidence.

Strategies with some supporting evidence

COMMERCIAL DIET-ORIENTED WEIGHT LOSS PROGRAMS

Data from some countries suggest that up to 13% of women and 5% of men participate in commercial weight loss programs (Latner, 2001). Because of commercial concerns, however, few results of these programs have been reported. One study compared the effects of self-help with the Weight Watchers program in overweight and obese men and women (Heshka et al., 2000). After twenty-six weeks, subjects in the commercial program had greater decreases in body weight (−4.8 vs. −1.4 kg) and waist circumference (−4.3 vs. −0.7 cm) than those in the self-help program. Although most commercial programs are oriented towards women, limited data indicate that male programs may have a higher success rate than female programs (Egger et al., 1996), although commitment is a limiting factor.

In summary, based on the available data, it seems that commercial weight loss programs can lead to modest weight losses and weight loss maintenance in some individuals. It would be speculative, but not unreasonable, to propose that existing commercial programs have most appeal to women who prefer a structured program with ongoing feedback through social or individual support.

SELF-HELP

For our purposes, self-help is considered to be those situations where no other structured person-to-person contact is made on an ongoing basis. By its nature, this is difficult to evaluate, but would include self-motivated lifestyle change, computer-assisted interventions, and packaged programs. Self-help has the advantages of increasing empowerment, self-efficacy and self-esteem. These can effect positive change to self-reliance, rated by individuals as one of the most effective strategies for effecting obesity (Furnham, 1994). Using the American National Weight Control Registry, Latner (2001) claimed that up to 45% of those who have lost weight and kept it off may have done so through self-help. Because diet books are ubiquitous, it must be assumed that these are a common form of self-help, although success is difficult to assess. Take-home kits, the internet and correspondence courses also claim moderate success (Egger et al., 1996). It is logical to think that directions from a knowledgeable clinician may also aid individuals suited to a self-help approach.

Recently, attempts have been made to use the internet as a self-help tool. Earlier programs have shown modest success but these have developed into more effective tools (Jonasson et al., 2007; see also www.professortrim.com). Such programs typically contain a self-monitoring section for detailing habits and physical activity; an interactive component used to design a personal program aimed at a reasonable weight loss over time; feedback; and coaching. Often, recipes, which can be adapted or modified, are included. Although the drop-out rate in such programs is high, it is reasonable to assume that they provide a very cost-effective way to treat obesity. They are cheap, available twenty-four hours a day, require a minimum of technical knowledge and are often seen as fun (Jonasson et al., 2007).

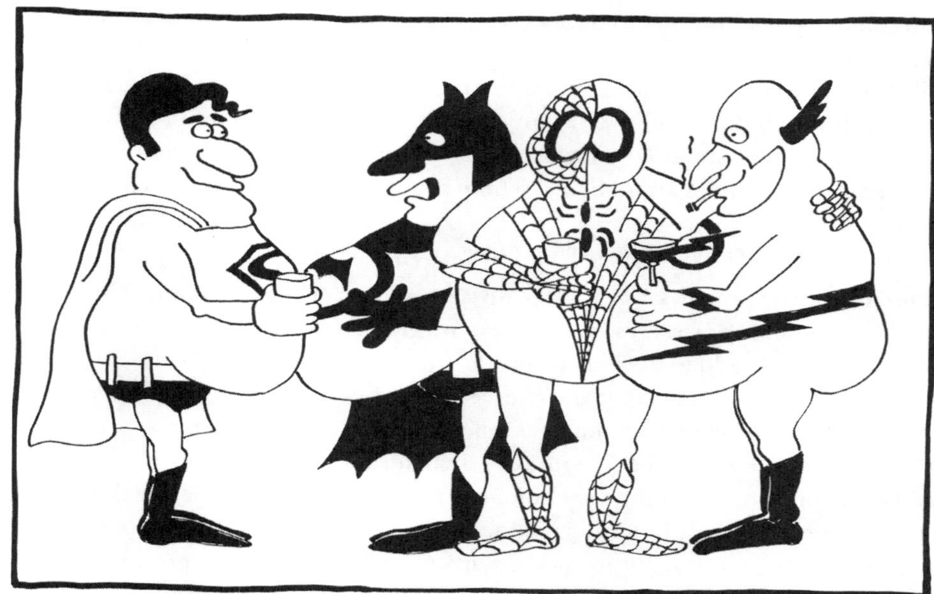

AT THE RETIRED SUPERHEROES CONVENTION.

Strategies with good supporting evidence

EXERCISE-BASED PROGRAMS

Physical activity and a hypocaloric diet form the basis of all effective weight loss programs and therefore must make up the generic component of any successful weight loss initiative. However, where exercise alone is the main consideration, the emphasis can vary according to requirement. There is little doubt that it is easier to modify energy balance in the short term by reducing EI than by increasing EE. A big person is more likely to be able to reduce EI (e.g. 1 000 kcal or 4 400 kJ per day in a 3–4 000 kcal or 13 200–17 600 kJ) per day diet) than to increase EE by the same amount (e.g. by walking an extra 10–12 km/day). Also, as efficiency increases (as a result of the improvements in aerobic capacity and decreases in body weight with regular exercise), absolute EE for a set task will decline, thereby reducing the effectiveness of a set unit of physical exertion.

Increases in physical activity have been found to be of particular value in maintenance (Elfhag and Rossner, 2005). Studies now show that exercise prescription (with diet) for weight loss should be for a minimum of around 150 min (2.5 hrs) or 2 500 kcal or 11 000 kj per week (Jacicic et al., 2001). Using a pedometer, this equates to around 10 000 steps/day in an 80 kg person. Exercise alone is unlikely to be effective for weight loss until around 200–300min (3–5hr) or 3 500 kcals (15 400 kj) per week (approximately 12 500 steps) is expended, with effects proportional to exercise volume. Data from the US National Weight Control Registry suggests that exercise for weight loss maintenance in the post-obese may need to be at about 60–80 mins/day of moderate activity, combined with a hypocaloric diet (Wing and Hill, 2001).

In summary, it seems that while exercise is a necessary component of any weight loss program, it is usually not sufficient (without diet) unless carried out at levels that are unlikely to occur as part of normal modern daily life and in obese individuals. Exercise programs through fitness or health centres that lack a nutritional input and/or are at a level insufficient to compensate for the negative energy balance inherent in a modern obesogenic environment are unlikely to have a lasting impact on weight control.

COUNSELLING AND BEHAVIOURAL APPROACHES

Counselling is the process of providing advice and guidance to a patient. This includes several behavioural approaches which, when integrated with dietary and exercise advice, have been shown to add to the long-term effectiveness of a program (Wing, 2004). These are based on the idea that eating and exercise behaviours are learned and therefore can be modified through such techniques as self-monitoring, stimulus control, problem solving, contingency management, cognitive restructuring, social support and stress management. Improvements in these techniques in recent years have added to their value as part of an integrated weight loss program, and a recent review of the data suggests that behavioural therapy does add to the benefits of other forms of weight loss treatment (NHMRC, 2003) and thus should be a part of all weight loss interventions.

PRE-PREPARED LOW ENERGY MEALS

There are a number of commercially available, pre-prepared, low energy meals available through retail outlets or direct. Pre-prepared meals, which are usually frozen for re-heating, are energy controlled for a meal and nutritionally balanced, enabling users to objectify their energy intake. Such meals may be used as a total or partial substitute for adlib eating. As such, they are useful not only for initial weight loss but also for use by a skilled clinician for 're-feeding' after more severe caloric restriction. A number of studies have shown positive benefits from pre-prepared meals (Metz et al., 2000), although their use in combination with other strategies has not yet been widely reported. They are most likely to appeal to individuals with time limitations or a lack of culinary skills or nutrition knowledge.

MEAL REPLACEMENTS (VERY LOW CALORIE DIETS)

Meal replacements in the form of very low calorie diets (VLCDs) provide balanced nutrition in powdered form mixed as a drink or 'shake'. These can be either low (e.g. fewer than 1200 kcals or 5 280 kJ per day) or very low (e.g. fewer than 800 kcals or 3 520 kJ per day) in energy and are usually used as a replacement for some, rather than all, meals or in combination with pre-prepared meals. Meal replacements can result in big, quick losses but can also be followed by rebound weight gains on their cessation, unless a maintenance program follows immediately afterwards.

They have been discouraged for personal use but can be effective with close clinical supervision, particularly to increase motivation in some patients. Recent research suggests that meal replacements are safe, can produce good losses, and can help reduce co-morbidities (NHMRC, 2003). One review suggested that almost everyone in the modern environment could benefit from the regular use of a meal replacement, because of excessive daily food intake (Egger, 2006).

What can be done in a brief consultation

If appropriate, take anthropometric measures (waist circumference, weight, bio-impedance).

Calculate and discuss ideal weight goals, using the formula given in *Professional resources*.

Ask whether the patient thinks diet, physical activity, or both are adding to weight gain.

Ask about stress in the patient's life and the general reaction to this. For example, does she or he eat more or less or move more or less when stressed?

Suggest the purchase or loan of a pedometer for measuring baseline activity levels (steps) over a week.

Provide information for the patient to complete the DAB-Q (Diet, Activity and Behaviour Questionnaire) (see www.professortrim.com/DAB-Q).

Explain the strategies available and the need for lifestyle modification in any weight loss.

Explain the chronic nature of obesity, the long-term basis of any treatment, and the importance of maintenance in contrast to initial loss.

MEDICATION

Although there is a considerable literature on prescribed weight loss medications (Atkinson, 2005), there are currently only a few options available, with many new versions currently being tested.

Sibutramine (Reductil) is a satiation enhancer which has been shown to add an average 5% extra weight loss when taken during a diet and exercise program. It also seems to have a slight thermogenic effect. It is likely to be most useful in those for whom hunger is a significant issue.

Orlistat (Xenical) is a gastric lipase inhibitor which reduces energy intake through the partial elimination of dietary fats. For this reason it can be used as a 'learning drug' in individuals who are unaware of the fat content of foods. About 30% of the fat consumed will be lost in the faeces. If patients adhere to a low fat diet, that is, less than approximately 67 g/day, this fat loss will not cause any clinical problems and the patient will lose weight both by fat restriction and the modest excretion of fat consumed. With higher fat intake, steatorrhea develops, which is unpleasant and reinforces better dietary habits. In that sense, orlistat has been termed an 'Antabuse' for fat over-consumption, because patients quickly learn how to adapt.

Phentermine (Duromine) is an adrenergic that is only available for short-term (three months) use. Phentermine is especially useful where quick weight loss is desired to increase motivation or to help break through plateaus. There are side effects of dysphoria and tachycardia in a small number of people, but these occur immediately and can be eliminated by discontinuing the drug. Close clinical supervision is also advisable on withdrawal to prevent a weight rebound.

Rimonabant (Acomplia) is a cannabinoid receptor blocker which has multiple effects in the brain, liver and gastrointestinal tract. It increases weight loss above placebo and also beneficially affects components of the metabolic syndrome. Rimonabant seems to affect various components of the energy balance system, leading to a negative energy balance. The chemical has even been tried in binge eating disorders, smoking cessation, and drug and alcohol abuse. So far, weight loss is the only clinical indication, but rimonabant appears to have intrinsic metabolic effects on fat and carbohydrate metabolism beyond that of weight loss. A side effect found in some studies, however, is depression.

Some antidepressant (SSRI) medications have weight loss effects while others tend to cause weight gain, possibly as a result of the patient's consumptive reaction to depression (i.e. those who eat more when depressed will lose weight when on antidepressants and those who eat less may gain weight). Antidepressants may have a particular benefit in relapse prevention.

In summary, prescribed medication is useful but should not be considered as mono-therapy in the absence of lifestyle modification.

SURGERY

In terms of potential weight loss, obesity surgery is clearly the most effective strategy available (NHMRC, 2003). Most bariatric surgery is performed laparoscopically. There are several types of bariatric surgery, the main forms of which (gastric banding, vertical banded gastroscopy and gastric bypass) involve the formation of a gastric pouch below the gastro-oesophageal junction. This was thought to reduce weight by restricting food ingested, but recent studies have shown that physical stimulation may induce hormonal hunger suppressant mediators. Laparoscopic banding ('lap banding') is now one of the most commonly used procedures, with good outcomes. Because of its intrusive nature, expense, and possible (although now extremely slight) risks, obesity surgery has been seen as a 'last resort' for intractable and life-threatening cases (NHMRC, 2003).

However, improvements in operative techniques have made it a preferred option in some less morbid cases. Postoperative treatment (and band adjustment in the case of lap banding) is the key to success and, like all other treatments, surgery is only effective when combined with a lifestyle change. A new treatment based on implantable gastric stimulation (IGS) is being tested and shows promise. Experimentally, multiple botulinus toxin injections into the ventricular wall have been tried in an attempt to prevent gastric motility and also show promise.

LIFESTYLE MODIFICATION

Lifestyle modification remains the focal point of all effective weight control strategies. It involves changing energy intake and/or energy expenditure but may also involve looking at *why* an imbalance has occurred (NHMRC, 2003). For best effect, lifestyle modification usually involves some of the other strategies outlined here, but patients need to be made aware that permanently changing some aspect of their current lifestyle is a necessary precursor to effective long-term weight loss. Specific lifestyle modifications are discussed in more detail in subsequent chapters.

COMBINING STRATEGIES

The practice of weight loss management requires creative interventions, as well as the selection of evidence-based strategies. Most effective treatments are likely to involve combining strategies and matching the right strategy to the characteristics of the patient. A literature review by Elfhag and Rossner (2005) produced a list of factors that influence weight loss and regain and these are shown in Table 4.4.

TABLE 4.4 Factors associated with weight loss maintenance and regain after intentional weight loss

Weight maintenance	Weight regain
an achieved weight loss goal	attribution of obesity to medical factors
more initial weight loss	perceiving barriers for weight loss behaviours
physically inactive lifestyle	history of weight cycling
regular meal rhythm	sedentary lifestyle
breakfast eating	disinhibited eating
less fat, more healthy foods	more hunger
reduced frequency of snacks	binge eating
flexible control over eating	eating in response to negative emotions and stress
self-monitoring	psychosocial stressors
coping capacity	lack of social support
capacity to handle cravings	more passive reactions to problems
self-efficacy	poor coping strategies
autonomy	lack of self-confidence
'healthy narcissism'	psychopathology
more confidence as a motivator	medical reasons as a motivator
stability in life	dichotomous thinking
capacity for close reasoning	

Source: Elfhag and Rossner, 2005

A key component of treatment is recognition of two main phases. The first is immediate weight loss and the second is long-term weight loss maintenance, and these invariably require different treatment emphases (NHMRC, 2003). The use of strategy mixes may also change between these phases. For example, a patient needing quick success for motivational purposes may be prescribed meal replacements or a prescription drug, then be gradually 're-fed' with pre-prepared meals or a balanced low energy diet with a graduated exercise program. Counselling and lifestyle modification would be continued throughout. A patient with less need for such a quick loss may be simply given an information-based program of diet and exercise. Packaged programs with clinical back-up can reduce the repetitive nature of discussing details with the patient and the time required of the clinician.

Summary

Many medical problems (such as appendicitis or pneumonia) call for a single treatment option (appendicectomy, antibiotics), which results in a definite cure of that particular medical problem. Chronic diseases with a lifestyle-based aetiology do not have a single treatment option. The skill of the clinician, therefore, is in matching the available, evidence-based options to the patient. As chronic diseases now account for 60% of the world's deaths and 47% of the global burden of disease, clinical management is increasingly more likely to require this kind of 'mixing and matching'. Obesity treatment could benefit from a re-conceptualisation in this light.

practice tips

PRACTICE TIPS: WEIGHT LOSS

	Medical practitioner	Practice nurse
Assess	Whether weight loss has been considered. Co-morbidities. Family history of weight/co-morbidities. Medication effects on weight. Contraindications for treatment options. Whether surgery or medication may be appropriate.	Body shape. Anthropometric measures. Stage of readiness to change. Goal weights/waist. Previous history of weight gain/loss. Smoking history. Diet and exercise (DAB-Q test; www.professortrim.com/DAB-Q). Treatment options. Other factors (e.g. stress, depression, early experience). Environmental influences.
Assist	By treating co-morbidities. By identifying potential short- and long-term goals. By reviewing progress of drug therapy for weight loss. By reviewing ongoing special dietetic programs such as meal replacements. By using templates as appropriate.	By educating about eating. Increases in basic physical activity; use a pedometer for monitoring steps; use appropriate tactics to move through stages of readiness to change. Time planning. By using templates as appropriate.
Arrange	Referral for co-morbidities where appropriate. List of other health professionals for a care plan.	Discussion of motivational tactics with other involved health professionals. Referral to a personal trainer, nutritionist or life coach if appropriate. Contact with self-help groups if appropriate.

key points

KEY POINTS FOR CLINICAL MANAGEMENT

- Do not automatically weigh and/or measure (at least at the start of a consultation) because this may impact negatively on some people.
- Try to determine the main contributing cause(s) to energy imbalance (e.g. food intake, energy expenditure).
- Within these, look for key factors (e.g. excess sweet or fat foods, portion size problems, fast foods only, emotional eating, night eating, sugar sweetened fluids, excessive computer use, more than fifteen hours of TV watching per week, weekend laziness).
- Consider/dismiss the impact of psychological factors such as stress, early abuse or 'compulsive/binge eating'.
- Use tools such as pedometers or questionnaires to encourage self-monitoring and feedback (see Chapter 6).
- Encourage regular visits (e.g. fortnightly/monthly), at least in the early stages, to assist with progress.
- Aim for long-term weight loss and maintenance but use short-term losses to motivate for ongoing lifestyle learning.

REFERENCES

AIHW (Australian Institute of Health and Welfare). (2006) *Australia's weight.* Canberra: AIHW.

Allison DB, Fonatine KR, Heshka S et al. (2001) Alternative treatments for weight loss: a critical review. *Cr Rev Food Sc Nut* 41(1): 1–28.

Atkinson RL. (2005) Management of obesity: pharmacotherapy. In Kopleman PG, Caterson ID, Dietz WH (eds). *Clinical obesity in adults and children,* 2nd edn, pp 380–93. London: Blackwell Publishing.

Egger G. (2006) Are meal replacements effective as a clinical tool for weight loss? *Med J Aust* 184(2): 52–53.

Egger G, Binns A. (2001) *The experts weight loss guide.* Sydney: Allen and Unwin.

Egger G, Swinburn B. (1996) An ecological model for understanding the obesity pandemic. *Brit Med J* 20: 227–31.

Egger G, Thorburn A. (2005) Environmental and policy approaches: alternative methods of dealing with obesity. In Kopelman PG, Caterson ID, Dietz WH (eds). *Clinical obesity in adults and children.* London: Blackwell Publishing.

Egger G, Bolton A, O'Neill M et al. (1996) Effectiveness of an abdominal obesity reduction program in men: the GutBuster 'waist loss' program. *Int J Obes* 20: 227–35.

Elfhag K, Rossner S. (2005) Who succeeds in maintaining weight loss? A conceptual review of factors associated with weight loss maintenance and weight regain. *Obes Rev* 13(6): 1070–76.

Furnham A. (1994) Explaining health and illness: lay perceptions on current and future health, the causes of illness and the nature of recovery. *Soc Sci Med* 39(5): 715–25.

Heshka S, Greenway F, Anderson JW et al. (2000) Self-help weight loss versus a structured commercial program after 26 weeks: a randomized controlled study. *Am J Med* 109(4): 282–87.

International Association for the Study of Obesity: www.iotf.org.

Jakicic JM, Clark K, Coleman E, et al. (2001) Appropriate intervention strategies for weight loss and prevention of weight regain for adults. *Med Sci Sports Exerc* 33(12): 2145–56.

Jonasson, Linné, Y, Neovius M Rössner S. (2007) An Internet-based weight loss program. *Scand J Publ Health* (in print).

King N, Caudwell P, Hopkins M et al. (2006) Plateaus in body weight during weight loss interventions. *Proceedings, 10th international Congress on Obesity,* Sydney, August 2006.

Latner J. (2001) Self-help in the long-term treatment of obesity. *Obes Rev* 2: 87–97.

Metz JA, Stern JS, Kris-Etherton P et al. (2000) A randomized trial of improved weight loss with a prepared meal plan in overweight and obese patients: impact on cardiovascular risk reduction. *Arch Intern Med* 160(14): 2150–58.

NHMRC (National Health and Medical Research Council). (2003) *National clinical guidelines for weight control and obesity management.* Canberra: Commonwealth of Australia.

Pittler MH, Ernst, E. (2004) Dietary supplements for body-weight reduction: a systematic review. *Am J Clin Nutr* 79(4): 529–36.

Richelsen B, Tonstad S, Rössner S et al. (2007) Effect of orlistat on weight regain and on cardiovascular risk factors following a very-low-calorie diet in abdominally obese patients. A three-year-randomized placebo controlled study. *Diabetes Care* 30:27–32.

Swinburn B, Egger G. (2004) The runaway weight gain train: too many accelerators, not enough brakes. *Br Med J* 329(7468): 736–39.

Thirlby RC, Randall J. (2002) A genetic 'obesity risk index' for patients with morbid obesity. *Obes Surg* 12(1): 25–29.

Vague J. (1947) La différentiation sexuelle, facteur déterminant des formes de l'obesité. *Presse Méd* 30: 339.

Welborn TA, Dhaliwal SS. (2007) Preferred clinical measures of central obesity for predicting mortality. *Eur J Clin Nutr* Feb 14; doi:10.1038/sj.ejcn.1602656.

Wing RR. (2004) Behavioural approaches to the treatment of obesity. In Bray GA, Bouchard C (eds). *Handbook of obesity: clinical applications. Second edition.* Marcel Dekker Inc: NY, pp 147–68.

Wing R, Hill JO. (2001) Successful weight loss maintenance. *Ann Rev Nutr* 21: 323–41.

World Health Organization: www.who.int.

professional resources

PROFESSIONAL RESOURCES: MEASURING BODY FAT AND FAT LOSS

Anthropometric measures

Weight Although a necessary measure, this does not always reflect body fat.
BMI (weight/height^2) Not a highly specific individual measure alone. Can be combined with waist circumference and body fat by other methods. Can discriminate against some muscular individuals.
Waist circumference (WC) A good measure in itself of metabolic risk. Can also be combined with other measures. Usually taken at mid-point between the bottom rib and the iliac crest but the umbilicus may be better for males.
Ideal weight Requires two simple measures and a calculator. The measures are weight, as measured by ordinary scales, and percentage body fat, as measured by Bio-Impedance Analysis (BIA) scales (these can be purchased economically from www.professortrim.com; they also measure weight).

The formula for ideal weight is:

(lean body mass [kg])/1 − percentage ideal body fat (in decimals)

where

lean body mass = weight − fat weight (kg)

fat weight = weight × percentage body fat

Ideal body fat percentage is 12−24% (men) or 15−35% (women). Knowing the variation in ideal body fat makes it possible to set different ideal weight goals, depending on starting body fat.

For example, a 100 kg man who is 30% fat will have 100 × 0.3 = 30 kg of fat weight and therefore 100 − 30 = 70 kg lean body mass. Goal 1 may be to get to 25% fat; hence, goal weight will be 70/1 − 0.25 = 93.3 kg. Goal 2 may be to get to 20% fat; goal weight will be 70/1 − 0.20 = 87.5 kg. Goal 3 may be to get to 18% fat; goal weight will be 70/1 − 0.18 = 85.4 kg. Goals 1, 2 and 3 might be short-term, medium-term and long-term goals.

Using this formula, goal weight is not only dynamic but is based on fat rather than weight, which is a less important measure.

Measures of genetic involvement in obesity

Genetics are often used as an excuse for overweight. The following test, developed by U.S. surgeons Thirlby and Randall (2002), provides an indication of whether genetics may be a factor in obesity.

Patient instructions: Answer the following four questions to see whether genetics can be blamed for your body weight. For measurement purposes, the term 'overweight' means having a Body Mass Index or BMI over 25, 'obese' means a BMI over 30, and 'very obese' a BMI over 40, where BMI is calculated by taking your weight (measured in kg) and dividing by the square of your height (measured in metres).

1. As far as you know, were either or both of your parents overweight or very overweight for most of their lives?

	Points	
	Obese	**Very obese**
Neither/don't know/no	0	0
Yes, one parent	7	14
Yes, both parents	14	28

2. Do you have any first degree relatives who have been obese for most of their lives?

Score 2 points for every obese first degree relative up to a maximum of 10 points.

3. How would you describe the average BMI of your siblings?

	Points
No siblings obese (BMI<30)	0
Average sibling obese (BMI>30)	6
Average sibling very obese (BMI>40)	12

4. When did you first become overweight and/or obese?

	Overweight	**Obese**
Never	0	0
Before age 10	20	30
Before age 20	10	20
Before age 30	5	10

Interpreting your score:

- 20: Your weight problem does not appear to be significantly genetically related. This means it is related to lifestyle and therefore should be quite easy to solve if you are committed to do so.
- 20–50: There appears to be a moderate hereditary component to your weight problem. This means you may find it a little harder to lose fat than some of your friends. You may need help from a dietitian but your problems should not be too difficult to overcome.
- 30–100: There appears to be a significant hereditary component to your weight problem. This means you may need special help and closer attention from a dietitian. With the proper approach and a long range plan, you should be able to overcome your bad start.

CHAPTER 5

The metabolic syndrome and diabetes

DAVID COLQHOUN, GARRY EGGER

The current epidemics of chronic disease are a result of discordance between our ancient genes and our modern lifestyle.

BOYD EPSTEIN

Introduction

Every year in the U.S., new medical developments are revealed in an eagerly awaited Banting Lecture. In 1988, the topic was slightly different. A Stanford University epidemiologist named Dr Gerald Reaven spoke about a cluster of disease risk factors occurring in people who had adopted a modern lifestyle and gone on to suffer major metabolic health problems, such as type 2 diabetes, stroke or heart disease. Reaven suggested this cluster included hypertension, hyperglycaemia, dyslipidaemia and abdominal obesity ('pot belly'). He called it syndrome X but, because of its link to metabolic problems, the cluster soon became known as the metabolic syndrome.

Reaven's findings were of moderate immediate interest and never really caught on until the metabolic syndrome began to burgeon during the rise in the obesity epidemic in the late 1990s. Increasingly, new measures were added, and by the middle of the first decade of the new millennium there were three official listings of symptoms of the metabolic syndrome. The most widely known definition of the metabolic syndrome comes from the National Cholesterol Education Program's *Adult treatment panel III report* (2002) and consists of any three of the following:

- fasting glucose >6.1 mmol/L
- waist circumference for Caucasian men >102 cm; for Caucasian women >88 cm
- triglycerides >1.7 mmol/L

- HDL cholesterol for men <1.0 mmol/L; for women <1.3 mmol/L
- blood pressure >130/85 mm Hg

It is ironic, therefore, that at this time, Reaven and other experts in the field had started to distance themselves from the syndrome, as such (Grundy, 2006; Reaven, 2006). The variable clustering of risk factors is undoubted, but whether they constitute a true medical syndrome is hotly debated. For Reaven, the immediate cause has always been insulin resistance and the proximal cause of insulin resistance in the modern age is clearly lifestyle and, more specifically, obesity and inactivity. Of course, individual risks may need to be treated, but it is clear that ignoring the underlying cause is not likely to result in the best outcomes.

The type 2 epidemic

The metabolic syndrome is a major signpost along the way to type 2 diabetes mellitus (T2DM) and other metabolic diseases. The journey may begin with abdominal fatness as the first visible sign, followed by an increase in insulin resistance and production. Then, when the pancreas fails to keep up that production, the BSLs begin to rise leading to prediabetes or overt T2DM. While much has been studied and written about the medical management of diabetes (near the end of this journey), this chapter looks at the contribution of lifestyle modification to the primary, secondary and tertiary management of the disease, particularly within the stage now referred to as 'pre-diabetes'. We leave detailed discussion of pharmacological management of diabetes to other forums.

The metabolic syndrome and diabetes

The metabolic syndrome is not a disease as such but rather a collection or clustering of cardiovascular risk factors. Often the first physical indicator is an increase in subcutaneous abdominal fat, which is accompanied by a rise in triglycerides (TG). Only 15–18% of obese people have none of the other factors that form the metabolic syndrome (Karelis et al., 2004a); on the other hand, 12–15% of lean people have more than one of these risk factors (Karelis et al., 2004b). The general tendency is for a clear association between risk and obesity, particularly abdominal obesity.

Although the pattern of risk also differs between individuals, an increase in insulin resistance (IR) is an early predictor (Krentz, 2002). This—and/or a rise in impaired fasting glucose (IFG) or impaired glucose tolerance (IGT) to the levels discussed below—has now been termed 'pre-diabetes' (Twigg et al., 2007). IFG and IGT represent different levels of metabolic disturbance. IFG (usually associated with hepatic insulin resistance) is defined as a BSL ≥6.1 mmol/L on fasting and <7.8 mmol two hours after a 75 g oral glucose load. IGT (usually associated with skeletal muscle insulin resistance) is defined as a BSL ≥7.0 mmol/L on fasting and 7.8–11.1 mmol/L after a two-hour load (Twigg et al., 2007). A typical pattern of development and a suggested role for lifestyle and conventional medicine is shown in Figure 5.1.

Progression from the first signs of pre-diabetes to fully diagnosed diabetes may take several years but can also occur rapidly. Generally, the quicker the rise from normal glucose tolerance (NGT) to IFG and IGT, the quicker the progression to full

FIGURE 5.1 Typical development of insulin resistance and type 2 diabetes and the role of lifestyle and conventional medicines

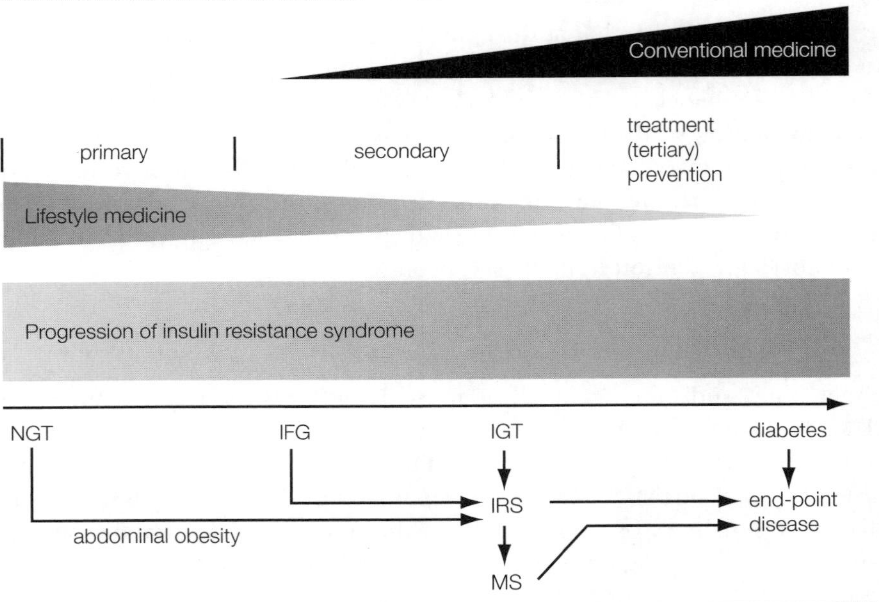

NGT = normal glucose tolerance; IFG = impaired fasting glucose; IGT = impaired glucose tolerance; IRS = insulin resistance syndrome; MS = metabolic syndrome

diabetes (Nichols et al., 2007), suggesting that progression may be linear in the early stages but becomes exponential with increasing deterioration. Either way, there is a window of opportunity for reversing the problem. Given that about 80% of people with T2DM will die from heart disease and many can go blind, require dialysis or amputation, and generally cause high costs to the community, it is important to understand what causes the disease and whether and how it can be prevented or reversed.

Causes of diabetes

T2DM is at the metabolic core of lifestyle medicine. The fact that it was almost unheard of a hundred years ago, is still rare or non-existent in populations living traditional lifestyles (International Association for the Study of Obesity), and has been reversed in urbanised indigenous groups by a return to their natural environment (O'Dea, 1984) clearly suggests that this is a 'disease of civilisation', with a primary aetiology in lifestyle. When more than 120 000 women were followed for over fifteen years by the Nurses Health Study researchers in America, 61% of the risk for T2DM was explainable by a BMI of >25 alone, 87% by a BMI >25 plus inactivity and diet, and 91% by a BMI>25 plus inactivity, diet and smoking (Hu et al., 2001). If, instead, a BMI of >23 was used as a cut-off, all of the above factors explained 96% of cases. While there is clearly a genetic factor involved, this is unlikely to manifest itself in the absence of any or all of these lifestyle risks.

T2DM has been predominantly a disease of the middle aged. However, as obesity levels have been rising in younger and younger age groups, it is now becoming increasingly prevalent in adolescents and children. Up to one-third of adolescents with diabetes in the U.S. now have the type 2 form of the disease, in contrast to the non-lifestyle related type 1, and the numbers are rising rapidly. Projections show that of those Americans born in the year 2000, about one-third can expect to develop diabetes in their lifetime, with an average annual cost to the community of approximately $AUD5 000, and a cost in their penultimate year estimated in 1998 dollars at about $15 000 (Brown et al., 2001). The risk rises enormously with the degree of overweight, with three-quarters of individuals with a BMI of >35 at 18 years of age expected to develop the disease in their lifetime, along with one-third of obese 65-year-olds (Narayan et al., 2007).

Early warning signs

Although it is diagnosed through elevated fasting plasma glucose, post-prandial glucose and/or a glucose tolerance test, there are other warning signs for T2DM that have now been verified. The classic textbook symptoms of manifest diabetes are polydipsia (excessive thirst), polyuria (excessive urination) and weight loss. However, most clinicians pick up T2DM cases in a routine or opportunistic screening because of other known risk factors, such as family history. Other indications that have been shown to precede diagnosis of the disease, in some cases by several years, include periodontal disease (including missing teeth), lack of sensitivity at the extremities, blurred vision, skin problems, dermopathy and, in men, sudden hair loss (androgenic alopecia). Snoring and sleep apnoea, excessive daytime sleepiness and decreased sexual function have also been shown to be potential indicators in a limited number of studies. Recognised predictive signs are age, family history, weight/waist changes and a high triglyceride/waist ratio (see *Professional resources*). These signs indicate an immediate need to act.

Early predictors

Recent research on birth weight and long-term metabolic outcomes has shown that both low and high birth weights indicate a future risk of the metabolic syndrome and other related chronic diseases. While the causes are not always clear cut, they are generally believed to be related to the mother's weight and glycaemic control. This underscores the importance of lifestyle medicine and best practice as far back as antenatal care. Interestingly, fetal malnutrition may manifest in later health problems.

From medication to motivation

The advantage of the lifestyle medicine approach to the management of T2DM is shown in the following graphs. Figure 5.2 shows a typical outcome from conservative management of hyperglycaemia, or the early stages of diabetes.

While diet and exercise is prescribed, along with mono-drug therapy in the early stages, this is often not complied with by the patient. Treatment escalates: medication is titrated upwards, poly-drug therapy is instituted, and finally insulin injections are required to maintain glycaemic control. Part of the reason for the inability to maintain tight glucose control can be seen in the long-term data from the UK

FIGURE 5.2 Traditional stepwise approach to the conservative management of type 2 diabetes

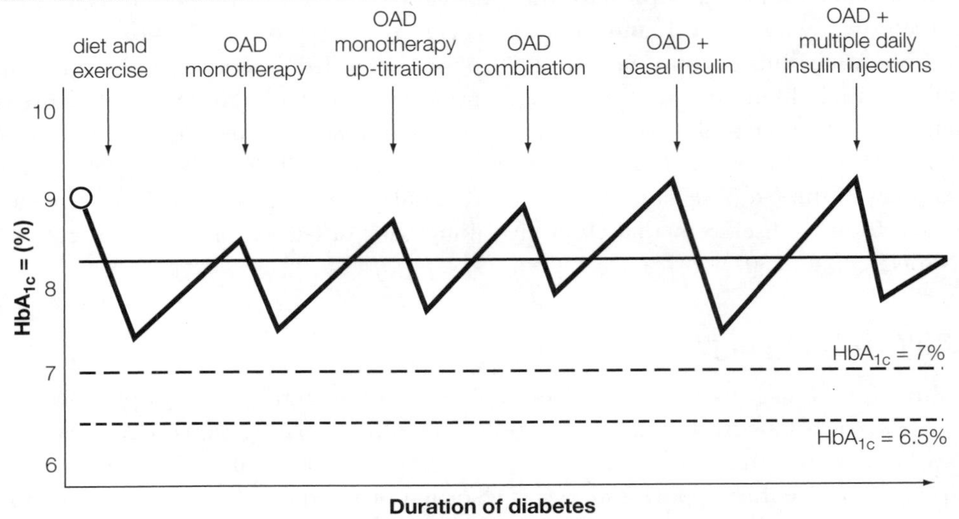

Prevention of Diabetes Study (UKPDS), shown in Figure 5.3. All of the medications used to treat T2DM, apart from the biguanides (e.g. metformin), used earliest in the process, cause weight gain. In general, the more advanced the treatment, the greater the weight gain. Yet weight gain has been convincingly shown to be one of the main causes of insulin resistance and hence less than optimal glucose control. Paradoxically, medication could be having a disease-causing (*iatrogenic*) as well as a disease-treating effect (Carver, 2006), resulting in a vicious cycle of treatment and outcome.

FIGURE 5.3 Weight gain with diabetes treatments

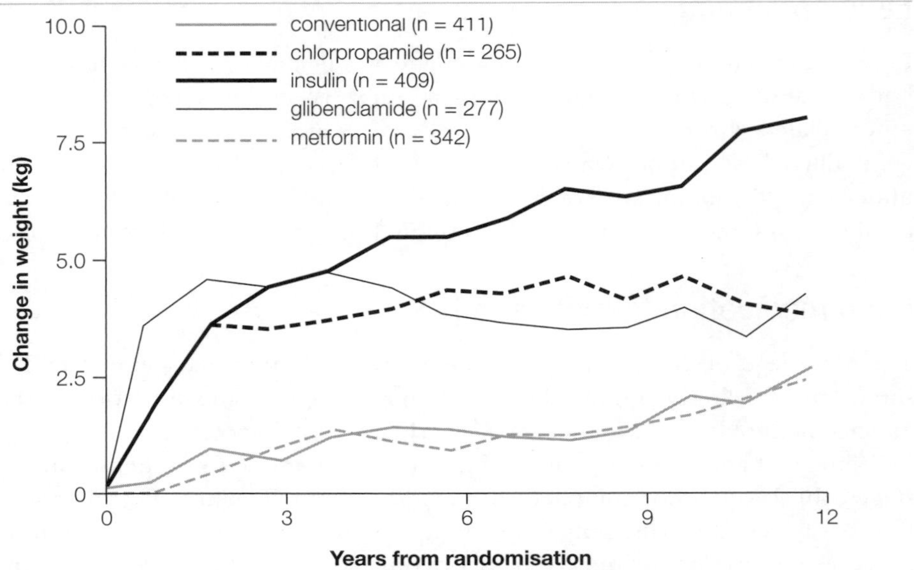

Source: Riddle et al., 2003

In a number of major prospective studies in different cultures, lifestyle change (particularly increases in physical activity) has been shown to increase glucose control and reduce, even reverse, early stage T2DM more successfully and more economically than pharmaceutical interventions (for a summary of these studies, see Tuomilehto, 2007). All have shown that weight loss (of approximately 5–10%), changes in nutrition (total energy reduction, reduced saturated fat, increased fibre) and increases in physical activity result in an average reduction in progression of about 60% compared to controls, with the effects remaining for up to seven years after intervention (Lindstrom et al., 2006). Where there is greatest compliance with intensive interventions for all risks (reduced body weight, decreased inactivity, decreased total energy intake, decreased saturated fat, increased mono-unsaturated fats, increased fibre intake), diabetes reduction approaches 100% (Hamman et al., 2007).

Figure 5.4 provides a personal, self-recorded report of a patient diagnosed with diabetes with a fasting plasma glucose of 9 mmol/L. Consistent with diabetes, his oral glucose tolerance test demonstrated a peak plasma glucose of 18 mmol/L. With a dedicated exercise program (shown by the increase in aerobic power in the graph) and change in diet leading to weight loss, lowering of fasting plasma glucose stabilised within the normal range after about 150 days. Why then, is this approach not given more than just a footnote in most treatment protocols?

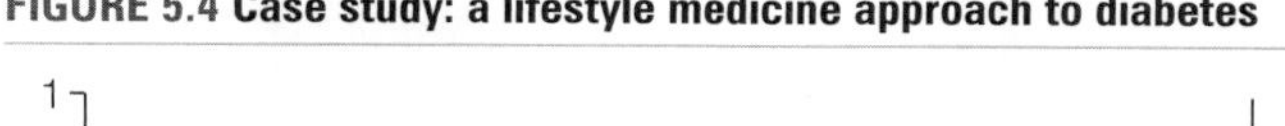

FIGURE 5.4 Case study: a lifestyle medicine approach to diabetes

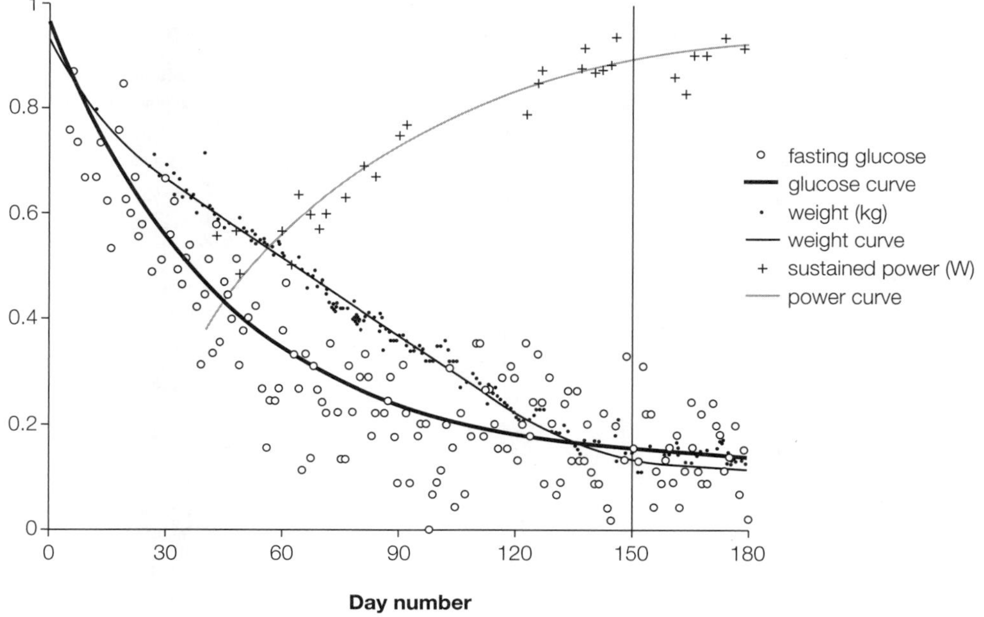

The answer is usually that it is 'too hard' in the modern obesogenic environment to motivate most patients to take this (reversion to 'normal') step of increasing activity levels and, to a lesser extent, modifying diet. Motivation is thus often the missing link between a clinician's prescription and a patient's cure. In the words of Dr Robert Rizza, president of the American Diabetes Association, 'Clinicians have the means to reduce serious diabetes complications by 60% . . . But to achieve it we need to re-organise our health system so that it rewards prevention and optimum care . . . To continue to pay for complications while refusing to pay for prevention is folly (Cherrington, 2006).'

Motivational strategies should include not only personal incentive and persuasion from a clinician but supportive public health approaches aimed at the hip pocket and other relevant 'nerves'. Using some of the techniques discussed in Chapter 3, we can look at the changes that need to be initiated by the clinician to prevent or reverse the diabetes epidemic.

Broadening treatment approaches

While treatment (and prevention) options for dealing with T2DM need to be broadened, tight glucose control—usually through a strict drug regimen—may be the best way of achieving this. This type of management is covered in standard medical texts and will not be reiterated here. Instead, we discuss aspects of lifestyle medicine that will contribute to such glucose control (shown in Table 5.1) and, in so doing, reduce the need for medication with its cyclical effects on the problem.

In recent times there have been several changes in emphasis when dealing with lifestyle factors in T2DM. Because the disease is reflected in a deficiency in

TABLE 5.1 Lifestyle medicine contributions to the phased treatment of metabolic disorders

	Metabolic syndrome	**Pre-diabetes**	**Early stage T2DM**	**Late stage (insulin dependent) T2DM**
Traditional/ conventional medicine	Screen for risks. Treat risks.	Measure risk. Treat comorbidities. Check regularly.	Medicate. Check for associated problems.	Add medication as required. Monitor medication. Treat associated problems.
	Implement motivational strategies.			
Lifestyle medicine (additions to conventional medicine)	Look for predictive signs. Educate about lifestyle change (see below). Treat behaviour.	Devise an exercise/diet plan. Devise a weight loss plan.	Involve an exercise physiologist/dietitian. Develop a dynamic exercise plan Devise a diet plan. Develop a weight loss program.	Involve an exercise physiologist/dietitian. Develop a specific exercise plan with progression. Provide a more intensive weight loss program.
Goals	1. Reduce risks. 2. Prevent progression. 3. Reduce medication.	1. Reduce risk. 2. Prevent the need for medication.	1. Control glycaemia. 2. Eliminate need for medication.	1. Tightly control glycaemia. 2. Reduce medication. 3. Prevent further complications.

metabolising glucose, the initial lifestyle prescription until around the 1980s was to decrease sugars in the diet, including through reduced alcohol. This was then superseded by advice to reduce dietary fats: by the 1990s it had become clear that dietary fat is causally involved, mainly because of its atherosclerotic properties and high energy density, which affects body weight (particularly in an increasingly sedentary population). Next, however, some fats (e.g. mono-unsaturates) were shown to have beneficial effects on T2DM prevention and progression—even moderate and regular alcohol intake was found to be beneficial. Diametrically opposite changes in dietary advice—for example, from avoiding coffee to advocating its moderate use (4 cups/d) or from reducing all carbohydrates to increasing low GI carbohydrates—have made nutritional prescription difficult to keep up with (McAuley and Mann, 2006; Twigg et al., 2007).

What can be done in a brief consultation

Discuss risk factors for T2DM and the preventable nature of this.

Measure waist circumference and explain the link between abdominal obesity and T2DM.

If appropriate, administer a diabetes check list (see *Professional resources*).

Explain how early stage pre-diabetes can be reversed with appropriate lifestyle changes.

Refer for blood tests: fasting plasma glucose, fasting lipids and liver function tests.

Provide information on diabetes prevention and reversal.

Recommend an exercise specialist with expertise in diabetes management.

In the meantime, there has been greater emphasis placed on the importance of physical inactivity as a causal factor, and consequently on increasing activity levels at all stages of treatment (Thomas et al., 2006). While weight loss is important (Bloomgarten, 2006), increased activity can be effective in achieving glycaemic control and end-point outcomes, even in the absence of weight loss (Brodney et al., 2000). The reasons for this are several and are now well documented (Sigal et al., 2006). Hence, physical activity prescription is now seen to be as important, if not more important, than nutritional prescription for T2DM prevention and control. Recent research also suggests that different forms of activity, such as resistance training (Eves and Plotnikoff, 2006) and increasing intensity of exercise, even to the extent of faster walking (Johnson et al., 2006), may have added benefits for T2DM control. This suggests a dynamic approach to exercise prescription from initial low levels of aerobic activity to increasing intensity to some resistance (such as circuit training) to increasing levels of resistance (see Chapter 7), together with the dynamic conventional approach.

A lifestyle medicine approach requires acknowledgment of the need for varied prescriptions according to the age of the patient. A thirty-five-year old male with recent T2DM and a BMI of 35 will clearly require more restructuring of his life than a sixty-five-year old woman with limited resources. The inclusion of an exercise specialist as part of a care plan is vital to help put this into practice.

Gestational diabetes (GDM)

Gestational diabetes mellitus (GDM), which develops in the middle stages of pregnancy, is also on the increase and also associated—almost totally—with lifestyle. About 3–5% of mothers will now develop GDM, and mothers who become diabetic during one pregnancy have a 50% chance of developing T2DM at some stage after delivery. This rises to almost 100% in those who develop the disease during three pregnancies (Hollander et al., 2007). However, several lines of research suggest that GDM is almost totally preventable. Pregnancy and pre-pregnancy body weight are proximal risk factors. Data from the Nurses Health Study shows that even pre-gravid activity levels are inversely associated with the risk of developing GDM in pregnancy (Zhang et al., 2006).

Exercise (even including resistance training) during pregnancy can reduce the risk (Brankston et al., 2004). There are also benefits in reducing weight and increasing activity levels before pregnancy and preventing excessive weight gain during pregnancy. Figure 5.5, for example, shows the reduced risk of GDM according to pre-gravid total and vigorous activity levels in more than 21 000 American nurses over eight years (Zhang et al., 2006). Obviously, the level of exercise and diet needs to be moderated by the demands of pregnancy and individual characteristics of the mother, and tight glucose control needs to be maintained through conventional methods if necessary. However, lifestyle changes before and during pregnancy and after parturition are likely to reduce the chances of progressing to later diabetes for both mother and offspring. Close supervision by an exercise specialist and dietitian as part of a care plan is advised for this.

FIGURE 5.5 Pre-gravid physical activity and risk of gestational diabetes

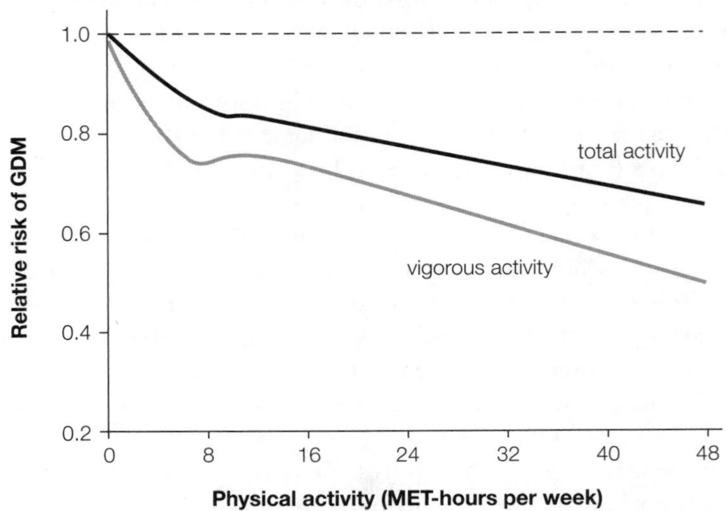

Source: Zhang et al., 2006

Summary

Type 2 diabetes mellitus (T2DM) is predominantly a lifestyle-based disease, often starting with abdominal obesity and progressing through the metabolic syndrome to insulin resistance, diabetes and end-point disease. Despite the enormous resources thrown at a pharmaceutical solution since the discovery of insulin in 1928, its treatment remains illusive. Epidemiological and physiological studies, however, now convincingly show that the solution lies in a limited number of lifestyle changes: reduced body weight, decreased inactivity, decreased total energy intake, decreased saturated fat and increased fibre intake. While pharmacological treatments will always remain necessary for severe cases of the disease, there is a desperate need for greater attention to lifestyle change in order to reduce what is fast becoming one of the biggest epidemics of the modern age.

practice tips

PRACTICE TIPS: MANAGING THE METABOLIC SYNDROME

	GP	**Practice nurse**
Assess	Membership of high risk groups; screen if necessary*. Need for blood tests. Level of risk. Co-morbidities and their treatment, including depression.	Potential signs of T2DM. Measurements. Diet, exercise and behaviour. Motivational factors.
Assist	By providing medication for risk reduction where appropriate. By identifying lifestyle changes required. By treating depression if present.	By discussing possible lifestyle changes. By negotiating reduction of barriers to this. By developing a strategy for putting this into action. By helping with depression if necessary.
Arrange	Referral to a specialist where indicated. List of other health professionals for a care plan.	Care plan if T2DM diagnosed. Contact with and coordination of other health professionals.

* High risk groups include certain ethnic groups (Indo-Asians, Afro-Caribbeans), people over 60 years of age, first degree relatives with diabetes, recurrent or major sepsis, obesity, peripheral skin breakdown (i.e. ulcers), personal history of gestational diabetes, coronary heart disease, autoimmune endocrinopathies (e.g. primary hypothyroidism), or organ-specific disorders (e.g. polycystic ovaries; androgenic alopecia) (www.lifescripts.com.au).

key points

KEY POINTS FOR CLINICAL MANAGEMENT

General

- Focus on reversal of early stage diabetes, particularly through aerobic exercise and weight loss.
- Have a clear focus to prevent progression of the disease.
- Focus on improving insulin sensitivity through regular exercise (increasing the intensity of aerobic exercise through to resistance training) in later stage diabetes.
- Prescribe (or work with an exercise specialist) to plan an individual and 'dynamic' exercise program.

Exercise

- While working on weight control, concentrate on fitness, with or without weight loss.
- Start with gentle aerobic activity (walking), working up to increased speed and, if possible, resistance training 2–3 times a week.
- Be aware of hypoglycaemic events; get the patient to carry readily digested carbohydrate while exercising.
- Be realistic in designing an exercise program for a big person.

Nutrition

- While high carbohydrate (45–60%), high fibre, low GI foods may be best, more moderate carb (approximately 40%) with higher protein diets may be more suitable for some.
- Vegetables, legumes, intact fruits and wholegrain cereals are the best forms of carbohydrates plus foods rich in fibre (approximately 30 g/day; preferably soluble) and low in GI.
- Reduce total free sugars to less than 10% of total energy.
- Increase the proportion of mono-unsaturated fats and reduce saturated and trans fats.
- Drink alcohol in moderation (i.e. 1–2 standard drinks/day); it is better if small amounts are drunk regularly.
- Regular coffee or tea may help prevent weight gain and can aid in the prevention of diabetes.

references

REFERENCES

Bloomgarden ZT. (2006) Weight control in individuals with diabetes. *Diab Care* 29(12): 2749–54.

Brankston G, Mitchell BF, Ryan EA et al. (2004) Resistance exercise decreases the need for insulin in overweight women with gestational diabetes mellitus. *Am J Obstet Gyn* 190: 188–93.

Brodney S, Blair S, Lee CD. (2000) Is it possible to be overweight or obese and fit and healthy? In Bouchard C. (ed) *Physical activity and obesity.* Champaign Ill: Human Kinetics.

Brown JB, Nichols GA, Glauber HS et al. (2001) Health care costs associated with escalation of drug treatment in type 2 diabetes mellitus. *Am J Health-Syst Pharm* 58(2): 151–57.

Carver C. (2006) Insulin treatment and the problem of weight gain in type 2 diabetes. *Diab Ed* 32: 910–17.

Cherrington AD. (2005) Presidential address: diabetes, past present and future. *Diab Care* 9: 2158–64.

Eves ND, Plotnikoff RC. (2006) Resistance training and type 2 diabetes. *Diab Care* 29(8): 1933–41.

Grundy S. (2006) Does a diagnosis of metabolic syndrome have value in clinical practice? *Am J Clin Nutr* 83: 1248–51.

Hamman RF, Wing RR, Edelstein SL et al. for the diabetes prevention group. (2007) Effect of weight loss with lifestyle intervention on risk of diabetes. *Diab Care* 29(9): 2102–07.

Hollander MH, Paarlberg KM, Huisjes AJM. (2007) Gestational diabetes: a review of the current literature and guidelines. *Obstet Gynaec Surv* 62(2): 125–36.

Hu FB, Manson JE, Stampfer MJ et al. (2001) Diet, lifestyle and the risk of type 2 diabetes mellitus in women. *NEJM* 345: 790–97.

International Association for the Study of Obesity: www.iaso.org.

Johnson ST, McCagar LJ, Bell GJ et al. (2006) Walking faster: distilling a complex prescription for type 2 diabetes management through pedometry. *Diab Care* 29: 1654–55.

Karelis AD, Brochu M, Rabas-Lhoret R. (2004a) Can we identify metabolically healthy but obese individuals (MHO)? *Diabet Metab* 30(6): 569–72.

Karelis AD, St-Pierre DH, Conus F et al. (2004b) Metabolic and body composition factors in subgroups of obesity: what do we know? *J Clin Endocrinol Metab* 89: 2569–75.

Krentz AJ. (2002) *Insulin resistance.* London: Blackwell Publishing.

Lindstrom J et al. on behalf of the Finnish Diabetes Prevention Study Group. (2006) Sustained reduction in the incidence of type 2 diabetes by lifestyle intervention: follow-up of the Finnish Diabetes Prevention Study. *Lancet* 368(9548): 1673–79

McAuley K, Mann J. (2006) Thematic review series: patient-oriented research. Nutritional determinants of insulin resistance. *J Lipid Res* 47(8): 1668–76.

Monnier L, Colette C, Boniface H. (2006) Contribution of postprandial glucose to chronic hyperglycaemia: from the 'glucose triad' to the trilogy of 'sevens'. *Diab Metab* 32(Spec No 2:2S): 11–16.

Narayan KMV, Boyle JP, Thompson TJ et al. (2007) Effect of BMI on lifestime risk for diabetes in the US. *Diab Care* 30(6): 1562–66.

National Cholesterol Education Program (NCEP) expert panel on detection. (2002) Third report of the National Cholesterol Education Program (NCEP) expert panel on detection, evaluation, and treatment of high blood cholesterol in adults (Adult Treatment Panel III). *Circulation* 106: 3143–21.

Nichols GA, Hillier TA, Brown JB. (2007) Progression from newly acquired impaired fasting glucose to type 2 diabetes. *Diab Care* 30: 228–33.

O'Dea K. (1984) Marked improvement in carbohydrate and lipid metabolism in diabetic Australian Aborigines after temporary reversion to traditional lifestyle. *Diabetes* 33: 596–603.

Reavin G. (2006) The metabolic syndrome: is this diagnosis necessary? *Am J Clin Nutr* 83: 1237–47.

Riddle MC, Rosenstock J, Gerich J on behalf of the Insulin Glargine 2002 Study Investigators. (2003) The Treat-to-Target Trial: randomized addition of glargine or human NPH insulin to oral therapy of type 2 diabetic patients. *Diab Care* 26(11): 3080–86.

Sigal RJ, Kenny GP, Wasserman DH et al. (2006) Physical activity/exercise and Type 2 diabetes. *Diab Care* 29(6): 1433–38.

Thomas DE, Elliott EJ, Naughton GA. (2006) Exercise for type 2 diabetes mellitus. *Cochrane Database of Systematic Reviews* Issue 3. Art. No.: CD002968. DOI: 10.1002/14651858.CD002968.pub2.

Tuomilehto J. (2007) Counter-point: evidence-based prevention of type 2 diabetes: the power of lifestyle management. *Diab Care* 30(2): 435–38.

Twigg SM, Kamp MC, Davis TM et al. (2007) Prediabetes: a position statement from the Australian Diabetes Society and Australian Diabetes Educators Association. *Med J Aus* 186(9): 461–65.

Zhang C, Solomon CG, Manson JE et al. (2006) A prospective study of pregravid physical activity and sedentary behaviors in relation to the risk for gestational diabetes mellitus. *Arch Int Med* 166(5): 543–48.

PROFESSIONAL RESOURCES: MEASURING DIABETES RISK

Diabetes risk measurement

Potential risk of diabetes can be indicated by the use of a pencil and paper test such as the Finnish Diabetes Risk Assessment Tick Test, shown here.

Measure	Score
age (years)	
45–54	2
55–64	3
BMI (kg/m2)	
>25–30	1
>30	3
waist circumference (cm)	
men 94–102; women 80–88	3
men ≥102; women ≥88	4
use of blood pressure medication	2
history of blood glucose	5
physical activity <4h/week	2
low daily consumption of vegetables, fruits or berries	1
TOTAL	

Individual scores are summed to give a single score that indicates risk:

- 0–3: very low risk
- 4–8: low risk
- 9–12: high risk
- 13–20: very high risk

Diabetes screening tests

There are a number of useful measures for monitoring metabolic disorders, including many of those listed in Chapter 2 (e.g. lipids, blood pressure, homocysteine), the anthropometric measures covered in Chapter 4, and the exercise measures covered in Chapter 6. Those discussed below are specifically for classification of pre-diabetes and diabetes.

- **Fasting blood glucose** (FBG) Provides an indication of borderline diabetes. FBG is defined by a fasting glucose of >6.1 mmol/L and levels of <7.8 mmol/L after a 2-hour challenge. Impaired glucose tolerance (IGT) is defined by a fasting glucose <7 mmol/L and levels of >7.8 mmol/L and <11.1 mmol/L after a 2-hour challenge. Fasting glucose >7 mmol/L and 2-hour glucose >11.1 is defined as diabetes.
- **Glucose tolerance testing** (GTT) has been used in the past, following a positive fasting plasma record. However, while the American Diabetes Education Association has now stopped recommending glucose tolerance testing in practice, it is still recommended in Australia if fasting blood glucose has been used in the past, following a positive fasting plasma record.
- **Haemoglobin A1C (HBA_{1c})** Provides a stable measure of blood glucose over time. Measures above 6% are indicative of T2DM. Comparisons of HBA_{1c} with FPG measures are shown in Table 5.2.

TABLE 5.2 HBA_{1C} equivalents in FPG

HBA_{1C} (%)	FPG (mmol/L)
6	7.5
7	9.5
8	11.5
9	13.5
10	15.5
11	17.5
12	19.5

- **The 'glucose triad' and the 'trilogy of sevens'** An overall picture of diabetes control can be based on an assessment of the 'glucose triad': HBA_{1C}; post-prandial glucose (PPG) and fasting plasma glucose (FPG). French researchers have suggested a 'trilogy of sevens', where diabetes is defined by the three measures over seven: $HBA_{1C} > 7\%$, PPG >7 mmol/L and FPG>7 mmol/L (Monnier et al., 2006).
- **Fasting lipids** See Chapter 2.
- **Waist circumference** See Chapter 4.
- **Weight** See Chapter 4.
- **Body fat percentage (Bio-Impedance Analysis)** See Chapter 4.

CHAPTER 6

Physical activity: generic prescription for health

GARRY EGGER, MIKE CLIMSTEIN

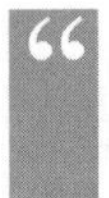

If we could give every individual the right amount of nourishment and exercise, not too little and not too much, we would have found the safest way to health.

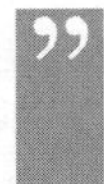

HIPPOCRATES

Introduction

According to the great Swedish exercise physiologist Professor Per-Olof Aastrand, if the whole of the history of *Homo sapiens* was a 400 metre race, a 100-year-old person living today would have participated only in the last 10 mm. For all but the last 2 mm, anyone participating in this race would have been active enough not to need gyms, swimming pools or fancy running shoes. Indeed, except for the very rich or elite (who had servants to do things for them), physical activity was part of the daily grind of staying alive.

This has led scientists to propose that a genome with genes selected for physical activity has 'fed forward' to healthy metabolism in humans over hundreds of thousands of years (Booth et al., 2002; Rowland, 1988) but this has been disrupted by the modern inactive lifestyle which began in the second half of the twentieth century and accelerated with the advent of advanced technologies (e.g. the internet) in its final years. Figure 6.1 illustrates the theoretical trend and possible reasons for changes in ambient activity levels in western populations over the last century. Estimates from this and other paleo-anthropological studies suggest a decrease in activity levels in recent times of up to 60% compared with about a hundred years ago. This is the equivalent of around 1000 kcal (4 400 kJ) per day less or walking about 16 km less each day.

FIGURE 6.1 Changes in activity levels over time

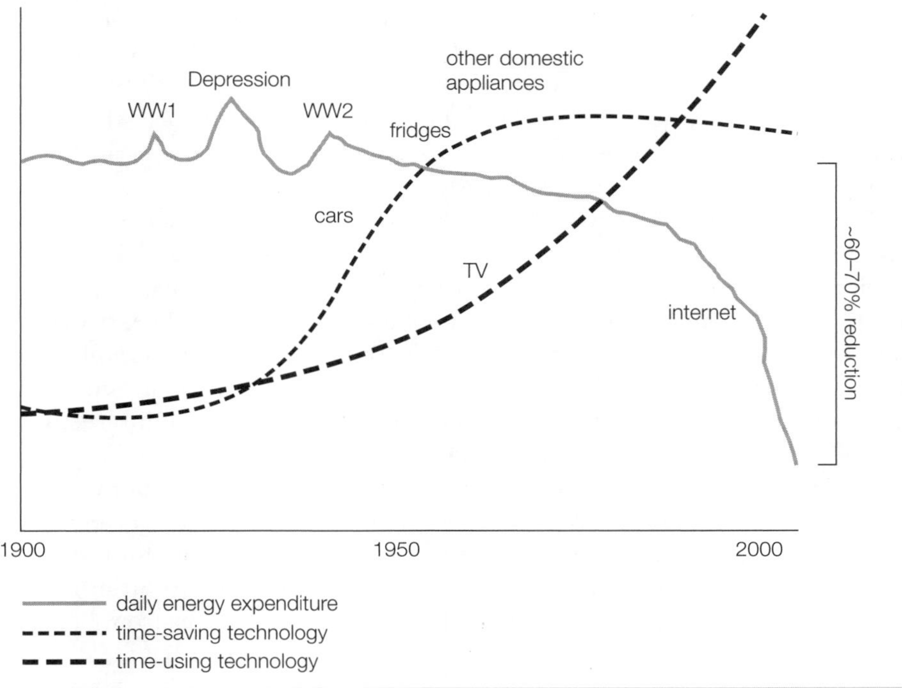

Source: Vogels et al., 2004

The disruption to healthy gene expression from this drastic change in energy expenditure has contributed to the rise of obesity throughout the world and its accompanying metabolic and mechanical pathologies (discussed in Chapter 4). According to Peters et al. (2002), this has resulted from a change in the environment that historically has 'pushed' humans to be active to one that requires 'pull', and hence a shift from 'instinct' to 'intellect' to attain a healthy gene expression. In other words, most humans now have to consciously plan extra-curricular physical activity in their daily lives because this does not happen naturally. Seen in this light, it is not the prescription of an unusual level of *exercise* that is required to reduce disease but the *reduction of inactivity* caused by industrialisation and modern technology. Similarly, it is not so much the benefits of exercise or physical activity (see box for the distinction between the two) that we need to promote as part of lifestyle medicine, but the dis-benefits of being sedentary or inactive.

Defining terms

Movement Any musculoskeletal activity of a person.

Physical activity Any musculoskeletal activity that involves significant movement of body or limbs.

Exercise A type of physical activity defined as a planned, structured and repetitive bodily movement done to improve or maintain physical fitness.

Fitness The capacity of the heart and lungs to pump blood to the working muscles and of the muscles to use this oxygen supply to carry out work.

Health Metabolic wellbeing as reflected in low risk levels of blood fats, blood pressure and body weight.

Activity levels, mortality, morbidity and wellbeing

Although physical activity has been seen as healthy since the days of Aristotle, the first modern evidence of its value came from a study of 31 000 London bus drivers by English epidemiologist Dr Jerry Morris in the 1950s (Morris et al., 1953). Morris established that bus drivers wore larger uniforms than conductors, who were much more active on the job. The drivers also had a higher incidence of heart disease, suggesting a link between heart disease, early death and inactivity.

Since then, the link between inactivity and early death, as well as a range of diseases and measures of wellbeing, has been clearly established in a number of major publications (for examples, see Bouchard et al., 1994; Warburton et al., 2006). Much of this work has come from the epidemiological research of Dr Steven Blair and his team from the Cooper Aerobics Institute in Dallas, Texas (for examples, see Blair et al., 2001; Lee et al., 2005). Blair's team measured the baseline fitness of large cohorts of men and women who attended the institute for health screening. They followed them for up to thirty years, measuring mortality and morbidity and relating these to measures of fitness and activity. Figure 6.2 illustrates mortality from cardiovascular disease in men and women categorised by tertiles of activity and fitness levels at baseline and follow-up. In general, the gradients are steeper for fitness than activity, but both are significant. This suggests that, while there are health benefits in being active over being inactive, there are even greater benefits from being aerobically fit, which comes from being vigorously active on a regular basis.

FIGURE 6.2 Mortality by fitness and physical activity categories

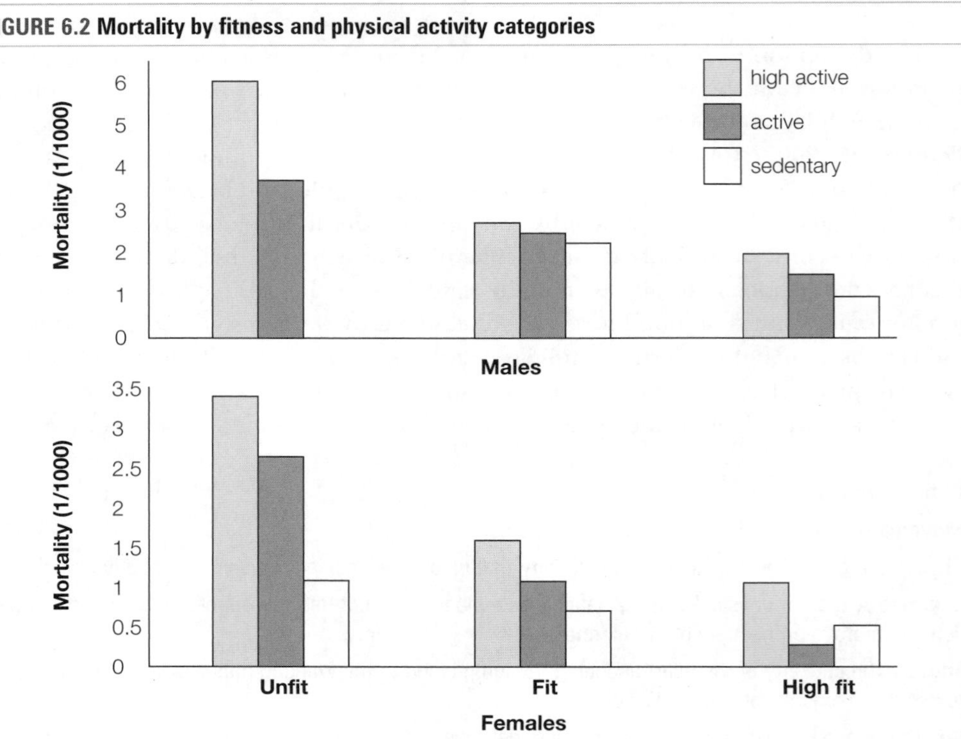

Source: Blair et al., 2001

This information has been used in developing the Australian *National Physical Activity Guidelines* (NHMRC, 2005), which have been adapted to provide a prescription which can be given to patients (as shown in Figure 6.3).

FIGURE 6.3 Physical Activity Guidelines

Name:______________________ D.O.B.:__________ Male / Female

1. Think of movement as an opportunity, not an inconvenience. Instead of using machines or other people, try adding the following to your day:

   (a) ______________________ (b) ______________________
   (c) ______________________ (c) ______________________

2. Be active every day in as many ways as possible: Try more of the following:

   ☐ Gardening ☐ Moving around the house ☐ Standing instead of sitting
   ☐ Doing things by hand ☐ Playing with the kids ☐ Playing games
   ☐ Active recreation ☐ Other

3. Put together at least 30 minutes of mild-moderate intensity activity on most, preferably all, days.

   ☐ Walking No. of steps/day:________ Other activity/ies:________ For this patient: Yes / No

4. If you can, also enjoy some regular, vigorous exercise for extra health and fitness.

   If yes, list activity/ies:______________________ Times/week: ☐ 1–2 ☐ 3–4 ☐ 5–7

Special requirements:______________________ **Review**: Next visit__________

Source: Adapted from NHMRC, 2005

The *Guidelines* provide a broad *generic* prescription for movement, physical activity, and exercise. This is summed up in a simple formula relating the health benefits of physical activity to the 'volume' of energy expended (the formula balances the one used in Chapter 8 for nutrition and originally discussed in Chapter 4):

volume of physical activity (energy expended) = **frequency** (how often) × **intensity** (how hard) × **duration** (how long)

In today's environment, there are two prescriptions for accomplishing this. The first is to do less passive activity (e.g. watching TV, using computers, searching the internet, playing video games). The second is to do more incidental activity or planned activity. 'Incidental' activity refers to physical effort that could otherwise be carried out by machines or other people (e.g. walking instead of driving, using stairs instead of the lift) and relates well to the first of the *Guidelines* shown in Figure 6.3. Clearly, incidental activity can contribute to the required energy volume for attaining health benefit(s). However, in the modern environment it is often quite difficult to achieve the required volume without some form of 'planned' physical activity, such as going for a walk, riding a bike or going to the gym.

Organisations such as the American College of Sports Medicine have also recently made use of widespread research findings to develop more *specific* prescriptions for a range of chronic diseases and disabilities (Durstine and Moore, 2003), from primary prevention to rehabilitation. A broad outline of these is given in Chapter 7, but before addressing specific exercise prescriptions for chronic diseases and disorders we will look at a system for analysing the different types of activities and their impacts on different areas of health.

Types of fitness: the four S's

Fitness is a broad, general term referring to the ability to carry out a physical task. In exercise science, this can refer to a number of different types of physical abilities ranging from agility to strength, many of which are related to skill or athletic ability. While important for sport scientists for improving athletic performance, these are of less concern for the health of the population. Health-related fitness can be loosely categorised into four S's: *stamina, strength, suppleness* and *size.* Although not strictly a type of 'fitness', size has been added here to indicate the importance of physical activity to body fatness in the modern environment and because it is a critical parameter in reducing falls in the elderly and improving glycaemic control in people with diabetes, as will be seen in the next chapter.

Stamina

Stamina is another term for aerobic or cardiovascular fitness. This refers to the capacity of the heart and lungs to pump oxygenated blood to the working muscles. Although there is a mountain of reference material describing how to increase this parameter of fitness (for examples, see Egger at al., 1999), our chief concern here is how to bring patients to a level of physical activity that is likely to be of benefit to their health. As described by Blair et al. (2001) and the *National Physical Activity Guidelines,* physical activity alone confers some benefits; however, fitness (from more intense activity or moderate to intense 'exercise') adds further benefit. In terms of the formula shown above, this suggests that *volume*—determined by frequent activity over long (preferably, continuous) periods at low intensity—will confer benefits for weight loss and health (and provide some level of fitness in the totally inactive). However, activity at a higher intensity, carried out less often and for less time, will provide added fitness *and* cardiovascular benefits.

At a population level, the greatest health gains will come from the most sedentary and inactive people in the population becoming even slightly more active. This is shown graphically in Figure 6.4. As can be seen, the benefits for the already active becoming even more active occur at a diminishing rate of returns. In other words, for a totally sedentary person, a daily walk around the block will significantly benefit his or her health, whereas an athlete exercising three hours a day may need an extra hour to attain even a minor increase in benefit. There is also undoubtedly a point beyond which injury risk and complications rise and tend to make added exercise less beneficial (O'Connor and Puetz, 2005).

As a generic prescription for stamina, aerobic activity (e.g, walking, jogging, cycling) should be carried out on most days of the week for 30–60 minutes (depending on intensity and desired outcome), or a minimum of around 2 500 calories or 11 000 kj of energy expended per week. At the lower end of intensity (see prescription for 'size', below),

FIGURE 6.4 Benefits of increasing physical activity

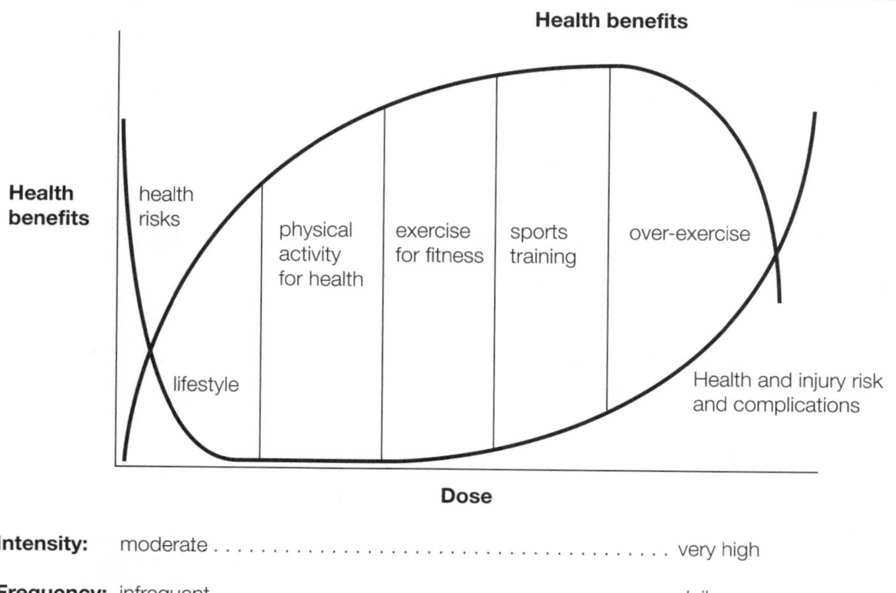

this can be accumulated over the course of a day and is determined by time spent or the distance covered in an activity that uses the large muscles of the body, such as walking, cycling, rowing or swimming. At this level, a measure of intensity, such as heart rate, is not necessary. For improvements in fitness, higher levels of intensity are required, and a heart rate training intensity of 60–80% of maximum heart rate (determined by the formula 220 − age) is recommended. An alternative to estimating exercise intensity via heart rate is to aim for a rating of 12–13 on a twenty-point scale of rating of perceived exertion (Borg, 1998), compared to around 8–10 for improved health.

Vigorous activity should not be recommended for those initiating exercise or for patients with cardiovascular risks or other problems and should be reached only after gradual progressive increases in intensity. While low intensity activity increases for health in the general population do not usually require specific precautions (people are normally carrying out this level of intensity in everyday activity), a qualified exercise physiologist should be involved in any exercise prescription for increased fitness.

Strength

Strength refers to the ability of the muscles of the body to contract against resistance. In the past, adequate strength was gained from daily living—lifting, carrying, working—however, as with aerobic exercise, this has decreased significantly as part of daily life because of technological developments. For this reason, and to increase muscle mass and reduce functional decline and fall-related injuries in older adults, the American College of Sports Medicine has set as a national goal of increasing to 30% by 2010 the proportion of adults who perform physical activities that enhance and maintain muscular strength and endurance on at least two days per week (up from 21.5%

in men and 17.5% in women in 2004) (Peters, 2006). Restoring the appropriate amount of muscular activity to prevent disease generally requires some form of 'planned' resistance training, where resistance can be in the form of:

- callisthenics (using the body as resistance, e.g. push ups, sit-ups),
- water (aquarobics),
- rubber straps or bands (as commonly used in physiotherapy),
- tins or bags of household goods (e.g. beans, rice),
- guided weight machines (pin loaded, hydraulic, pneumatic), or
- free weights (barbells and dumbbells).

Although planning a resistance training program can be complicated, it should be individualised to ensure it is safe and clinically effective and is thus generally best left to an exercise specialist. The general principles outlined below will apply to most regimens.

RESISTANCE TRAINING AIMS AND TERMS

Resistance training can be used to increase muscular strength and power, muscular endurance, cardiovascular fitness (and produce weight loss) and (body bulk (i.e. lean muscle mass), or a combination of these. Training involves the following:

- **Repetitions (reps)** The number of times an exercise is repeated.
- **Sets** The number of groups of repetitions.
- **Speed** Speed of contraction (generally slower on lowering, or 'eccentric', exercise).
- **Rest** Rest time between sets.
- **Load** The amount of weight or resistance used.
- **Repetition maximum (RM)** The amount of weight able to be lifted a set number of times (i.e. 80% of 10 RM is 80% of the weight that can just be lifted ten times).

RESISTANCE REGIMENS

Generic regimens for improving strength/power and endurance are outlined below. Muscle bulking will not be considered here because this is generally not associated with health outcomes. Regimens need to be individualised for specific purposes and conditions.

- **Strength/Power** Regimens generally involve low reps (4–6) and sets (2–3) with relatively heavy weights (i.e. 60–80% RM) and 1–2 minute rest between exercises. This requires a gradual progression from the endurance regimen discussed below. Power outcomes involve greater speed of contractions and are generally used by athletes to improve performance.
- **Endurance** Regimens are based around higher reps (10–20) and fewer sets (1–2) with lighter weights (40–60% RM) and minimal rest between exercises. This can include 'circuit training', which involves moving quickly through a number of different exercises involving different muscle groups.

Most resistance training exercises are completed in a bilateral manner, meaning both arms or legs are completing the repetition at the same time. However, for patients who are on prescribed antihypertensive medications, have a history of stroke, or have low ejection fractions, it is recommended they complete (if appropriate) all resistance training exercises unilaterally (i.e. one arm or leg at a time). The rationale for this recommendation is that the increase in blood pressure (systolic and diastolic) is directly related to both the intensity of the weight lifted and the amount of muscle mass involved. The intensity of the weight lifted can be reduced to minimise the effect on blood pressure by making the movement unilateral, essentially reducing the active muscle mass by 50%.

EXERCISES

There are a large number of resistance exercises available for different muscle groups, and these are found in various publications (e.g. Egger et al., 1999). In general, they are split into 'compound' exercises, involving large muscle groups or several major muscles, and 'isolation' exercises, which isolate single muscle group(s). For health and fat loss purposes, compound exercises are likely to be more effective because they involve more muscle mass and hence greater total energy use. Isolation exercises are used more often for rehabilitation of specific muscles.

While resistance training has typically been used for strength and power sports and for body bulking, there is recent empirical evidence for its application in middle-aged and older people to enhance functional living (Henwood and Taaffe, 2006). Falls, for example, make up the single biggest cause of injury in older adults. Resistance training has been shown to reduce fall injuries and hence health costs (Liu-Ambrose et al., 2004). Resistance training, in some form, for all elderly people is likely to become a trend of the future.

Suppleness (flexibility)

Flexibility is important to maintain musculoskeletal integrity and to reduce the likelihood of injury to muscles in athletes. Its main value in health is in maintaining muscle length in muscle groups that may be strengthened but not lengthened from aerobic and resistance exercise, thus preventing injury due to sudden tearing of these muscles. Flexibility is improved by stretching and holding muscles (without pain) for up to 15 seconds at a time. Three main forms of stretching useful for lifestyle medicine are:

- **Static stretching** A muscle is stretched and held for 10–15 seconds, and this is repeated a number of times.
- **Ballistic stretching** This is a dynamic form of stretching which involves a 'bouncing' movement of the muscle in preparation for sport. This is not recommended for general health.
- **Proprioceptive neuromuscular facilitation (PNF) stretching** This is a two-phase process where a muscle is stretched and held for 8–10 seconds, then relaxed. Next, the opposing muscle is isometrically contracted for 8–10 seconds, then relaxed, before the original muscle is stretched further. This 'tricks' the stretched muscle to extend further through the complicated recruitment of neural mechanisms designed to prevent over-stretching and over-contraction. PNF stretching leads to the greatest gains in flexibility (Sharman et al., 2006).

MUSCLE GROUPS FOR STRETCHING

Although it is functional to stretch all major muscle groups, this is often difficult for overweight people. The goal of a lifestyle medicine program is to stretch, at a minimum, those muscles likely to be shortened and/or strengthened through aerobic or strength work. The main functional muscles here are the hamstrings, peroneal muscles at the front of the leg, and gastrocnemius (calf) muscles at the back of the leg. Simple stretches to recommend and demonstrate to patients as a minimum to accompanying an aerobic exercise program are shown in Figure 6.5.

FIGURE 6.5 Some basic stretches for increasing suppleness

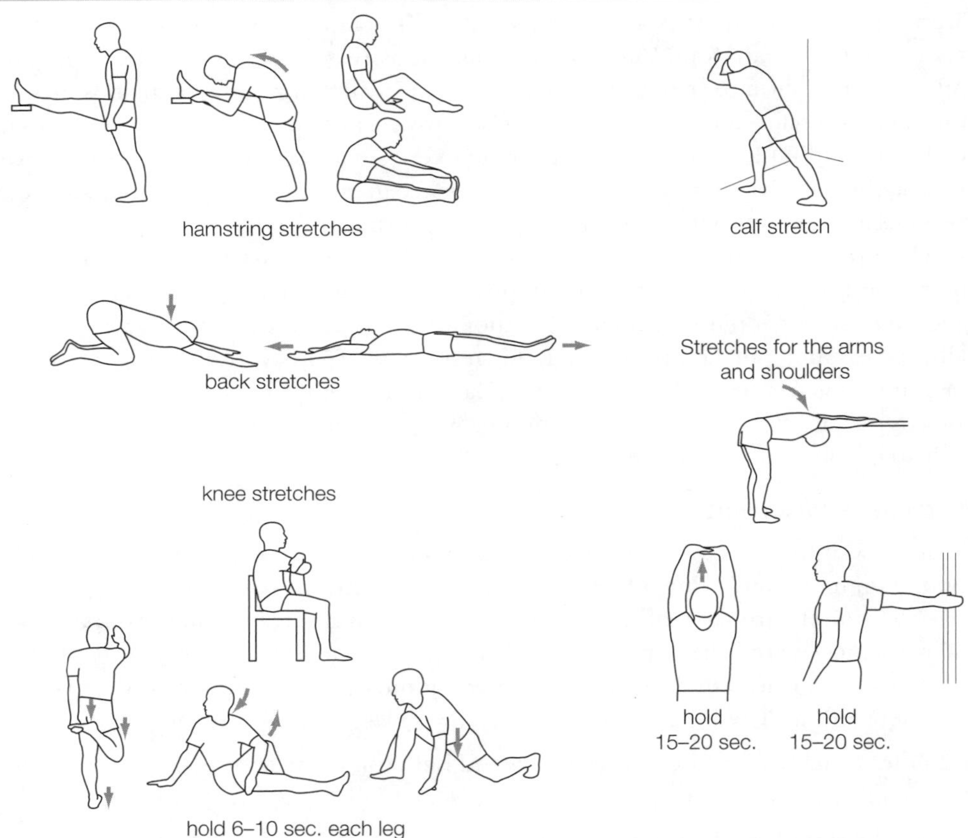

For best effect, muscles should be stretched after a brief period of 'warming up'. This is analogous to stretching chewing gum while it is still moist compared with stretching it after it has dried and is likely to tear. Patients should complete a 5–10 minute brisk walk prior to completing stretching exercises.

Size

Size, in the context in which it is used here, refers to excess body fatness. Reducing this can be accomplished by either stamina (aerobic) or strength (resistance) exercise, using the formula for exercise 'volume' described earlier. The development of stamina and strength, however, and the added cardiovascular benefits, requires systematically increasing the intensity of an exercise. Reductions in size (body fat) are influenced more by the total *volume* of physical activity.

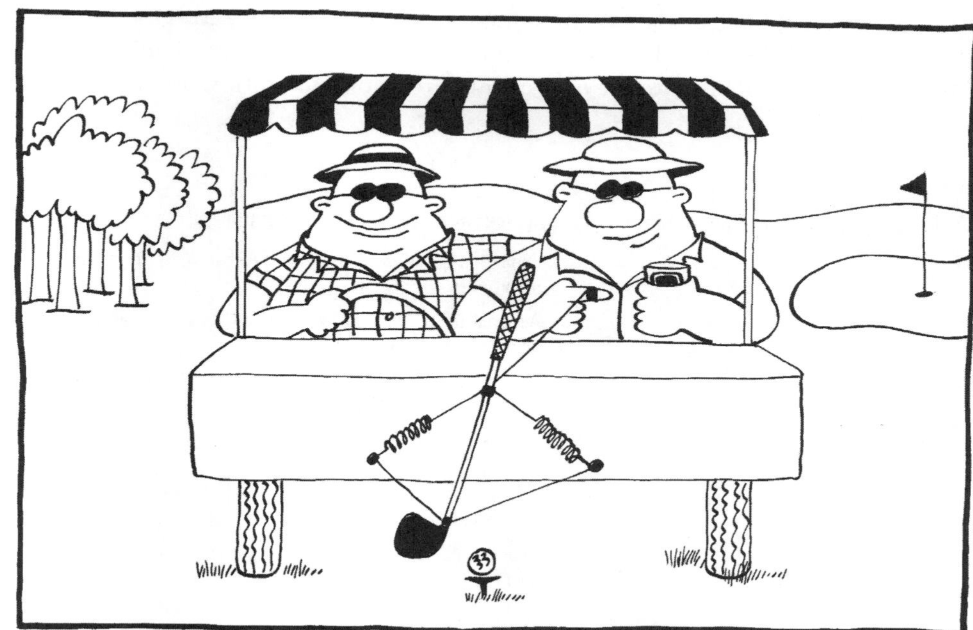

ERIC THE IDLE TESTS HIS LATEST ENERGY SAVING INVENTION.

Weight loss (at least theoretically) is a linear function of physical activity volume (although this does not necessarily happen in practice, as described in Chapter 4, because of physiological adjustments that occur with changing energy balance). The best types of activities are the aerobic, weight-bearing activities (e.g. walking, jogging, skiing), in contrast to those where the body weight is supported (e.g. cycling, rowing, canoeing). For the majority of the inactive population, the greatest benefit in fat reduction will come from increased daily walking. Because this is influenced by volume and not intensity, it does not need to be continuous but can be accumulated over the course of a day.

Pedometers are ideal tools for measuring this in steps, irrespective of length or speed of stride. As an average 80 kg man will burn roughly 1 kcal (4.4 kJ) for every twenty-five steps, relatively precise calculations can be made for total daily or weekly step counts by body weight. A recommended table of steps used in the Professor Trim's Weight Loss Program for Men is shown in Table 6.1.

TABLE 6.1 Recommended weekly steps by body weight

Body weight	Minimum steps/day	Optimum steps/week
70–80	8 500	>100 000
81–90	7 500	>100 000
91–100	7 000	>90 000
101–110	6 500	>80 000
111–120	6 000	>70 000
120–130	5 500	>60 000
>130	5 000	>50 000

A weekly stepping goal is recommended, in contrast to the daily goal often suggested for health benefits, because this allows for 'good' days and 'bad' days when time may be limited. Broad activity recommendations for different outcomes are discussed in Table 6.2.

TABLE 6.2 Suggested recommendations for physical activity and size reduction

General	Combine exercise with a hypocaloric diet. Increase 'incidental' as well as 'planned' exercise.
For preventing weight gain	Accumulate 30 mins of added moderate intensity activity per day (approximately 50 000 steps/week).
For weight loss	Accumulate 30–60 mins of added moderate intensity activity per day (approximately 70 000 steps/week).
For weight loss without changing diet	Accumulate 3 500 kcals (15 400 kJ) of moderate intensity activity per week (100 000 steps/week).
For weight loss maintenance (post-obese)	Accumulate 60–90 mins of moderate intensity activity per day (>100 000 steps/week).
	Alternatively, measure baseline activity and increase progressively by 30%.

Resistance training can add to the benefits of aerobic exercise for fat loss. Because work against resistance results in the maintenance or growth of muscle tissue, and because muscle is more metabolically active than fat, resistance training can result in a raised metabolic rate with a consequent increase in daily energy expenditure. In the early stages of a fat loss program, however, this may not be reflected in weight loss because muscle is over two times more dense (and therefore heavier) than fat: hence, fat loss can actually occur in the presence of weight gain (from increased muscle bulk). For this reason, and because resistance may result in maintenance or increases in total body mass, resistance training is recommended after an initial period of fat loss through a hypocaloric diet and aerobic activity.

Progression of exercise training

For best effect, a physical activity program should be dynamic, changing to suit the needs of an individual as she or he becomes more fit. This requires ongoing supervision and attention in most cases where specific prescription is required. Even in the case of generic exercise prescription, ongoing supervision and attention is recommended to guarantee compliance and motivation. This can be done with the enlistment of an accredited exercise physiologist (consult www.aaess.org.au).

Purpose, meaning and physical activity

In an important paper published in 2001, Dr William Morgan suggested that the missing factor in exercise prescription—what he calls Factor P—is a purpose for being active (Morgan, 2001). Morgan claimed that in the past, activity was tied to survival and so had meaning and purpose. The reason adherence to exercise prescription today is so low is because of a lack of meaning and purpose in exercise for exercise

What can be done in a brief consultation

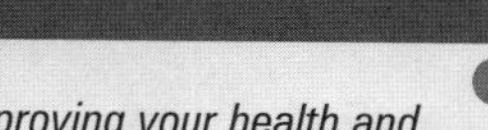

Ask, *Do you ever engage in physical activity for the sole purpose of improving your health and fitness?* to get an indication of fitness level.

Measure waist circumference, weight and body fat (if possible), and relate these to physical activity involvement.

Explain the difference between exercise for fitness and movement for fat loss.

Suggest an immediate program of accumulated (preferably weight-bearing) activity for health benefits.

Lend, rent or suggest the purchase of a pedometer to measure activity level baseline and to provide step goals.

Work through the four Physical Activity Guidelines prescription (see Figure 6.3) and give the prescription to the patient.

Provide written material on lifestyle areas identified.

sake. Morgan admitted that exercise can develop its own meaning and that a goal of exercise prescription may be to get to the point of exercise 'addiction'.

Other writers in this field have suggested that there are phases people go through in reaching a level of fitness that is intrinsically rewarding and thus provides purpose in an otherwise non-purposeful environment. In the early stages of fitness development, however, this is unlikely, and other purposes (with extrinsic forms of reward) should be sought. Morgan refers to a quote by Norwegian psychiatrist Dr Egil Martinesen that 'if the patient is considering the purchase of an exercise machine, a dog would make for a good selection'. Lifestyle-related activities, instead of those developed as part of a non-purposeful regimen, have been shown to work best in this respect.

The clinician's role

Physical activity has typically been regarded in a 'motherhood' light, with a clinician's exhortation to 'do some exercise' thought to require no further elaboration. With the rapidly changing ambient exercise environment of the twenty-first century, however, this is no longer sufficient. Doctors and allied health professionals all now require at least a partial knowledge of the fundamentals of generic exercise prescription and an understanding of the requirements for referral for specific prescription. More importantly, because there is no pharmaceutical substitute for exercise, there is a need for a detailed understanding of what will best motivate a patient to become more active, not only for the short term but for the rest of his or her life in an environment which demands some form of intellectually driven activity plan. While doctors may recognise the need for this, and practice nurses or other health professionals may help assess and measure this need, the best support in the long run is going to come from involving qualified exercise physiologists or personal trainers, at least until the point where intrinsic motivation can stimulate the patient to continue.

Summary

Because the human body has evolved in an environment of regular activity, this has 'fed forward' to a healthy metabolism. However, the decrease in activity in the modern environment is now reflected in metabolic abnormalities. Re-establishing a regular pattern of physical activity is thus imperative for metabolic health. The four S's of fitness—stamina, strength, suppleness and size–summarise exercise needs. Together, these provide a generic prescription for activity for most people. Individual prescription may then be needed for dealing with specific problems, and this is the basis of the next chapter.

PRACTICE TIPS: PRESCRIBING PHYSICAL ACTIVITY AND EXERCISE FOR HEALTH

	Medical practitioner	**Practice nurse**
Assess	Need for increased activity (e.g. with an active question; see *Professional resources*). Need for more detailed fitness testing (i.e. graded exercise test). Need for more specific prescription. Factors limiting activity (contraindications and/or limitations).	Need for activity/exercise. Factors limiting activity. The four S's; do a basic step test if needed. Need for advanced testing. Need for referral.
Assist	By identifying activity goals with the patient (short term and long term). By recommending a generic program. By suggesting a type of program. By suggesting types of alternatives (e.g. gym, exercise physiologist, personal trainer).	By providing of a generic exercise prescription (see *Professional resources*). Removal of impediments to movement. Areas for improvement in the four S's. By developing motivational goals. By planning of an exercise regimen. By providing ongoing support/encouragement.
Arrange	An exercise physiologist. Referral to a specialist if required for injury (e.g. podiatrist, orthopaedic specialist, physiotherapist).	Consultation with an exercise physiologist to develop an exercise plan. A personal trainer if detailed care and motivation required. A local fitness centre membership if desired.

KEY POINTS FOR CLINICAL MANAGEMENT

- Generic prescription for physical activity is vital for all patients; specific prescription may require more skilled and ongoing input by referral to and working with an exercise physiologist.
- Consider motivational levels and ongoing commitment to being physically active, not just immediate commitment.
- Suggest small changes that may stimulate compliance.
- If possible walk (or exercise) before breakfast for optimal weight loss (unless diabetic) because this recruits fat into the energy cycle earlier than if food is used for energy.
- Exercise lightly clad in cooler months because the body is required to used more energy to maintain core body temperature.

- Vary the type/intensity/duration of physical activity for fat loss to reduce the effects of 'efficiency' and hence reduce energy requirement.
- Exercise before a main meal to reduce hunger and therefore overeating.
- For weight loss, use weight-bearing exercise such as walking where possible.
- If joint or other problems do not allow weight-bearing exercise, carry out weight-supportive exercise such as walking in water, swimming, cycling or rowing over longer periods.

REFERENCES

Blair SN, Cheng V, Holder JS. (2001) Is physical activity or physical fitness more important in defining health benefits? *Med Sci Sports & Ex* 33(6 Suppl 2): S379–99.

Booth FW, Chakravarthy MV, Gordon SE et al. (2002) Waging war on physical inactivity: using modern molecular ammunition against an ancient enemy. *J Appl Physiol* 93: 3–30.

Borg G. (1998) *Borg's perceived exertion and pain scales*. Champaign, Ill: Human Kinetics.

Bouchard C, Shephard R, Stephens T (eds). (1994) *Physical activity and health: international proceedings and a consensus statement*. Champaign, Ill: Human Kinetics.

Durstine JL, Moore GE. (2003) *ACSM's exercise management for persons with chronic disease and disabilities*. Champaign, Ill: Human Kinetics.

Egger G, Champion N, Bolton A. (1999) *The fitness leader's handbook. Fourth edition*. London: Simon and Schuster.

Henwood TR, Taaffe, DR. (2006) Short-term resistance training and the older adult: the effect of varied programmes for the enhancement of muscle strength and functional performance. *Clin Physiol & Funct Imag* 26(5): 305–13.

Lee S, Kuk JL, Katzmarzyk PT, Church TS, Ross R. (2005) Cardiorespiratory fitness attenuates metabolic risk independent of abdominal subcutaneous and visceral fat in men. *Diab Care* 28(4): 895–901.

Liu-Ambrose T, Khan KM, Eng JJ et al. (2004) Resistance and agility training reduce fall risk in women aged 75 to 85 with low bone mass: a 6-month randomized, controlled trial. *J Am Geriat Soc* 52(5): 657–65.

Morgan WP. (2001) Prescription of physical activity: a paradigm shift. *Quest* 53: 366–82.

Morris JN, Heady JA, Raffle PA. (1953) Coronary disease and physical activity of work (part 2). *Lancet* 265: 1111–20.

NHMRC (National Health and Medical Research Council) (2005). *National physical activity guidelines.* Canberra: Australian Government Press. Available from www.health.gov.au/internet/wcms/Publishing.nsf/Content.

O'Connor PJ, Puetz TW. (2005) Chronic physical activity and feelings of energy and fatigue. *Med Sci Sports & Exer* 37(2): 299–305.

Peters JC. (2006) Obesity prevention and social change: what will it take? Perspectives for progress. *Ex Sport Sc Rev* 34(1): 4–9.

Peters JC, Wyatt HR, Donahoo WT et al. (2002) From instinct to intellect: the challenge of maintaining healthy weight in the modern world. *Obes Rev* 3: 69–74.

Rowland TW. (1998) The biological basis of physical activity. *Med Sci Sports & Ex* 30(3): 392–99.

Sharman MJ, Cresswell AG, Riek S. (2006) Proprioceptive neuromuscular facilitation stretching: mechanisms and clinical implications. *Sports Med* 36(11): 929–39.

Vogels N, Egger G, Plasqi G et al. (2004) Estimating changes in daily physical activity levels over time: implications for health interventions from a novel approach. *Int J Sports Med* 25: 607–10.

Warburton DE, Nicol CW, Bredin SS. (2006) Health benefits of physical activity: the evidence. *Can Med Assoc J* 174(6): 801–09.

Wizen A, Farazdaghi R, Wohlfart B. (2002). ICO Conference, Brazil, 2002.

professional resources

PROFESSIONAL RESOURCES: MEASURING FITNESS

A simple screening question

Ask *Do you ever engage in physical activity for the sole purpose of improving your health and fitness?* to get an indication of fitness level.

Professor Trim's clinical test battery

This is a brief test battery for measuring the four S's and involving a ten-minute fitness test. Individual scores are given for each of the six tests. There is also a total score for comparison with later results. With the exception of tests 1 and 2, all should be added to give a total score; tests 1 and 2 scores should be multiplied before being added to the other scores.

Size: Tests 1 and 2

Measure Bio-Impedance Analysis using body fat scales.

Measure waist circumference, measured at the mid-point of lowest rib and iliac crest *or* umbilicus for men and mid-point for women. Measures should be consistent.

Measurement	Score	
Test 1. BIA (%)	Score out of 5	see table below
Test 2. Waist circumference (cm)	Score out of 6	see table below
Combined size score (BIA × waist circumference)	Score out of 30	see table below

Explanation: BIA (Bio-Impedance Analysis) measures body fat through a process of electrical conductance. Normal ranges for men are 12–24% and for women 15–35%. Waist circumference is a measure of fat distribution. For best health, Caucasian men should be <100 cm and women <90 cm around the waist. Cut-offs for Indians and Asians are 10 cm less and for Pacific Islanders 10 cm more. The size score (BIA × WC) gives a measure of medically dangerous fat distribution.

How to calculate a score for these tests:

	Men	Women	Contribution to total score
BIA (%)			
Good	<24%	<32%	5
OK	24–30%	32–35%	4
Poor	>30%	35%	3
Waist circumference (cm)			
Good	<90	<80	6
OK	90–100	80–90	3
Poor	>100	>90	1

Stamina: Tests 3 and 4

Take a resting pulse over a minimum of 15 seconds to get a score per minutes.

Do the Scale of Physical Activity Level (SPAL) Questionnaire (Wizen et al., 2002), i.e.:

Which is the highest level activity on the scale which you are able to carry out for 30 minutes or more?

1. Sit
2.
3. Walk slowly
4.
5. Walk at normal pace/cycle slowly
6.
7.
8. Jog/cycle
9.
10. Run
11.
12. Run fast/cycle fast
13.
14.
15. Run very fast (>15 km/hr)
16.
17.
18. Perform aerobic activity at a professional level (women)
19.
20. Perform aerobic activity at a professional level (men)

The measures here are in METs (1 MET = 1 metabolic unit, or the amount of energy burned at rest). For greater precision the following formula (METpred) is available for corrections with age:

$$\text{METpred} = 7.37 + (0.595 \times \text{MET}) - (0.057 \times \text{age})$$

Test 3. Pulse (beats per minute)	Score out of 8	} see table below
Test 4. SPAL (METS)	Score out of 34	

Explanation: Pulse is a rough measure of physical fitness and hence receives a low overall score. SPAL is a pencil and paper measure of aerobic fitness. Measures are in METS, or multiples of metabolism at rest. Average scores for men are 6–9 METS and for women 5.5–8.5. High scores indicate better fitness.

How to score for these tests:

	Men	Women	Contribution to total score
Resting pulse (bpm)			
Good	<65	<75	8
OK	66–95	76–105	5
Poor	>95	>105	0
SPAL			
Very good	>12	>11.5	34
Good	9.0–11.9	8.5–11.4	28
OK	6.0–8.9	5.5–8.4	17
Poor	3.0–5.9	2.5–5.4	12
Very poor	<3.0	<2.5	6

Suppleness (sit-and-reach or sit-and-stand test): Test five

Lower back flexibility can be measured with a sliding flexibility rule or a ruler placed between the centre of the feet. The procedure is then as follows:

1. Warm up the body before measuring.
2. Sit on the floor with legs straight and feet in the foot holes provided on the flexibility rule (or with ruler between the feet).
3. Slowly bend forward at the trunk with legs straight and measure the distance that can be reached with finger tips either before or beyond the feet (maximum +15 cm; minimum −15 cm).
4. If the finger tips do not reach the feet, the measure is regarded as a minus score. If the finger tips pass the feet, the measure is regarded as a plus score.
5. Check the score in the table provided and get a total contribution score.

Test 5. Sit and reach (cm)	Score out of 16

Explanation: This test measures the flexibility of hamstrings and lower back, which is a good indication of overall flexibility. Low flexibility suggests possible musculoskeletal problems. Higher scores are better than lower and lower limits for people under 40 years old are +4 cm and for people over 40 year olds, −1 cm.

How to score for this test:

	Age <35 years	Age >35 years	Contribution to total score
Very good	>15	>7	16
Good	+15 to +5	+7 to 0	12
OK	−1 to +4	0 to −10	8
Poor	−1 to −10	−11 to −5	4
Very poor	less than −10	less than −15	2

Strength (sit-ups or stand-ups): Test 6

In relatively active people, sit-ups to measure abdominal strength over 20 seconds is the preferred test. This is done by counting the number of completed sit-ups that can be done in a set period (in this case 20 seconds). The procedure is:

1. Lie on your back on the floor with feet on a standard height chair so that the knees are bent at right angles.
2. Fold the arms in front of the chest with elbows pointing forward.
3. Raise the shoulders off the ground in a 'crunch' position until the elbows touch the thighs. Return then to the position of shoulders flat on the ground.
4. Carry out as many complete sit-ups as possible in a 20-second period. If the elbows do not touch the thighs, or the shoulders are not returned to the flat-on-the-ground position, the sit-up is not counted.
5. Check the number of sit-ups completed in the table provided and get a total contribution score.

For the more frail and the extremely overweight or injured, a sit-and-stand test, rising from a chair to full extension of the legs is an alternative. Scores are similar.

Test 6. Stand-ups (numbered)	Score out of 12

Explanation: Abdominal strength as measured by the sit-up test and leg strength as measured by stand-up test are good measures of overall body strength. Acceptable levels for people under 30 years old are twelve sit-ups and stand-ups in 20 seconds; for people aged 30–39, eleven; and for people over 40, ten.

How to score for this test:

	Age <29	Age 30–39	Age >40	Contribution to total score
Good	>17	>15	>13	12
OK	12–17	11–15	10–13	8
Poor	<12	<11	<10	4

Total fitness score

The total fitness score (out of 100) = (test 1 × test 2) + test 3 + test 4 + test 5 + test 6. The total score indicates fitness level:

- 0–20 Very poor: needs to be considerably improved
- 21–40 Poor: needs work on all areas
- 41–60 Average: can be improved for better results
- 61–80 Good: improvements possible in some areas
- 81–100 Very good: fitness is generally not a concern

Weaknesses which could be improved:

- body fat
- aerobic fitness
- flexibility
- strength
- total fitness

Patient handout

Reducing body fat

There is no best single way to lose fat. Some people benefit from one approach while others benefit from another. The one thing we can say is that if you make changes that cannot be maintained for life, it's not likely to help you reduce weight long term—and that's what it's all about. Check with your doctor to see what is likely to be the best approach for you to lose weight out of about a dozen techniques available.

Increasing aerobic fitness

In the first instance this is not hard. It just requires increasing the amount of movement you do over the course of a day. You can use a pedometer to measure the number of steps you do each week, and then try to increase this over the next few weeks by 30% or more. If you want to lose weight, you should try to accumulate >70 000 steps a week or more. But 'accumulate' means this doesn't have to be all in one go. Once you have started to increase the amount of movement you do, you may then want to increase your fitness a little more by increasing the intensity of the movement. Having a personal trainer or using an accredited gym can be other ways of increasing fitness.

Increasing flexibility

Flexibility is important to prevent stiffness and muscle and joint pain. Flexibility is increased by stretching muscles as shown in the diagram (see Figure 6.5). Do not stretch to a point of pain, and hold the stretch for 8–10 seconds before relaxing and repeating. You can also increase flexibility through yoga, Pilates and a range of similar programs.

Increasing strength

Strength is increased by carrying out exercises against resistance. This can be resistance against your own body weight (called callisthenics), resistance against water (such aquarobics), using large rubber bands or other heavy objects, or becoming involved in a weight training program at a gym or with a personal trainer. Resistance training helps to maintain muscle mass and reduce body fat. This type of exercise is vital for older people to prevent falls and muscular weakness.

CHAPTER 7

Physical activity: specific prescription for disease management and rehabilitation

MIKE CLIMSTEIN, GARRY EGGER

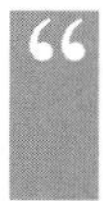

It seems to me that we need to begin thinking about exercise prescription and the problem of adherence to physical activity in a very different sort of way.

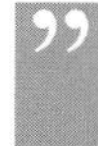

MORGAN, 2001

Introduction

In the summer of 2005, while exercise physiologists around the world were 'bunkered down' in their expensively equipped research laboratories, Dr Heinz Drexel and his colleagues from the Vorarlberg Institute for Vascular Investigation at Feldkirch, Austria, were out in the Alps, handing out lift passes and measuring a group of volunteers' reactions to walking up or down steep ski slopes (Drexel, 2006). After a month of training half the group to walk up and half to walk down a ski run daily for a month, catching the lift the other way, the researchers measured changes in their subject's blood chemistry. They then switched the groups for a month and measured their reactions to this.

To the surprise of many, the responses were different. The concentric contraction of muscles walking up hill (shortening under load) caused a significant decrease in triglycerides in the blood (a risk factor for heart disease) whereas the eccentric contraction of muscles required in walking downhill (lengthening under load) caused a greater decrease in blood sugars (a risk factor for diabetes). Low density lipoprotein (LDL) cholesterol was reduced by approximately 10% in both cases.

The significance of these findings is in the specificity of the metabolic responses to various types of physical activity. For a long time, it was thought that a generic prescription for exercise for health was adequate. In fact a consideration of historical landmarks in physical activity research (Figure 7.1) illustrates that while the ambient environment in earlier times necessitated activity for survival, humans required little extra exercise. Exercise prescription in the mid-twentieth century and before was based mainly in the interests of getting young men 'fit for war'; during the 1970s and, '80s, the concentration was on training for athletes and sportspeople; and only since the publication of the US Surgeon General's *Guidelines* in 1994 has the orientation changed to physical activity for health (US Surgeon General, 1996).

FIGURE 7.1 Historical landmarks in physical activity research

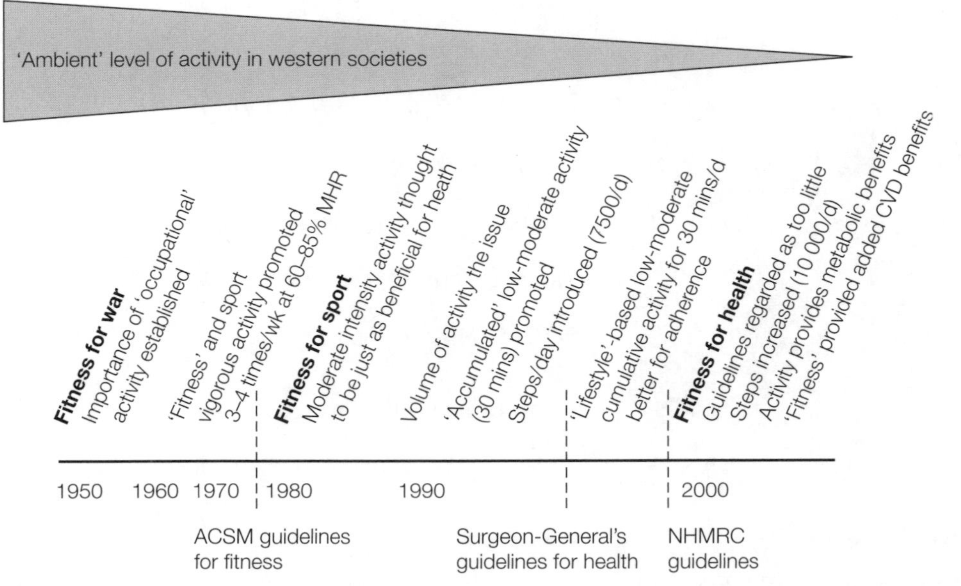

These shifts in direction resulted in the development of new national physical activity guidelines in several countries, including Australia (NHMRC, 2005; shown in prescription form in Figure 6.3). There has been an even greater decrease in ambient activity levels since the Australian guidelines were first published in 1999, the result of the internet. The recent American College of Sports Medicine's (ACSM) manual *Exercise management for person's with chronic diseases and disabilities* (Durstine and Moore, 2003) suggests the need for a modified series of guidelines (shown in Figure 7.2), with some additions to the standard guidelines as well as a different dimension for specific prescription.

While the generic prescription shown in Figure 7.2 is absolute, more specific prescription of exercise for metabolic health is now also indicated. This has been illustrated in a number of reviews (e.g. Pedersen and Saltin, 2006), meta-analyses (e.g. Snowling and Hopkins, 2006), and other reports from meetings (e.g. Bouchard et al., 1994). The ACSM report lists more than forty medical conditions for which there is evidence of benefit from regular exercise for prevention or therapy (Table 7.1).

FIGURE 7.2 Potential additions to the 1999 *National guidelines for physical activity* including specific prescriptions for disease management

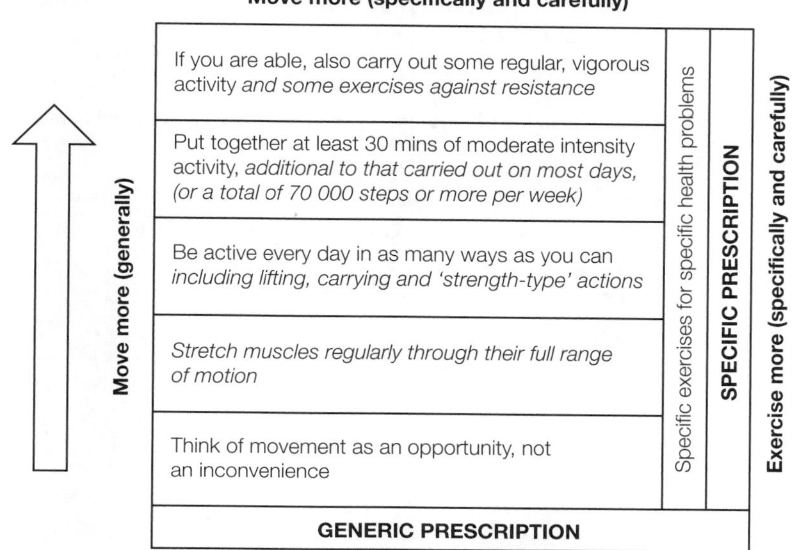

Source: Adapted from NHMRC, 2005

TABLE 7.1 Medical conditions with evidence regarding the benefits of regular exercise for prevention of therapy

AIDS	chronic pain	mental health (anxiety, depression)	premenstrual syndrome
ageing: physical frailty	diabetes	migraine	renal transplant
ankylosing spondylitis	haemophilia	multiple sclerosis	sarcopenia
arthritis (rheumatoid, osteoarthritis)	hypercholesterolemia	myasthenia gravis	sickle cell anaemia
cancer (breast, colon, prostate)	total cholesterol	obesity	sleep disorders
cardiac transplant	HDL	osteoporosis	stroke
congestive heart failure	LDL	Parkinson's disease	urinary incontinence
coronary heart disease	VLDL	peripheral vascular disease	
chronic fatigue	triglycerides	physical disability	
chronic obstructive pulmonary disease (COPD)	hypertension	post-polio syndrome	
	low back pain		

Source: Durstine and Moore, 2003

This points to the importance of involving skilled exercise personnel as an integral part of any allied health team presenting lifestyle medicine, while still acknowledging the importance of generic prescription for general metabolic health outlined in Chapter 6. The present chapter is designed to illustrate some of the major areas where specific prescription may be indicated and how and when to involve an accredited exercise physiologist in the allied health team.

Exercise and disease management

Table 7.2 outlines a small sub-sample of the ailments listed in Table 7.1, with asterisks indicating the level of evidence for potential benefit from each of the four forms of fitness (the four S's) discussed in Chapter 6 for prevention and/or treatment.

TABLE 7.2 Evidence for specific benefits of different types of exercise prescription in management of ten major diseases

	Stamina		Strength		Suppleness		Size	
Disease	Prevent	Treat	Prevent	Treat	Prevent	Treat	Prevent	Treat
Alzheimers	–	*	–	*	–	–	–	–
anaemia	–	*	–	*	–	–	–	–
arthritis	*	*	*	**	*	***	**	**
asthma	–	**	–	**	–	–	*	*
CHD	**	***	*	**	–	*	**	**
COPD	*	**	–	*	–	*	*	*
chronic fatigue	–	**	–	--	–	–	–	–
diabetes	***	***	*	**	–	–	**	***
frailty	*	*	*	*	*	*	–	–
fibromyalgia	–	*	–	–	–	*	*	*
hyperlipidaemia	*	**	*	*	–	–	**	*
hypertension	**	**	–	*	–	–	**	**
lower back pain	–	–	*	*	*	*	*	*
obesity	***	***	*	**	–	–	***	***
Parkinson's	–	*	–	*	–	*	–	–
stroke	**	**	–	**	–	*	*	*

– = no evidence; * = limited evidence; ** reasonable evidence; *** strong evidence

Source: Adapted from Durstine and Moore, 2003

No attempt is made here to cover all of the ailments that benefit from exercise or the fine detail of prescription: discussion is confined to a small number of commonly occurring problems with predominantly lifestyle-based aetiologies that are discussed in detail elsewhere throughout this book. Each condition is considered in the context of the four S structure discussed in Chapter 6 and the 'volume' equation outlined in Chapter 4. For more details on specific programming, readers are referred to the ACSM manual *Exercise prescription for disease management* (Durstine and Moore, 2003), *Clinical exercise physiology* (Ehrman et al., 2003) and other publications in the references at the end of this chapter.

Exercise and diabetes

Exercise has now emerged as one of the key treatment options for type 2 diabetes mellitus (T2DM), even in the absence of weight loss (Thomas et al., 2006), with effective and progressive exercise protocols being evolved for dealing with different stages of the disease. According to Nieman (1998), 'with optimum diet and exercise therapy, and achievement of ideal body weight, only about one in ten type 2 diabetes patients would require any medication'. Paffenbarger et al. (1997) showed that diabetes develops progressively and that for every 500 kcal (2 200 kJ) increase in energy expenditure per week, the risk of T2DM is reduced by 6%.

Exercise prevents diabetes through a number of different mechanisms, many of which duplicate the effects of insulin in glucose disposal (Signal et al., 2004). Aerobic exercise on a daily basis (including increased incidental exercise) should be encouraged as the basis of management. Increased frequency, duration and intensity results in greater glycaemic control (Boule et al., 2003). However, resistance training has also been shown to be highly effective (Dunstan et al., 2003), and a progression from light aerobic exercise through to more intensive resistance training in a motivated patient is likely to have optimum benefits. Resistance training exercises should be completed on two to three days per week. Potential types and kinds of training for general T2DM management are shown in Table 7.3. Prescription needs to take account of the specific requirements of the patient and any limitations or contraindications the patient may have pertaining to exercise (Eves and Plotnikoff, 2006).

TABLE 7.3 Typical exercise needs for type 2 diabetes management

Exercise type	Examples	Frequency	Intensity	Duration	Cautions
Size and stamina	walking cycling aquarobics walking in water incidental exercise	Preferably daily. Don't miss two consecutive days.	mild-moderate: 40–65% HR_{max} or <13 on an RPE scale, increasing with fitness	30–60 mins accumulated More is better. 8–10 000 steps/d or increase 30% from baseline	Effort should be predictable. Monitor medication. Check extremities with neuropathy.
Strength	resistance weights circuit training (large muscle groups)	2–3 days/week	1 set, 10–15 reps, 60% of 1 RM, increasing weight with strength	8–10 exercises, until complete	eye pressure gradual progression
Suppleness	static stretching yoga, PNF	before and after aerobic exercise, extra if needed	Don't stretch to the point of pain.	until complete	over-stretching

A recent position statement has been released by the American Diabetes Association (ADA, 2006), which recommends the following for physical activity:

- One hundred and fifty minutes per week of moderate-intensity aerobic physical activity (50–70% of maximum heart rate) is recommended and/or at least 90 minutes per week of vigorous aerobic exercise (>70% of maximum heart rate). The physical activity should be at least three days/week, with no more than two consecutive days without physical activity.
- In the absence of contraindications, people with T2DM should perform resistance training exercise three times a week, targeting all major muscle groups, completing three sets of 8–10 reps at a weight that cannot be lifted more than 8–10 times.

According to the ADA position statement, vigorous exercise may be contraindicated for individuals with diabetic retinopathy and non-weight bearing exercise is recommended for people with diabetic peripheral neuropathy. The ACSM position statement for diabetes states that increased intensity, additional sets, or a combination of volume and intensity may produce greater benefits and may be appropriate for certain individuals (Albright et al., 2000).

Exercise has also been found to be effective for both the prevention and treatment of gestational diabetes mellitus (GDM). While the precautions of normal exercising during pregnancy apply, resistance exercise (using elastic or rubber bands) has been found to be effective in reducing GDM into the second trimester of pregnancy (Brankston et al., 2004). There is also an inverse association between pre-gravid activity (amount and duration) with later GDM, suggesting a role for exercise in management of GDM before and throughout pregnancy (Dempsey et al., 2004).

Precautions

Generally, the danger associated with not exercising in diabetes is greater than that from exercising, although special and individual cautions do apply. Because exercise reduces blood sugars, consistent self-monitoring of blood glucose levels prior to, during and after exercise is required to avoid hypoglycaemia. For additional recommendations for exercise and diabetic patients, refer to the ACSM's *Guidelines for exercise testing and prescription* (Durstine and Moore, 2000). Special care also needs to be taken with peripheral neuropathy (weight-bearing exercise is generally contraindicated) and blood and eye pressure during resistance training. Increases in blood pressure may be minimised by having the patient complete all resistance training exercises unilaterally and using lighter intensity (i.e. 40–50% of 1 RM).

Exercise and heart disease

There is strong scientific evidence to support exercise in the prevention (Giannuzi et al., 2003) and rehabilitation of coronary heart disease (Scrutinio et al., 2005). The identified benefits include improving coronary risk factors, reducing symptoms and reducing the risk of new coronary events. Furthermore, exercise has been shown to reduce overall and cardiovascular mortality by approximately 25% (Giannuzi et al., 2003).

Cardiac rehabilitation

Comprehensive cardiac rehabilitation is appropriate for many patients with heart disease, including post-revascularisation (CABG, coronary stents, angioplasty), post-AMI, angina, heart failure, heart transplantation, valve replacement/repair, cardiomyopathy and pacemaker insertion. The concept of comprehensive cardiac rehabilitation was developed in the 1950s and includes a medical evaluation, prescribed exercise, education and counselling. Cardiac rehabilitation traditionally consists of three phases:

- **Phase 1** is conducted in hospital and initiated within the first 24–48 hours. Exercise is generally limited to range of motion (ROM) exercises and self-care activities multiple times per day. With progression, walking is included, generally limited to an exercise intensity of resting heart rate +20 bpm.
- **Phase 2** is also generally provided in hospital and initiated 2–6 weeks post event. Exercise is generally completed three days per week with constant monitoring

(ECG and BP). Educational lectures pertaining to medications, heart disease, risk factor reduction (smoking cessation, stress management) and exercise are also an important component of the program. This phase of rehabilitation generally lasts from four weeks to six months.

- **Phase 3** is generally conducted in a community setting in health and fitness facilities. Exercise that is deemed clinically effective and safe may include treadmill walking, cycling, rowing, swimming and resistance training. A clinical exercise physiologist generally prescribes exercise routines, with progress reports provided to both the patient and referring doctor on a regular basis.

Doctors are advised to contact their local hospitals for phase 1 and 2 cardiac rehabilitation programs available in their area; contact local health and fitness facilities for structured phase 3 programs, ensuring that they meet recognised guidelines and are staffed by suitably qualified exercise physiologists. Emergency equipment including a defibrillator should also be available.

The beneficial effect of rehabilitative exercise for patients with diagnosed coronary heart disease is well established (Jolliffe et al., 2000). Pederson and Saltin (2006) reported that exercise-based cardiac rehabilitation reduced all-cause mortality by 20% and cardiac mortality by 26%.

Resistance training has also been found to be beneficial in acute myocardial infarction patients. Elhke (2006) summarises the recommendations for resistance training in this population:

- frequency: 2–3 days/week
- intensity: initially, 50% of 1 RM, progressing to 60–70% 1 RM
- volume: 8–12 reps in younger adults, 10–15 in the elderly
- progression: upper body, 1–2 kg; lower body, 2–4 kg
- recovery: 30–90 seconds between sets and >48 hours between sessions.

Resistance training may be contraindicated in patients with unstable angina, exertional angina or low ejection fractions. Consult with the patient's cardiologist for the appropriateness of resistance training in the rehabilitation program. Rehabilitative exercise recommendations for heart disease and related disorders are quite diverse, but Adams et al. (2006) have shown that most resistance exercises are safe for most cardiac patients and that the American Cardiology Association suggestion that patients should not 'lift anything greater than 5 lbs' is totally unrealistic and based on a lack of scientific evidence. Medical professionals are advised to seek the advice of their local exercise physiologist or cardiac rehabilitation programs.

Exercise and arthritis

Arthritis is one of the most common forms of musculoskeletal problems in modern society. Figures from the U.S. suggest that 22% of the adult population have medically diagnosed arthritis and around 8% have arthritis-attributable activity limitations. (Hootman et al., 2006). The two main forms of the disease are osteoarthritis and rheumatoid arthritis, but there are more than a hundred other forms, making a universal prescription difficult. Nevertheless, in most cases—and often contrary to popular opinion—exercise in some form, with supervision, can improve the progression of the disease.

TABLE 7.4 Exercise recommendations for arthritis

Exercise type	Examples	Frequency	Intensity	Duration	Cautions
Suppleness	ROM* and PNF* stretching of affected joints warm water exercises mild yoga and tai chi if appropriate	1–2 sessions/ week	Very mild, moderated by pain	As long as it takes	Avoid over-stretching. Warm up slowly.
Strength	circuit training machines rubber bands isometric exercise	2–3 days/week with at least one day's rest	Start mild with gradual increases.	2–3 reps to begin, building to 10–12 reps	Avoid medial/lateral forces, high reps and high resistance.
Stamina and Size	large muscle aerobic activities combine full, partial and non-weight bearing aquarobics	3–5 days/week	40–60% HR_{max}	5 min session building to 30 mins	Increase duration, not intensity, with progression.

ROM = range of motion; PNF = proprioceptive neuromuscular facilitation (see Chapter 6)

Basic exercise parameters for arthritis are shown in Table 7.4. While vigorous exercise is contraindicated in the presence of acute joint inflammation, the more common presentation is of subacute or chronic joint symptoms. Specialist advice should first be sought about the value of an exercise intervention, noting that the most immediate benefit may be to diminish the ill-health effects of inactivity, as much as improving the problem. Low impact activities should be selected, with the emphasis on suppleness and joint range of motion. Aquarobics or warm water exercise can be used for stamina, flexibility and weight loss. Resistance training should aim to stabilise the musculature around affected joints and, while the load may need to be reduced if pain or swelling occurs, this should not mean eliminating the exercise per se. Speed of movement is not an issue and exercise dose can be accumulated during several sessions throughout the day.

Exercise and hypertension

A diagnosis of hypertension often leads to a recommendation not to exercise because it can raise blood pressure. However, while this is true in the acute phase, chronic exercise has been shown to reduce both systolic and diastolic blood pressure by up to 10 mm Hg in Stage 1 or 2 hypertension, as defined by the NHMRC. This can halve the risk of cardiovascular death and, together with the reduced risk from lowered body weight, can have significant benefits for the one in three adults known to have higher-than-recommended blood pressures. The benefits shown most commonly come from aerobic exercise, with or without weight loss (Pedersen and Saltin, 2006). However, recent evidence has also identified improved blood pressure from resistance training exercise (Fagard, 2006). With the exception of circuit training, which involves an aerobic component, chronic strength or resistance training has not been shown consistently to lower BP. As stated previously, all hypertensive patients carrying out resistance training exercises should complete all of the exercises in a unilateral manner and at a lower intensity.

TABLE 7.5 Exercise recommendations for hypertension

Exercise type	Examples	Frequency	Intensity	Duration	Cautions
Size and Stamina	large muscle endurance activities (e.g. walking, cycling)	3–7 days/week	mild-mod (40–60–80% HR_{max})	Can be accumulated for weight loss. 30–60 min session for BP	Don't use HR if on beta-blockers. Alpha-blockers may cause post-exertional hypertension. Not for Stage 3 hypertension.
Strength	possibly, circuit training if desired	3–4 days/week	high reps, low resistance	30–60 mins	Avoid isometrics. No high intensities.
Suppleness					Only as related to aerobic and strength exercises.

As shown in Table 7.5, some precautions need to be taken. The benefits for those with Stage 3 or essential hypertension may not be direct but may come from reduction of other risk factors. However, this is also likely to require ongoing medication.

Exercise and dyslipidaemia

Because exercise enhances the ability of muscles to oxidise fat, it is a primary recommendation for the correction of dyslipidaemia, including hypertriglyceridaemia and raised sub-fractions of cholesterol. Because many patients with this problem also have hypertension or symptomatic heart disease, the recommendations for exercise prescription need to be quite specific. This prescription follows recommendations for the general public, but the amount of physical activity needs to be increased and there may be some benefits in different forms of exercise for different dyslipidaemic states (Table 7.6). The benefits in hypercholesterolemia are primarily attained from aerobic exercise, however, it is recommended that both aerobic and resistance training exercises be completed (Kim and Lee, 2006).

Aerobic exercise has been shown to have less effect in lowering LDL cholesterol, for example, than in lowering triglycerides or raising HDL (although there is some suggestion that raising HDL may be better done through resistance training). Inclusion of a low fat diet and weight loss can enhance the effects, and inactive patients are likely to benefit most from increases in activity levels.

TABLE 7.6 Exercise recommendations for dyslipidaemia

Exercise type	Examples	Frequency	Intensity	Duration	Cautions
Size and stamina	weight loss with low saturated fat diet large muscle aerobic exercises for raising HDL and lowering TG	daily	mild–mod (40–70% HR_{max})	40–60 mins Frequency and duration are more important than intensity.	Exercise may potentiate the propensity for statin-related muscle damage.
Strength	resistance training to lower LDL	2–3 days/week with at least one days rest	Start mild with gradual increase.	2–3 reps building to 10–12 reps	Changes may require several months.
Suppleness					Only as related to aerobic and strength exercises.

As with other ailments where medication is necessary, exercise should be regarded as adjunct to drug therapy, except in mild cases where it may be sufficient in itself. One particular disadvantage with the use of statins—which are used effectively for lipid correction—is an increased risk of myalgia and this appears to be even greater in heavy exercisers (Thompson et al., 2003). The implications of this are discussed further in Chapter 21.

What can be done in a brief consultation

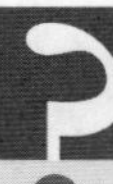

Check on the different types and levels of exercise currently carried out.

Advise that there are different exercise requirements for specific health problems (the four S's; see Chapter 6).

Ask about factors limiting potential exercise involvement (e.g. sore joints, muscular pain, time).

Where risk factors may be mild, prescribe aerobic exercise (e.g. walking) for a short period and check effects before using medication.

Consider simple measures such as flexibility or strength exercises.

Refer to an exercise physiologist for specific exercise prescription.

Exercise, stress anxiety and depression

Stress imposes a threat on the body and elicits a set of 'flight or fight' neuroendocrine responses, mobilising energy and inducing a state of insulin resistance in the body. Although this was essential in ancient times for survival, such threats have largely been overtaken in modern society by psychosocial threats. Identical stress responses are initiated by emotional or psychological stressors, but the energy mobilised is not used up and can be stored as visceral fat in the body. Tsatsoulis and Fountaoulakis (2006) suggest that physical activity should be the natural means for preventing or ameliorating the metabolic and psychological co-morbidities induced by chronic stress. Physical alleviation of the body's reaction to stress can come through either aerobic ('flight') or resistance ('fight') activity; the level of specificity has not been detailed.

Current recommendations for dealing with stress are to follow standard exercise prescription protocols for the general population. Because anxiety (a possible outcome of stress) can create a heightened level of arousal, 'dampening down' of the sympathetic nervous system through more intensive activity—either stamina or strength based, and carried out earlier in the day to maintain reduced sympathetic tone—may be the most effective approach. Given that a redistribution of energy substrates occurs to visceral stores, endurance activities such as walking or jogging may have the greatest effects on metabolic homeostasis, as well as anxiety moderation. Flexibility activities like yoga or tai chi can add a relaxation component to this.

Similarly, there is no clearly defined exercise prescription for depression, although there is clear evidence that this may be as effective as modern antidepressant medications (Motl et al., 2005), with the added benefit of improving physical functioning (Brenes et al., 2007). Recent research suggests a close and possibly even causal link between inactivity and depression (see Chapter 13) and a consistent effect of exercise that is as effective as medication over the long term (e.g. Pedersen and Saltin, 2006). Remaining active even in the absence of significant weight loss has also been shown to result in less depression, after accounting for potential confounders (Craig et al., 2006). Increased aerobic intensity with time may also be a factor, with training used as a supplement to medical treatment, except in the case of mild depression where it may be sufficient in itself.

Singh and colleagues (2005) investigated the effectiveness of two intensities of progressive resistance training exercise compared to normal GP care in patients with diagnosed clinical depression. Middle-aged patients with either major or minor depression were randomised into either high intensity progressive resistance training (80% of 1 RM), low intensity progressive resistance training (20% of 1 RM) or normal GP care. The exercise groups completed the exercises three days per week for eight weeks. Investigators found the high intensity progressive resistance training was more effective than either low intensity progressive resistance training or GP care in the treatment of these patients.

Further support for the benefits of progressive resistance training in patients with depression was reported by Motl et al. (2005), who studied the effects of six months of walking or resistance training exercise in older adults. They found depressive symptom scores significantly decreased following initiation of the exercise therapy and there was a sustained reduction for up to five years after both treatments.

Other conditions

As well as the diseases and disease risks mentioned above, there are a number of common conditions where specific exercise prescription can improve or optimise health.

Guidelines for exercise in **pregnancy**, for example, are now available through a number of peak bodies, including the American College of Obstetrics and Gynecology (Artal et al., 2003). These include recommendations for protecting the fetus and health of the mother through the various stages of pregnancy, with a decrease in exercise volume and weight-supportive exercise during the last trimester. Particular attention needs to be paid to appropriate, rather than excessive, maternal weight gain and the specific needs of those at risk of or with gestational diabetes. All of the four S's are important, but should be achieved using particular precautions and individual specifications.

Studies with **older people** have shown the importance of emphasising strength to reduce the sarcopenia (muscle wastage) that occurs with ageing and to protect against falls. Suppleness or flexibility training is also recommended in this group, with less emphasis on stamina and the need for weight loss.

Perhaps counterintuitively, a graduated program of light to moderate aerobic exercise has therapeutic effects for **chronic fatigue syndrome**. Exercise and sleep are related, and recent research indicates a possible association between decreased sleep and obesity, with a possible link through increased inactivity (this is discussed more in Chapter 16).

Recently, attention has turned to exercise during **menopause** as an alternative to hormonal therapy. As well as protecting against **osteoporosis**, a structured stamina and strength-training program can assist in reducing menopausal symptoms (Fugate and Church, 2004). Appropriate exercise during the perimenopausal stage can also help ameliorate the weight gain that often occurs in menopause. Suppleness training is indicated for middle-aged people, as is an appropriate hypocaloric diet and exercise program to maintain body weight.

Some other common problems and possible exercise solutions are shown in Table 7.7.

TABLE 7.7 Common problems and possible exercise solutions

Problem	Possible exercise prescription
cramping	regular contractions (concentric and eccentric) of affected muscles, with and without resistance
constipation	endurance or extended aerobic exercise
fatigue	gentle endurance exercise in the mornings; increasing duration and intensity as tolerated
incontinence (stress)	Kegal pelvic floor strengthening mobility improvement with endurance, balance and resistance training as needed
insomnia	endurance or resistance exercise in the early or mid-afternoon
lower back pain	resistance training to strengthen back extensor muscles (specific instruction required) strengthening of rectus abdominis and hip extensor muscles
recurrent falls, gait and balance disorders	lower extremity resistance training for hips, knees and ankles, including, for example, lateral movements, balance training and tai chi
weakness and sarcopenia	moderate to high intensity resistance training for all muscle groups

Summary

While a generic prescription for all patients to 'move more' is appropriate in the modern environment, there are some conditions where more specific exercise prescription may provide added benefits. These include exercise regimens for rehabilitation, as well prevention where familial and biological risks indicate a propensity toward certain problems (e.g. dyslipidaemia). The level of specialty required for this necessitates the use of a qualified exercise physiologist as part of the allied health professional team.

PRACTICE TIPS: EXERCISE PRESCRIPTION FOR SPECIFIC PURPOSES

	Medical practitioner	Practice nurse
Assess	Whether a specific exercise prescription is appropriate. General fitness level. Aspects of the four S's that may need attention. Special precautions that may be needed/provided to exercise specialist. Possible drug contraindications for exercise.	Basic aspects of the four S's that may need attention: stamina, suppleness, strength and size.
Assist	Understanding of the importance of exercise. By obtaining regular updates on progress.	By increasing motivation to undertake specific exercise. By providing feedback about interest in prescribed programs and specialists.
Arrange	Referral for specific exercise prescription advice where required. List of other health professionals for a care plan (ensure exercise specialists have details about medical history and drug use).	Close consultation with an exercise physiologist to devise a program. Contact with gym or fitness centre for ongoing exercise program if appropriate.

KEY POINTS FOR CLINICAL MANAGEMENT

- Where specific exercise prescription and ongoing supervision is required, refer to an accredited exercise physiologist (see www.aaess.com.au).
- While basic exercise testing can be conducted in the clinical situation, this should only be used as the basis for more detailed testing and prescription carried out by a testing specialist.
- Regularly monitor exercise routines and ensure changes to exercise parameters as appropriate for the progression and goals of the program.
- Communicate regularly with an exercise specialist to ensure matching of medical and exercise goals.
- The exercise prescription must be individualised to ensure it is safe and clinically effective.
- Exercise intensity poses the greatest risk to any patient. Always ensure either the maximal exercise exertion (RPE on the Borg scale) or maximal exercise HR is set for each patient to ensure his or her safety during exercise. An accredited exercise physiologist can assist using the results of a recent graded exercise test.
- Telemetry heart rate monitors (i.e. Polar heart monitors, www.polar.fi/polar/entry.html) are particularly useful in helping patients ensure they do not overexert themselves during exercise.
- It is good practice to require all cardiac patients to complete a hospital-conducted cardiac rehabilitation program prior to having them exercise in a community setting (i.e. gym or fitness centre).

REFERENCES

ADA (American Diabetes Association). (2006) Standards of medical care in diabetes. *Diab Care* 29; S4–S42. Available from http://care.diabetesjournals.org/cgi/content/full/29/suppl_1/s4.

Adams J, Clin MJ, Hubbard M et al. (2006) A new paradigm for post cardiac event resistance exercise guidelines. *Am J Cardol* 97: 281–86.

Albright A, Franz M, Hornsby G et al. (2000) American College of Sports Medicine position stand: exercise and type 2 diabetes. *Med Sci Sports Exerc* 32: 1345–60.

Artal R, O'Toole M, White S. (2003) Guidelines of the American College of Obstetricians and Gynaecologists for exercise during pregnancy and the postpartum period. *Brit J Sports Med* 37: 6–12. Available from http://bjsportmed.com/cgi/reprint/37/1/6.

Bouchard C, Shephard RJ, Stephens T (eds) (1994) *Physical activity, fitness and health: international proceedings and consensus statement.* Champaigne, Ill: Human Kinetics.

Boule NG, Kenny GP, Haddad E et al. (2003) Meta-analysis of the effect of structured exercise training on cardio-respiratory fitness in type 2 diabetes mellitus. *Diabetologia* 46: 1071–81.

Brankston GN, Mitchell BF, Ryan EA et al. (2004) Resistance exercise decreases the need for insulin in overweight women with gestational diabetes mellitus. *Am J Obstet Gynecol* 190: 188–93.

Brenes GA, Williamson JD, Messier SP et al. (2007) Treatment of minor depression in older adults: a pilot study comparing sertraline and exercise. *Ageing & Mental Hlth* 11(1): 61–68.

Craig CL, Bauman A, Phongsavan P et al. (2006) Jolly, fit and fat: should we be singing the 'Santa Too Fat Blues?' *CMAJ* 175(12): 1563–66.

Dempsey JC, Sorensen TK, Williams MA et al. (2004) Prospective study of gestational diabetes risk in relation to maternal recreational physical activity before and during pregnancy. *Am J Epidem* 159(7): 663–70.

Drexel H. (2006) Different forms of walking and effects on blood chemistry. *Am Heart Assoc 2006 Scientific Sessions abstract 3826.*

Dunstan D, Zimmet P, Slade R et al. (2003) *Diabetes and physical activity. International Diabetes Institute position paper.* Melbourne: International Diabetes Institute.

Durstine JL, Moore GE. (2003) *ACSM's Exercise management for persons with chronic diseases and disabilities.* Champ Ill: Human Kinetics.

Durstine JL, Moore GE. (2000) *ACSM's guidelines for exercise testing and prescription.* Champaigne Ill: Human Kinetics.

Ehrman JK, Gordon PM, Visich PS et al. (2003) *Clinical exercise physiology.* Champaigne Ill: Human Kinetics.

Elhke, E. (2006) Resistance exercise for post-myocardial infarction patients: current guidelines and future considerations. *Nat Strength & Condit Assoc J* 28(6): 56–62.

Eves ND, Plotnikoff RC. (2006) Resistance training and type 2 diabetes. *Diab Care* 29: 1933–41.

Fagard RH. (2006) Exercise is good for your blood pressure: effects of endurance training and resistance training. *Clin Exp Pharmacol Physiol* 33(9): 853–6.

Fugate SE, Church CO. (2004) Nonestrogen treatment modalities for vasomotor symptoms associated with menopause. *Ann Pharmacother* 38(9): 1482–99.

Giannuzzi P, Mezzani A, Saner H et al. (2003) Physical activity for primary and secondary prevention. Position paper of the Working Group on Cardiac Rehabilitation and Exercise Physiology of the European Society of Cardiology. *Eur J Cardiovasc Prev Rehab* 10(5): 319–27.

Jolliffe JA, Rees K, Taylor RS et al. (2000) Exercise-based rehabilitation for coronary heart disease. *Cochrane Database Syst* Rev 4-CD001800.

Hootman J, Bolen J, Helmick C et al. (2006) Prevalence of doctor-diagnosed arthritis and arthritis attributable activity limitation—United States, 2003–2005. *MMWR* 55(40): 1089–92.

Kim NJ, Lee SI. (2006) The effects of exercise type on cardiovascular risk factor index factors in male workers. *J Prev Med & Pub Hlth* 39(6): 462–68.

Morgan WP. (2001) Prescription of physical activity: a paradigm shift. *Quest* 53: 366–82.

Motl RW, Konopack JF, McAuley E et al. (2005) Depressive symptoms among older adults: long-term reduction after a physical activity intervention. *J Behav Med* 28(4): 385–94.

NHMRC (National Health and Medical Research Council). (2005) *National physical activity guidelines.* Canberra: DoHA. Available from www.health.gov.au/internet/wcms/Publishing.nsf/Content.

Nieman DC. (1998) Exercise immunology: integration and regulation. *Int J Sports Med* 19(Suppl 3): S171.

Paffenbarger RS Jr, Lee IM, Kampert JB. (1997) Physical activity in the prevention of non-insulin-dependent diabetes mellitus. *World Rev Nutr Diet* 82: 210–18.

Pedersen BK, Saltin B. (2006) Evidence for prescribing exercise as therapy in chronic disease. *Scand J Med Sci in Sports* 16(Suppl 1): 3–63.

Scrutinio D, Bellotto F, Lagioia R et al. (2005) Physical activity for coronary heart disease: cardioprotective mechanisms and effects on prognosis. *Monaldi Arch Chest Dis* 64(2): 77–87.

Signal RJ, Kenny GP, Wasserman DH et al. (2004) Physical activity/exercise and type 2 diabetes. *Diab Care* 27(10): 2518–35.

Singh NA, Stavrinos TM, Scarbek Y et al. (2005) A randomized controlled trial of high versus low intensity weight training versus general practitioner care for clinical depression in older adults. *J Gerontol. Series A, Biol Sci & Med Sci* 60(6): 768–76.

Snowling NJ, Hopkins WG. (2006) Effects of different modes of exercise training on glucose control and risk factors for complications in type 2 diabetic patients: a meta-analysis. *Diab Care* 29(11): 2518–27.

Thomas MC, Zimmet P, Shaw JE. (2006) Identification of obesity in patients with type 2 diabetes from Australian primary care: the NEFRON-5 study. *Diab Care* 29(12): 2723–25.

Thompson PD, Clarkson P, Karas, RH. (2003) Station-associated myopathy. *JAMA* 289(13): 1681–89.

Tsatsoulis A, Fountoulakis S. (2006) The protective role of exercise on stress system dysregulation and comorbidities. *Ann NY Acad Sci* 1083: 196–213.

US Surgeon General. (1996) *Physical activity and health: a report of the Surgeon General.* Atlanta, GA: Department of Health and Human Services Centres for Disease Control.

Vogels N, Egger G, Plasqi G et al. (2004) Estimating changes in daily physical activity levels over time: implications for health interventions from a novel approach. *Int J Sports Med* 25: 607–10.

PROFESSIONAL RESOURCES: INDICATIONS FOR DEFERRING OR TERMINATING PHYSICAL ACTIVITY

According to the Australian Association for Exercise and Sport Science, there are several indications for deferring activity and having a medical review:

- unstable angina
- uncontrolled cardiac failure
- severe aortic stenosis
- uncontrolled hypertension or grade 3 (severe) hypertension (e.g. blood pressure ≥180 mm Hg systolic or ≥110 mm Hg diastolic)
- symptomatic hypotension <90/60 mm Hg
- acute infection or fever or feeling unwell (including, but not limited to, acute myocarditis or pericarditis)
- resting tachycardia or arrhythmias
- diabetes with poor blood glucose control (e.g. blood glucose < 6 mmol/L or >15 mmol/L)

There are also indications for terminating activity:

- squeezing, discomfort or typical pain in the centre of the chest or behind the breastbone with or without spreading to the shoulders, neck, jaw and/or arms, or symptoms reminiscent of previous myocardial ischaemia
- dizziness, lightheadedness or feeling faint
- difficulty breathing
- nausea
- uncharacteristic, excessive sweating
- palpitations associated with feeling unwell
- undue fatigue
- leg ache that curtails function
- physical inability to continue
- for people with diabetes: shakiness, tingling lips, hunger, weakness, palpitations

For more information, see the association's website: www.aaess.com.au.

CHAPTER 8

Nutrition for the non-dietitian

JOANNA McMILLAN PRICE, GARRY EGGER

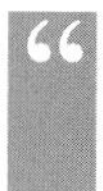

Research about diet and nutrition seems to contradict itself with aggravating regularity.

WALTER WILLET, 2005

Introduction

Peruse the pages of any mix of popular media and you will consistently find one thing: a lack of consistency on the supposed health benefits of different aspects of nutrition. One week we are told that coffee causes cancer, the next that it prevents it. All fat was once thought to be dangerous; now we are advised to eat more of some types to prevent heart disease. Dairy products were thought to be fattening; now they are actually promoted for weight loss.

So what is going on? Why is it so hard for scientists to reach a definitive conclusion on good nutrition? And how do we know that what we are promoting now is not likely to change in the future?

The science of nutrition

Nutrition is a comparatively young science, with much to be discovered. Because of the wide range of ingredients in foods and the multidimensional physiological responses to this, research can be tedious and demanding. Progress is made in stages, with inevitable controversies in small issues but a gradual evolution of understanding of major health-related factors.

To discuss nutrition and health in a single chapter in the context of lifestyle medicine is therefore a daunting task. Consequently, we have chosen to focus only on those aspects of nutrition that are relevant to metabolic health and, in particular, obesity and weight control (and the extent to which these influence other aspects of metabolic health). Even here, we cannot hope to cover the full range of information available, so we have chosen to concentrate on those new and practical findings that have implications for lifestyle medicine. Again, this is not meant as a substitute for competent professional advice, but to complement such information.

We look first at calorific volume in food and the factors contributing to this, then turn to new findings relating to specific aspects of the major nutrients and the implications of these findings for metabolic health. We have assumed a knowledge of nutritional components, and so do not elaborate on the basics. More detailed recommended nutritional reading is contained in the *References* and *Professional resources*. Energy intake from fluids and the influence of eating behaviours are considered in subsequent chapters.

The concept of (energy) volume

It has long been known, at least for animals, that longevity is increased with relatively low total energy intake over the course of a lifetime. Why this may be so is not clear. Because of ethical considerations in doing the research, it is also not clear whether the same applies to humans, although the indications are that it does. Several hypotheses have been proposed as to why this may be so (Civitarese et al., 2007; Morgan et al., 2007). It is also not known whether a restriction of all or just some types of calories may be important (Heilbronn and Ravussin, 2006). Nevertheless, while there are diet books on just about every component of nutrition, the truth is that the most significant component of nutrition for weight control (and metabolic health) is its (calorific) volume (Rolls, 2007).

Volume, as outlined in Chapter 4, in energy input is made up of three components:

energy density (how rich) × **portion size** (how much)
× **frequency of eating** (how often)

This determines total energy input and, therefore, potential energy imbalance.

Energy density

In the past, the main concern for weight control has been dietary fat in food. This was based on the notion that fat contains 9 kcal/g (38 kJ/g) whereas carbohydrate and protein are less than half of this (alcohol, which is 7 kcal/g or 30 kJ/g, has a more confusing story and is discussed in Chapter 9). Hence, while reducing fat in a diet can significantly reduce total energy input more than an equivalent weight reduction of other nutrients, this is not the only component of food that determines total energy.

Food manufacturers in the 1990s capitalised on science's obsession with fat by promoting products as being a particular percentage 'fat free', having replaced the fat with sugar and other carbohydrates. Paradoxically, the end result was often an increase in calories per gram or energy density (ED) of the food. Energy density, it has recently been realised, is the most significant component of energy intake, and attempts are being made to quantify levels that may be recommended for weight loss and good health.

Based on figures by Dr Barbara Rolls and colleagues from Penn State University (Rolls et al., 2006), an upper limit cut-off of around 3 kcals/g (approximately 13 kJ/g) has been determined for those with a weight concern (Cameron-Smith and Egger, 2002). Other cut-offs are shown, with some food examples, in Table 8.1. ED can be easily calculated from food labels by dividing the energy per 100 g by 100. ED in fluids is related to mL of fluid, with recommendations for cut-offs of this given in Table 9.1 in Chapter 9.

The principal factors decreasing ED in foods are fibre and water; the principal factors increasing it are fats and sugars. Hence, foods such as fruits, vegetables, pastas

TABLE 8.1 Recommended energy density (ED) cut-offs for food intake

Energy Density	Measure	Recommendation	Examples
low	<7.5 Kj (1.8 kcals)/g	Eat freely.	fruit, vegetables, cereals, baked beans, several fish, bread, pasta, cereal grains, porridge, lean meats (e.g. kangaroo)
medium	7.6 kJ (1.81 kcals)/g–13 kJ (3 kcals)/g	Eat sparingly.	low fat ice creams, gelato, avocado, fruit pies/muffins, jelly sweets, coconut milk
high	>13 kJ (3 kcals)/g	Eat only occasionally (if at all).	fatty meats, full cream dairy products, cheeses, spreads (butter/margarine), chocolate pastries/pies/cake/biscuits, fried foods, potato crisps/thin chips, snack foods, coconut oil, ghee

and cereal usually have a low ED whereas full cream dairy products, many processed foods, and those with added sugars, have a high ED.

Of course, the ED of a food does not tell one anything about its nutritional value. For example, foods containing healthy fats may have a high ED but should still be included in a healthy diet. Information on ED must, therefore, be taught alongside other relevant nutrition information on aspects such as healthy fats and quality carbohydrates. Nevertheless, a reduction in the ED of foods in the diet is the first way to reduce total energy input.

However, without any other changes, successful weight loss is unlikely. The next step is to reduce portion size.

Portion size

The size of a meal is obviously a relevant factor in total energy intake and it is apparent that meal sizes have increased in recent times. The size of a standard McDonald's meal in the 1950s was 75 g of fries with 200 mL of Coke—by 2001, this had become 200 g of fries with 950 mL of Coke. Neilsen and Popkin (2003), in a survey of portion sizes in meals eaten at home, in restaurants or as take-aways from 1977–1998, found that most meals, including those cooked at home, increased in size over time, some by more than 50%.

Larger meals can be eaten as part of a weight loss program if the energy density of the individual ingredients and the portion sizes of these ingredients is kept low. This is the secret of the Mediterranean diet, which is composed of low ED, high–fibre foods eaten in reasonable amounts. However, even low ED foods, if eaten in large enough amounts, can make weight control difficult. This is illustrated in the differences in the average body weight of the French, who eat relatively small but high ED meals, compared to the Americans and Australians, who tend to eat lower fat but larger meals. Portion sizes are therefore important and should ideally be reduced by choice, but they can be manipulated by behavioural factors such as the size of a meal plate (see Chapter 10).

Rolls and colleagues (2006) have found that food intake, at least in a laboratory situation, is clearly dependant on ED and portion size, as shown in Figure 8.1. Larger portion sizes (and higher ED meals) tend to be eaten in company and where food is served at restaurants and external sources. Hence, advice as to how to manage portion size and choice of meals in such settings needs to be provided.

FIGURE 8.1 Influence of energy density and portion size on food intake

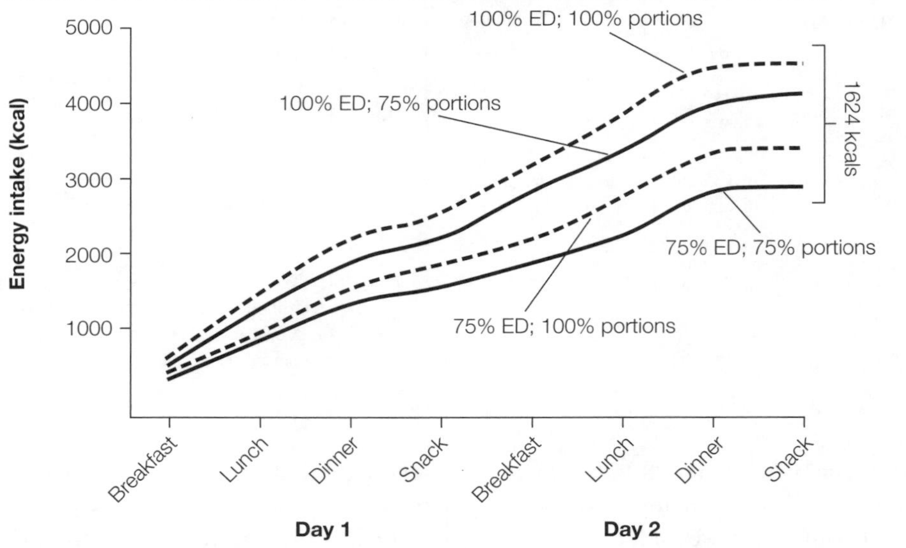

Source: Rolls et al., 2006

Eating frequency

The third factor in total energy input is the frequency of eating. Given that there is energy expenditure involved in digesting food, this can be relevant (depending on the total amount of energy consumed during the course of a day). Although controversial, some research suggests that it takes more energy for the body to digest and metabolise several small meals across the course of the day than one large meal containing the same amount of calories. Figure 8.2 provides a theoretical display of this.

FIGURE 8.2 Energy expenditure associated with food frequency

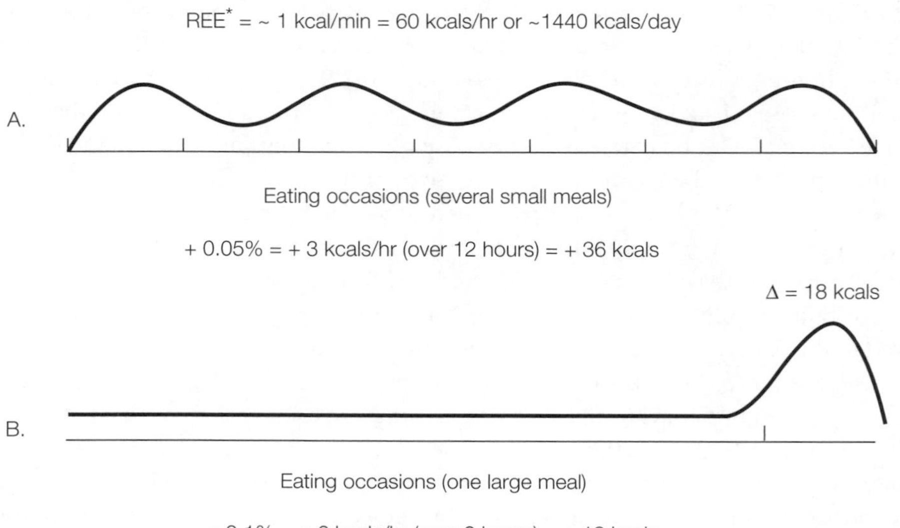

*resting energy expenditure

If average energy expenditure (EE), expressed as a resting metabolic rate of about 1 kcal (4.2 kJ) per minute in an average-sized (80 kg) person, the rate of increased EE associated with the thermogenic effect of an average meal intake has been calculated at 0.05%. If several small meals are eaten during the day, as shown in the top scale in Figure 8.2, then this would account for an extra 36 kcals/day (150 kJ). Assuming that thermogenesis increases by twice as much after a single, larger meal (0.1% metabolic rate) and that this has an effect lasting for up to three hours, the difference between graphs A and B account for about 18 kcals/day (76 kJ). It must be stressed that this is purely theoretical, but it does show the relevance of eating frequency, provided total energy intake is constant.

The important point here, however, is that increasing eating frequency only works if the total (calorific) volume of energy intake remains the same. In practice, people are accustomed to eating a certain quantity of food at each meal and advice to eat more often can simply result in eating more. People struggling with their weight usually need structured advice about their eating, with information on what to eat and how much to eat at each meal or snack. A further advantage of eating regularly is that it prevents excessive hunger that can result in overeating. A useful clinical tip here is to advise patients not go for more than about four hours without something (healthy) to eat.

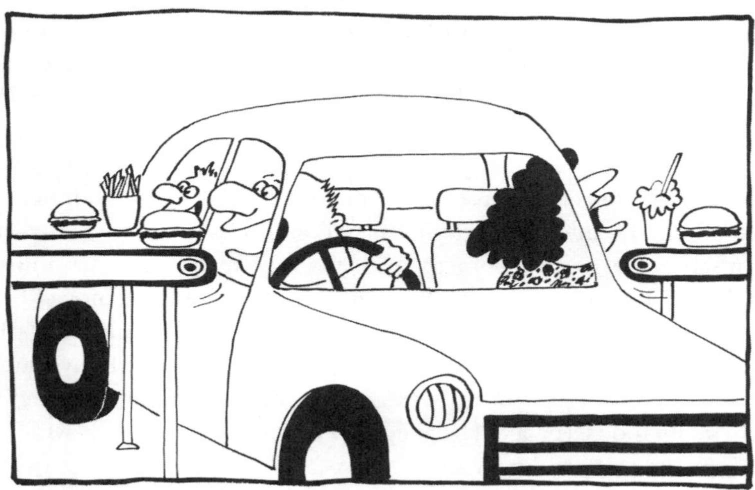

FAST FOOD – THE NEXT STEP

Recent developments in nutrient understanding

In simple terms, a 'volume' approach to nutrition suggests that foods that are low in energy density and eaten in small portion sizes, frequently, are likely to have weight control and metabolic health benefits. Within this, there is value in looking at the nutritional and metabolic components of certain nutrients.

Protein

Protein has perhaps been undervalued in nutrition in recent times because of the concentration on obesity and the influence of more obesogenic nutrients such as carbohydrate and fat. Protein and its component amino acids have an essential anabolic function in the building and replacement of muscle. Muscle, in turn, according to a recent review (Wolfe, 2006), has probably also been under-appreciated for its key role in health and disease.

Studies of hunter-gatherer humans calculate protein intakes of 19–35% of energy (Cordain et al., 2002) in Paleolithic times. This has dropped to an average of 13–15% in modern societies, largely as a result of increases in fat and carbohydrate. There is now a shift back towards increased protein intake for metabolic and obesity benefits. Increasing protein is proving to be a successful strategy for weight loss, particularly maintaining weight loss over time. This is most likely due to several key factors: protein has more than three times the thermic effect of either fat or carbohydrate; it is the most satiating macronutrient; it has a relatively low energy content (4 kcal/g or 17 kJ); and it requires considerable energy loss for storage as fat (25%). Like other nutrients, however, protein has been found to come in a wide variety of forms.

Recently, this has been dichotomised into 'fast' and 'slow' protein, where the former is digested quickly and, through action on the portal circulation, appears to send satiety signals that result in early cessation of eating (Layman and Baum, 2004). This is obviously advantageous for those looking for weight loss or maintenance, because of the reduced total energy intake likely to occur over the course of a day. The combination of 'fast' protein and calcium also appears to increase faecal energy loss, adding to the weight loss benefits. While forms of fast protein are still being tested, it appears that dairy products such as whey, with high concentrations of the amino acid leucine, are some of the best. Other potential fast proteins are seafood, soy proteins, and perhaps lean wild game meats, although this is not currently known (Westerterp-Platenga and Lejeune 2005).

While the advice to eat more protein, like our hunter-gatherer ancestors, is valid, it is not easy to do. This is because of the major differences in the modern food supply. For example, the meat from domesticated animals is far higher in total and saturated fat and lower in essential omega-3 fats than the meat from wild animals eaten in the past. Many popular commercial high protein diets are far removed from our evolutionary diet and there are major health concerns from many such plans. An increased intake of protein need not be accompanied by a low carbohydrate intake or a high fat intake. For weight control and good health, a high protein diet should also be rich in plant foods (particularly vegetables and fruit) and provide a moderate amount of quality carbohydrates and healthy fats.

Nevertheless, an increase in protein content in the diet (preferably at the expense of decreased fat and high GI carbohydrate, see below) is likely to have health and weight control benefits in the general population. An alternative way of doing this may be through meal replacements (such as those discussed in Chapter 4) where a high protein, calcium and other nutrient content can be contained in small energy packets.

Carbohydrate

Carbohydrate has also come in for its fair share of attention over the last decade or so, particularly in relation to weight control. Reducing carbohydrate intake is the basis of the Atkins Diet, one of the most popular weight-loss programs of recent years. Yet research in the late twentieth century shows that carbohydrate is far from a homogeneous nutrient. Traditionally classified into 'simple sugars' or 'complex carbohydrate' based on saccharide chain length, the assumption was it is better to consume complex carbohydrates and reduce the intake of sugars. More recent analysis shows that this classification is not useful in telling us how the carbohydrate affects us physiologically.

The Glycaemic Index (GI) has emerged as a better criterion because it measures directly the impact of foods on blood glucose. The GI is a ranking of foods on a scale of 100, using a standard measure of glucose for reference. While initially met with scepticism, particularly regarding its practical application, there is now growing evidence for a role of GI in preventing and treating diabetes, reducing the risk of cardiovascular disease and certain cancers, and weight control (McMillan-Price and Brand-Miller, 2006).

Two features of low GI foods (defined as those with a GI value ≤55) are potentially beneficial for weight control: their satiating qualities and their ability to promote fat oxidation at the expense of carbohydrate oxidation. Both of these characteristics stem from slower rates of digestion and absorption—and correspondingly lower glycaemic and insulinaemic post-prandial responses—of low GI compared to high GI foods. However, not all studies have agreed on the impact of the GI on weight loss. Part of the problem may be in knowing the GI of individual foods. While much research has gone into providing GI values, there are numerous foods yet to be tested. In general, low GI foods are those that have had less human interference or processing, although this is not always the case. Wholegrain products do not always have a low GI; for example, brown bread and the majority of breakfast cereals have a high GI. Similarly, many processed, high fat and sugar products have a low GI, but this does not mean they should be recommended. Rather, the GI is a tool to help reduce the glycaemic and insulinaemic impact of the diet. It should not be used in isolation but in accordance with other key nutrition messages.

Both the GI and the total amount of carbohydrate in a food affects the absolute blood glucose response. It has therefore been suggested that glycaemic load (GL), defined as the GI/100 × grams of carbohydrate, is more useful. However, this has limited practical utility because it is clearly dependent on the serving size of the meal. In practice, reducing the GI of carbohydrate foods in the diet is effective in reducing the overall GL of the diet.

In essence, the GI is useful as a concept and can help improve the quality of carbohydrates in the diet, but obsession with the numbers should be avoided. GI values for individual foods can be obtained from www.glycemicindex.com.

What can be done in a brief consultation

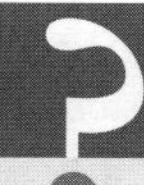

Ask patients where they see deficiencies in their current nutrition.

Provide information for completing the DAB-Q questionnaire (see *Professional resources*).

Discuss the concept of calorific volume and its components for nutrition.

Explain energy density and how to read labels for this.

Advise on the importance of breakfast and regular meals (every four hours) to prevent gorging.

Provide specific nutritional information for health risks (e.g. reduced saturated fats for lipid lowering).

Recommend a good nutrition website, such as www.healthyeating.com.au.

Fat

The biochemistry and epidemiology of fat in human health is extremely complicated, and we will confine ourselves to the three main forms of dietary fatty acids: saturated (SFA), mono-unsaturated (MUFA) and poly-unsaturated (PUFA), so named because of the relative degree of saturation of carbon atoms with hydrogen. All three are natural to food sources. Trans fatty acids are those that are created by the hydrogenation of these fats, primarily in food processing. Trans fats have been shown to be dangerous for health, are now being restricted worldwide, and will not be discussed further here.

Fat has been the 'bad guy' in nutrition for many years. Because all fats, irrespective of type, have an energy content of 9 kcals/g (38 kJ), a reduction in all forms from around 40% of dietary energy to 30% has been recommended for cardiovascular disease (CVD) prevention and weight control. As the average intake of fat in Australian men is around 110 g a day and women around 90 g a day, this means a reduction to around 80 g and 70 g respectively. However, recently it has been found that not all fats have the same health or weight control properties (Khor, 2004). SFAs have been consistently shown to have the most atherogenic properties and hence should be reduced to less than 10% of total energy in the diet. MUFAs and some PUFAs, on the other hand, have actually been shown to have protective effects against CVD.

Because of this, recommendations have moved away from the rather simplistic 'eat less fat' to more specific advice on the type of fat that is best to eat. MUFA intake should be maintained or recommended in place of SFA. MUFAs are found in olive and canola oils, many nuts and their oils including peanuts, almonds and macadamias, and in meat from wild game such as kangaroo, crocodile and in venison. PUFAs can be split into the omega-6 and omega-3 fractions and the ratio of these two types of fat seems to be important. Our hunter-gatherer ancestors ate far more omega-3 and far fewer omega-6 fats than we do today, and this is likely to have played an important role in preventing CVD (Cordain et al., 2005). The long chain omega-3 PUFAs are particularly important and are only found in oily fish (e.g. salmon, herring, mackerel, trout, tuna), or seafoods and dietary supplements made from fish liver (e.g. cod liver oil). Short chain omega-3s do not have the same beneficial effects but can be elongated in the body to some degree and are also recommended. Linseed (sometimes called flaxseed) and green leafy plant food (especially seaweeds) are the best sources. Since a high intake of the omega-6 PUFAs prevents maximum absorption and use of the omega-3s, it is important to reduce these fats at the same time to achieve the desired balance. This means fewer PUFA margarines and most seed oils, including sunflower, safflower and corn oil.

While these recommendations apply for CVD health, recent work particularly by Dr Kerin O'Dea and colleagues at Monash University has shown paradoxically that isocaloric diets high in mono-unsaturated fats compared to saturated fats can also help reduce body fat, particularly abdominal fat (Piers et al., 2003). As this goes against a law of thermodynamics, one explanation may be that energy expenditure is increased somehow on a high MUFA diet (such as the Mediterranean diet), possibly because of increased feelings of wellbeing. Alternatively, there may be differences in the absorption and utilisation of MUFA and SAFA that may explain such results. Regardless, it appears that the best recommendations on dietary fats now are:

- a reduction in total fats to 25–30% of energy in the total diet;
- a reduction in saturated fats to <10% of energy in the total diet;

- a maintenance of mono-unsaturated fats in proportion;
- a reduction of some poly-unsaturated fats, particularly seed oils; and
- an increase in omega-3 PUFAs, particularly from fish and seafood.

Salt

Modern western diets are relatively high in sodium even without the addition of extra salt. However, adding salt is often part of a meal and this brings total salt intake to well above the 154 mmol per day which has been indicated for good health. In the past, salt has been implicated as a cause of high blood pressure, but findings relating to this have been variable. More recently, it has been found that salt sensitivity tends to have a genetic component and that salt intake in some families is likely to have more of an impact on blood pressure than in others.

Only recently has salt been considered as a factor in obesity. This does not relate to its energy content but to other appetite factors in salt. Because it increases thirst, a high salt intake in children, in particular, is likely to lead to a high fluid intake. And because a large proportion of the fluid intake of children in modern western societies is in calorific form, this is likely to increase energy intake over the course of a day. Salt, whether it be sodium chloride, potassium chloride or MSG, is also known to decrease satiation of food and therefore lead to greater energy intake and increase hunger. But salt may also have an effect on the learned aspects of nutrition discussed in Chapter 10. The craving for salty foods can be learned, leading to a desire for an increase in those foods; for example, salted peanuts are craved more and are able to be eaten in much larger quantities than unsalted nuts (consuming them with alcohol adds to the total energy intake because alcohol can have a decreased inhibitory effect).

Specific dietary requirements

It is beyond the scope of this chapter to discuss dietary requirements for specific health issues; referral to a qualified dietitian is recommended. Dietary advice based on estimates of energy intake and calorie reduction is also not considered here because it is not generally necessary, except in specific cases where more skilled dietetic input may be involved.

The basic dietary advice considered above is applicable to weight control and good metabolic health in general. A generic dietary approach for weight loss and diabetes management is shown in Table 8.2, although it should be stressed that individual dietary advice may be required for the management of specific diabetes cases.

Assessing food intake

Food intake can be assessed through a number of means: skilled clinical questioning, dietary diaries or food frequency questionnaires. None are perfect because they require the recall or honesty of the patient in an area where psychological barriers can play a role.

In the first instance, if an energy imbalance has occurred through food intake, it is useful to consider *why* and *how* this may have happened. Some typical reasons why are:

- an obesogenic environment encouraging over-consumption;
- genetic influences, such as hunger and substrate utilisation;

TABLE 8.2 General dietary recommendations for weight loss and diabetes management

	Healthy normals	Diabetes	Weight loss
Total energy	Reduce to balance EE	—Reduce to cause energy deficit — (e.g. 250–500 kcals/day)	
Fat			
Saturated	Reduce to <10%	——Reduce to <10%——	
Polyunsaturated	Reduce to <10%	——Reduce to 10% or less——	
Monosaturated	Maintain or increase to >10%	10–16% if not overweight	Reduce to 10%
Carbohydrate	~50%	40–50% but reduce total amount if weight still a problem after fat reduction Increase low GI and decrease low GI carbs	
Sweeteners	Not necessary	Use if weight is still a problem after fat reduction	
Alcohol	2–4 drinks /day	——Reduce if weight is still a —— problem after fat reduction	

- medications leading to hyperphagic behaviour (see Chapter 21);
- life stages, such as adolescence, pregnancy or menopause;
- life events, such as quitting smoking or early abuse; and
- age and its influence on food consumption.

How excess energy intake occurs can be through a range of means such as:

- too much total food,
- too much fat,
- too much high energy density food,
- too much high GI food,
- binge eating/night eating/excessive dieting,
- holiday eating/social eating/feasting,
- too much alcohol/food with alcohol,
- too much soft drink,
- too little fibre,
- lack of awareness of intake,
- the 'eye–mouth gap', and
- the 'exception rule'.

The 'eye–mouth gap' refers to the finding that overweight individuals tend to underestimate their food intake (Lissner, 2002). The 'exception rule' describes a tendency in some patients to discount days of excess as exceptions, although they are quite common. Determining the factors common to an individual patient is tantamount to recommendations to correct this.

The DAB-Q (dietary, activity and behaviour questionnaire)

The advent of computers and the internet have aided dietary measurement in recent times. Several computerised dietary analyses are available, but these generally require skilled interpretation and prescription by a dietitian. One self-help assisted program for patients was developed by Egger et al. (2006): the DAB-Q (Dietary, Activity and Behaviour Questionnaire) enables patients to complete a number of questionnaires at a public website (www.professortrim.com/DAB-Q) and bring printouts to the clinician for discussion and negotiation about change. These rank items and behaviours that are frequently consumed or carried out and that are potent in causing weight gain but can reasonably be modified.

Summary

Nutrition is a relatively young science which is constantly changing in response to ongoing research. The key aspects of nutrition for metabolic health are the total volume of energy consumed and the nutrient composition mix. New findings suggest that protein, carbohydrate and fat need to be examined in terms of specific properties, such as speed of digestion, substrate utilisation and rate of metabolism. Finally, salt is a significant component of modern foods and may have an effect on weight control through its effect on overconsumption of other energy-dense fluids and foods.

PRACTICE TIPS: PROVIDING NUTRITIONAL ADVICE

	Medical practitioner	**Practice nurse**
Assess	Whether diet is a significant contributor to ill-health. Potential dietary influences on risk. Why dietary imbalance may have occurred. How dietary imbalance may have occurred.	Food intake through such processes as the DAB-Q (see *Professional resources*) or a diet diary. Impact of ED, portion size or frequency.
Assist	By treating dietary-influenced co-morbidities. By identifying general nutritional goals. By reviewing progress of drug therapy for weight loss/metabolic treatment. By reviewing ongoing special dietetic programs such as meal replacements. By using templates as appropriate.	General education about eating. By providing good nutritional literature. Monitoring food intake if possible. By using appropriate tactics to move through stages of readiness to change.
Arrange	Referral for specific dietary advice where required. List of other health professionals for a care plan.	Discussion of motivational tactics with other involved health professionals. Consultation with a dietitian/nutritionist. Contact with self-help groups.

KEY POINTS FOR CLINICAL MANAGEMENT

- Use tests such as the DAB-Q (see *Professional resources*) to quantify incorrect eating and activity patterns.
- Ascertain which aspect of food volume may be important for a particular patient.
- Teach cut-offs for energy density (at least 'high' cut-off).
- Discuss ways of reducing portion size in the patient's environment.
- Stress importance of ED and portion size together.
- Advise on frequent, low ED food intake (i.e. every four hours).
- Change nutrient proportions for weight loss.
- Suggest low GI carbohydrates for diabetes management and possibly weight control.
- Reduce saturated and some poly-unsaturated fat but maintain the proportion of mono-unsaturated fats.
- Check on salt intake and reduce if necessary.

REFERENCES

Cameron-Smith D, Egger G. (2002) *The ultimate energy guide*. Sydney: Allen and Unwin.

Civitarese AE, Carling S, Heilbron LK et al. for the CALERIE Pennington team. (2007) *PLoS Medicine* 4(3): e76 doi:10.1371/journal.pmed.0040076.

Cordain L, Boyd Eaton S, Brand-Miller J et al. (2002) The paradoxical nature of hunter-gatherer diets: meat-based, yet non-atherogenic. *Eur J Clin Nutr* 56(Suppl 1): S42–52.

Cordain L, Boyd Eaton S, Sebastian A et al. (2005) Origins and evolution of the Western diet: health implications for the 21st century. *Am J Clin Nutr* 81: 341–54.

Egger G, Pearson S, Pal S. (2006) Individualising weight loss prescription: a management tool for clinicians. *Aust Fam Phys* 35(8): 591–94.

Heilbronn LK, Ravussin E. (2005) Calorie restriction extends lifes span–but which calories. *PLoS Med* 2(8): 231.

Khor GL. (2004) Dietary fat quality: a nutritional epidemiologist's view. *Asia Pac J Clin Nutr* 13(Suppl): S22.

Layman DK, Baum JI. (2004) Dietary protein impact on glycaemic control during weight loss. *J Nutr* 134: 968S–73S.

Lissner L. (2002) Measuring food intake in studies of obesity. *Pub Hlth Nutr* 5(6A): 889–92.

McMillan-Price J, Brand-Miller J. (2006) Low-glycaemic index diets and body weight regulation. *Int J Obes* 30: S40–S46.

Morgan TE, Wong AM, Finch CE. (2007) Anti-inflammatory mechanisms of dietary restriction in slowing aging processes. *Interdiscp Top Geront* 35: 83–97.

Nieslen SJ, Popkin BM. (2003) Patterns and trends in food portion sizes. *JAMA* 289(4): 450–53.

Piers LS, Walker KZ, Stoney RM et al. (2003) Substitution of saturated with monounsaturated fat in a 4-week diet affects body weight and composition of overweight and obese men. *Br J Nutr* 90(3): 717–27.

Rolls B. (2007) *The volumetrics eating plan: Techniques and recipes for feeling full on fewer calories*. NY: Harper.

Rolls BJ, Roe LS, Meengs JS. (2006) Reductions in portion size and energy density of foods are additive and lead to sustained decreases in energy intake. *Am J Clin Nutr* 83: 11–17.

Westerterp-Plantenga MS, Lejeune PGM. (2005) Protein intake and body weight regulation. *Appetite* 45(2): 187–90

Wolfe RR. (2006) The under appreciated role of muscle in health and disease. *Am J Clin Nutr* 84: 475–82.

RECOMMENDED READING

Cardwell G. (2003) *Gold medal nutrition. Third edition*. Perth, Australia: Nutrition Impact Pty Ltd.

Ruppel Shell E. (2002) *The hungry gene. The science of fat and the future of thin*. NY: Atlantic Monthly Press.

Schlosser E. (2001) *Fast food nation*. Boston: Houghton Mifflin.

Saxelby K. (2006) *Nutrition for life*. South Yarra, Victoria: Hardie Grant Books.

Stanton R. (2002) *Good fats bad fats*. Sydney: Pub Group West.

Willett WC. (2001) *Eat, drink and be healthy*. NY: Simon and Schuster.

PROFESSIONAL RESOURCES: MEASURING NUTRITION

DAB-Q (Diet, Activity and Behaviour Questionnaire)

The Diet, Activity and Behaviour Questionnaire (DAB-Q) is a simple, free, online questionnaire to help patients determine the best way to lose weight. The DAB-Q asks about eating and activity patterns. There are five tests, covering:

- foods eaten in excess;
- foods that could be increased;
- passive activities carried out in excess;
- activities that could be increased; and
- eating behaviour.

Results are scored on frequency, weight gaining potential and changeability (i.e. the ease with which this food or activity could be changed by this patient), giving a maximum score out of 100. High scoring items are then targeted for change.

The DAB-Q is available from www.professortrim.com/DAB-Q. More information is available from Egger et al. (2006).

CHAPTER 9

Fluids, fitness and fatness

GARRY EGGER, SUZANNE PEARSON

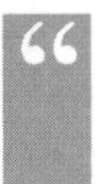

Let them drink Coke.

VARIATION ON A THEME FROM A MODERN MARIE ANTOINETTE

Introduction

During the early stages of the obesity epidemic in the 1980s and '90s, having excess fat was attributed to eating excess fat. This made sense, because it was well known that dietary fat is twice as energy dense as carbohydrate or protein in physical terms and possibly even more in biological terms (i.e. less energy is required to store fat as fat than to store carbohydrate or protein as fat). Hence, reducing fat, for most people, would result in a reduction of total energy intake and a decrease in body weight. However, this diverted our attention away from high-energy containing beverages. As a result, soft-drink manufacturers were emboldened when marketing their products.

As indicated in Chapter 8, it has become clear that fat, alone, is not solely responsible for the obesity epidemic. It is the energy density of foods and beverages, together with portion size and frequency of consumption, that tends to increase total energy intake and, in the absence of a high-energy output, contribute to the growing waistlines of the population. This applies to the calories in each millilitre of drink as much as to the calories per gram of food. In fact, it could be more so with beverages, because of the likelihood of 'passive over-consumption' of fluid energy, due to its non-satiating effect. This is compounded by the fact that soft-drink varieties and consumption have doubled over the last twenty years and constitute more than 50% of the increase in energy intake since the 1970s (Popkin et al., 2006). The spotlight has thus turned on the obesogenic and other health effects of beverages, as well as foods.

In this chapter, we look at some of the different types of beverages now available and the effects of these, mainly on energy intake but also on other aspects of health.

As with other chapters, we focus only on fluids for general health. We do not look at fluid needs for specific diseases, such as heart failure or renal insufficiency, or specific purposes, such as endurance sports.

How much fluid is required?

A common misconception is that humans require eight glasses of water, each with eight ounces of fluid (227.2 mL), every day for survival and good health. In a considered review of this, Valtin (2002) found no scientific basis for this suggestion. Fluid requirements have a wide number of influences, including age, size, activity level and temperature, so a generic prescription is of little value. While eight glasses of water may be adequate for an individual of middle age and average size in a temperate climate, the same may not be true for an active older adult in a hot climate or an inactive adolescent in a cool but moist climate. In general, it is believed that a range of fluid intake of about 1–4 L a day is required (Popkin et al., 2006). The average intake in the U.S. in 1998 was 2.18 L. This represents an increase of approximately 30% from the mid-1970s, largely as a result of increases in the consumption of bottled water, soft drinks (doubled), alcoholic beverages and juices (2.5-fold) (Valtin, 2002).

It is important to remember that fluid is obtained from many different sources. In addition to water, tea, coffee and other beverages, fluid is a component of most foods, especially fruits and vegetables. Hence, the volume of fluid consumed as beverages does not necessarily reflect the total daily fluid intake. Furthermore, water is produced in the body as a 'waste product' during the breakdown of nutrients.

In general, fluid requirements are well controlled by thirst in a natural environment (Kleiner, 1999). Though low-level dehydration is not uncommon in many older people (defined as a >2% decrease in body fluid), over-hydration is difficult to achieve in healthy people. Consequently, a recommendation to maintain fluid intake is unlikely to be deleterious. It is therefore the *type* of fluid that is most relevant for health and energy intake.

How much energy in fluid is recommended?

A healthy diet does not require fluids to contain energy or nutrients—potable water is adequate to provide all the fluid needs of humans. As explained in Chapter 8, energy density is a prime determinant influencing daily energy balance. As the energy in fluids can be passively over-consumed, excessive intake is of great concern for preventing weight gain and associated problems. The energy density of beverages and their intake recommendations are shown in Table 9.1.

Recommended fluid intakes

Currently, about 20% of the total dietary energy intake in countries such as the U.S. and Australia is derived from beverages. As a general guideline, it is recommended this figure be reduced to around 10%. Current and recommended levels of six different categories of fluids designed to get to this level are shown in Figure 9.1. These are based

TABLE 9.1 Recommended energy-density cut-offs for fluids (beverages are categorised here by energy-density alone, not on nutrient content or nutritional value)

Energy density	Measure	Recommendation	Examples
low	<1 kJ (0.2 kcal)/mL	drink freely	water tea/coffee low calorie soft drinks/cordials some iced teas skim milk vegetable juice
medium	1 kJ (0.2 kcal)/mL–1.49 kJ (0.3 kcal)/mL	drink sparingly	low fat milk (unflavoured) some sports drinks alcohol (with provisos) some iced teas
high	>1.5 kJ (0.4 kcal)/mL	drink occasionally (if at all)	sweetened soft drinks fruit juice full cream milk kids 'energy' drinks sports drinks flavoured milk

Source: Cameron Smith and Egger, 2002.

on the findings of a Beverage Guidance Panel (Popkin et al., 2006) formed in the U.S. While some criticism of these guidelines has been made (Weaver et al., 2006), the suggestions given below provide a broad outline of recommended fluid requirements.

Suggested changes in beverage intakes

BEVERAGES THAT CAN BE INCREASED OR MAINTAINED

Level 1—Water should be increased from about 40% to at least 50% of total fluid intake (or to 2–16 glasses a day depending on factors such as age and climate).

Water is and always has been the staple fluid. Historically, it has been consumed from the source of catchment, with variations in mineral quality depending on run-off surfaces and other geographical conditions. To cater for larger populations in more recent times, water has been stored and maintained over longer period with additives (such as fluoride in some areas as a public health measure to prevent dental decay). Other minerals are also often found in water, including calcium, magnesium and numerous trace elements.

Water is becoming a scarce commodity in some parts of the world, including southern, eastern and western Australia, and this has led to an increased mineralisation of the water supply in these areas. The increased calcification (hardness) of water, which is natural in these areas, has been shown to have a protective effect for cardiovascular disease. However, increased salination, which results from a rising of the water table in some areas, can have adverse effects on blood pressure in some people.

Commercially sold bottled water has become popular in recent times, satisfying consumer anxieties about increasing contamination of water supplies. The lack of fluoride in bottled water helps alleviate worries about added fluoride. This, however, now means that bottled water may lack the protection against dental decay that comes from fluoride. In most areas of the developed world, transport and production of

FIGURE 9.1 Current and recommended fluid intakes

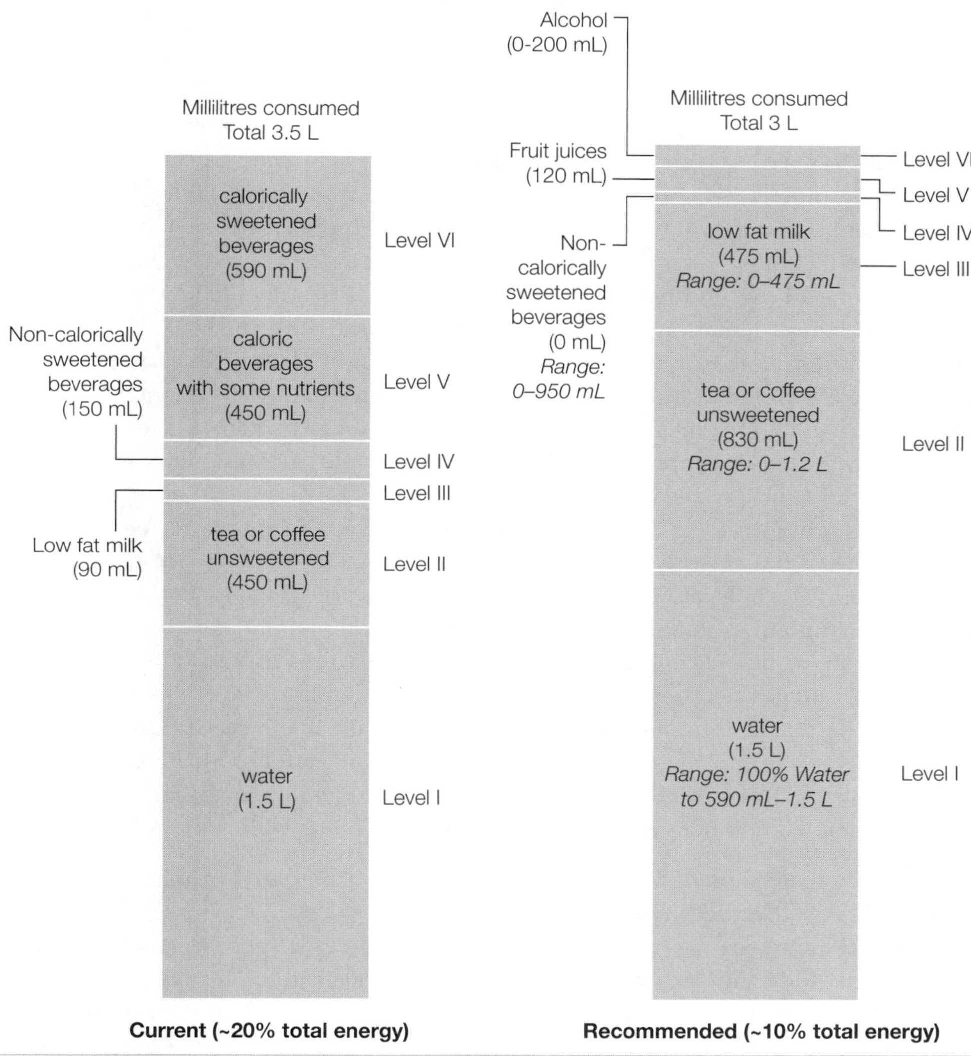

Source: Popkin et al., 2006

bottled water is a waste of natural resources, and this water does not provide any additional health benefits.

Level 2—Tea/coffee can be increased from 13% to about 30% of total fluid intake, or up to 6–8 cups/day.

There is an inverse link between tea consumption and heart disease, with both green and black tea having health benefits, particularly in the prevention of cardiovascular disease. A moderate consumption of coffee has also been shown to have health benefits, particularly in the prevention of type 2 diabetes (Greenberg et al., 2006), although it is not clear whether this is due to components in the coffee or to weight loss, which may also be a minor benefit of coffee consumption. Whether the benefits are related to caffeine in coffee or other components is also not clear, given that decaffeinated coffee has also been shown to have health and weight loss benefits. Caffeinated drinks without added sugar (i.e. artificially sweetened cola drinks) or fat (i.e. low fat milk added to coffee/tea) have a zero or very low energy content and therefore add little or nothing to total energy balance. Teas or coffees made with whole milk or cream, however, lose the low energy advantage.

The limitation of tea/coffee consumption seems to be in the level of caffeine consumed, which may adversely affect some people. A limit of 400 mg of caffeine a day for most people (about 3–4 cups of strong coffee or 6–8 of tea) and 300 mg in pregnant women has been suggested. As an indication of caffeine quantity, a standard cup of brewed coffee contains around 150 mg caffeine, a cup of tea around 80 mg and a glass of cola about 40 mg. 'Caffeinism'—which is characterised by anxiety, nervousness, sleep disturbance, irritability, agitation and gastrointestinal disturbances, and which can cause withdrawal symptoms such as headache and irritability—can result from high doses of caffeine, the level of which may be individually determined. A daily intake level of about 1000 mg (1 g) of caffeine is thought to be a cut-off for this. Withdrawal from caffeine, where this may be contraindicated (such as in anxiety), can be achieved gradually to reduce any withdrawal effects, which disappear within a few days.

Recent studies show a genetic interaction with caffeine metabolism. A gene identified as CYP1A2 has been implicated in adverse effects of caffeine consumption for heart disease (Cornelis et al., 2006). While not necessarily related, about 50% of the population respond to caffeine intake with increased sympathetic nervous system activity (for example, an ability to sleep after drinking coffee) that others do not appear to be affected (and can sleep soundly after caffeine). The implications of this are not clear, but it may be that the thermogetic, lipolytic and metabolic effects of caffeine may be greater in some people than in others, explaining why caffeine intake can facilitate moderate weight loss in some people. Regardless, low energetic caffeinated drinks can be recommended in moderation in most people without a health risk.

Level 3—Low fat/skim milk and soy beverages can be increased from 3% to approximately 15% of total fluid intake, or 1–1.5 full glasses a day.

Dairy products have had a mixed press over recent years, largely because of the high levels of saturated fat in dairy products from domesticated cattle. The dairy industry has been quick to correct this through technological advances that allow the production of most dairy products at different levels of fat content. This has reduced the energy content while maintaining the nutritional value of dairy foods.

Low fat dairy is a particularly good source of calcium and vitamin D. Because whey, the main protein source in milk, is regarded as a 'fast' protein (see Chapter 8), it may have value in increasing satiety and thus assisting weight loss. Another mechanism for weight loss through dairy products may be the combination of whey protein and calcium, which has been shown to increase faecal energy loss (Lorenzen et al., 2007). The weight loss benefits of low fat dairy products have been verified in several, but not all, recent studies on dairy products and weight loss. Dairy product intake has also been found to be inversely related to the metabolic syndrome. Soy beverages have health benefits but contain less calcium than dairy.

Level 4—Non-calorically sweetened beverages (diet drinks) currently form 4% of total intake but can be lowered to 0%, or raised to 30%, or up to 0–3 glasses a day, if replacing levels 5 and 6.

Non-calorically sweetened beverages are those that are artificially sweetened with aspartame or sucralose. 'Diet' beverages have traditionally had a slightly different taste to versions sweetened with sugars. However, new developments in food technology have allowed the molecular restructuring of artificial sweetener molecules to provide a much more similar taste.

While there are no real health benefits from consuming such drinks, their use as a 'treat' or as an alternative to high energy and sweetened drinks is likely to continue, so these would be recommended over other caloric beverages. Widely published scare campaigns regarding the use of artificial sweeteners are not supported in the scientific literature, although there are known effects on dental caries if they are consumed regularly and in large quantities (see Chapter 19). The artificial sweeteners used may also increase a desire for sweet foods, although this is currently unproven.

BEVERAGES THAT SHOULD BE REDUCED AND/OR DRUNK SPARINGLY

Level 5—Caloric beverages with some nutrients should be decreased to less than 3% of total fluid intake, or 1 glass or less, a day.

Caloric beverages with some nutrients include fruit juices, milk and alcohol. Fruit juices do provide some of the nutrients of their natural source, but their high concentration of fruit sugars contributes to their having an energy density equivalent to that of sweetened soft drinks. According to Popkin et al. (2006), 'There is no specific need to consume fruit juice and consumption of whole fruits should be encouraged for satiety and energy balance.' Fruit 'smoothies' and drinks from the new type of 'juice bars' are usually high calorie versions of fruit drinks and are therefore also not recommended.

Vegetable juices are generally lower in energy than fruit juices and so are better than fruit juices in terms of energy balance. However, processed vegetable juices can have high levels of added sodium, making consumption of whole vegetables preferred. Whole milk is both energy dense and high in saturated fat. Sports drinks usually contain about 50–90% of the energy of sweetened drinks but (sometimes) contain some minerals that are advantageous for endurance events. The high energy content of most sports drinks, however, suggests they should be used sparingly.

Alcohol is also energy dense, but the biological value of this energy is not as clear as with other drinks. Alcohol may have some other health benefits, which will be discussed in greater detail below.

Level 6—Calorically sweetened beverages should be decreased to less than 3% of total energy, or 0–1 glass/day.

Sweetened soft drinks are those least recommended for beverage intake because they add a high-energy burden, have a low nutrient value, can be passively over-consumed, and may contribute to other deleterious health concerns (e.g. dental caries; see Chapter 21). While consumption of these fluids is likely to remain high in some communities, soft-drink manufacturers including Coca Cola and Pepsico are aware that this is a diminishing overall market. At least 40% of their total markets in 2007 came from low energy drinks or water, and market growth in these products far exceeds that of sweetened beverages.

Unlike water, where intake is finely regulated by thirst, sweetened beverages can be craved and consumed in the absence of thirst. Conditioned learning can be the cause of this (see Chapter 10), such that people who drink soft drinks when thirsty tend to then crave their sweet taste rather than water in subsequent thirsty states. Encouraging the drinking only of water when thirsty may help de-condition this learned process; if sweetened drinks have to be taken, they can be used as a treat when people are not thirsty.

Although not the case in Australia, fructose from corn syrup is used to sweeten soft drinks in some parts of the world, including the U.S. This not only has the effect of increasing energy density (as with sucrose) but could have an even greater role in obesity through the special effects of fructose on the metabolism of fat in the liver. Spanish scientists have shown that when fructose affects a specific nuclear receptor (PPAR-alpha), the liver's ability to degrade the sweetener is decreased, leading to even greater fat deposition (Roglans et al., 2007).

Soft drinks can also have a corrosive effect on teeth. However, in a novel study examining to what extent this occurs, researchers measured the weight of enamel lost with various types of soft drinks (Jain et al., 2007). This showed that non-cola soft drinks are more corrosive than cola drinks but that, within cola drinks, the full sugared versions are more corrosive than the diet versions, supporting even further the use of non-sweetened soft drinks if these have to be consumed. There appears to be no health justification in recommending any level of calorically sweetened beverages as part of a normal diet.

What can be done in a brief consultation

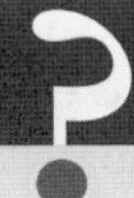

Check on soft drink, fruit juice and cordial consumption.

Administer a fluids questionnaire (see *Professional resources*), if appropriate.

Explain the importance of fluid intake in energy consumption and weight gain.

Discuss when and how much alcohol is consumed.

Discuss the high-energy value of fruit juice, full cream milk, and sports drinks.

Provide a hand-out on fluids and health, such as the one shown in Figure 9.1.

Recommend a good nutrition website, such as www.healthyeating.com.au.

Alcohol

Alcohol is obtained from the fermentation of carbohydrate from a variety of plant sources. In energetic terms, alcohol is measured in a bomb calorimeter as containing 7 kcals (31 kJ) per gram. However, due to the complex metabolism of alcohol, it is controversial as to whether, when and how this 'physical' energy is utilised biologically.

There are three biochemical cycles for the metabolism of alcohol, none of which result in its conversion to fat or other nutrients, but all of which involve conversion to energy in some form. As a toxin, alcohol has priority in the energy cycle and will displace other nutrient sources. Hence, foods high in energy density will be 'spared' if consumed with alcohol, meaning that the 'beer gut' in men is probably more of a beer-and-peanuts or beer-and-chips gut than a beer gut per se. The

MEOS (myethylated oxygenated system) of alcohol metabolism in the liver results in a greater futile cycle of energy wastage from alcohol in big, regular drinkers, but losses of alcohol from heat, urine, breath and sweat may also reduce the biological value of alcohol energy, even in casual drinkers. Epidemiological studies consistently show an inverse association between alcohol consumption and weight gain, which would tend to support this. A further possible effect of alcohol on weight gain is through stimulating appetite. However, a review of studies carried out in this area also indicates this is not the case (Gee, 2006). Hence, the inconsistent biochemical and clinical evidence and the possibility of intra-individual differences mean a firm conclusion on alcohol and weight gain cannot yet be drawn (Mattes, 2005).

While the metabolic value of alcohol is disputed, there is no dispute about the energetic value of alcoholic mixes. Mixes made with sweetened soft drinks, fruit juice or full cream dairy products provide the energy of the mix as well as some of the energy from the alcohol itself. Because alcohol is metabolised differently, however, the level of fermentation of a carbohydrate source (and thus the alcohol content) may influence the energetic value of a drink. Consequently, a low carbohydrate beer may contain less metabolisable energy, although greater alcohol, than a high carbohydrate version.

Alcohol also has been shown to have health benefits for atherogenesis and the prevention of cardiovascular disease and type 2 diabetes when consumed in moderation. It has been proposed that this is due in part to the antioxidants contained in alcohol (Tolstrup et al., 2006). Red wine, in particular, has been suggested as a high source of a polyphenol antioxidant called resveratrol, which has been found to have health benefits in humans, particularly in raising HDL cholesterol levels, as well as delaying the ageing process in mice sustained on a 'junk food' diet (Sinclair and Guarente, 2006). However, comparisons between French drinkers of red wine and Irish drinkers of anything (Marques-Vidal et al., 1996) suggest that all alcohol may have a protective effect.

All this means that alcohol may need to be considered differently to other beverages. There are apparent health advantages from its consumption in moderation but also potential risks (see Table 9.2). There are also quite obvious social disadvantages from alcohol abuse. Overall, this suggests caution in the recommended use of alcohol. The World Health Organization guidelines of a maximum of four standard alcoholic drinks a day for males and two for females, with 1–2 alcohol-free days, are a good basis for recommendations until further evidence is forthcoming.

TABLE 9.2 Health advantages and disadvantages of alcohol consumption

Advantages (moderate consumption): decreased	Disadvantages (high consumption): increased
mortality	birth defects
heart disease	breast cancer
stroke	cirrhosis
kidney disease	hypertension
type 2 diabetes	atrial fibrillation

Summary

Fluids provide a significant contribution to total energy intake and need to be carefully considered and managed in any lifestyle-based program. The general prescription of eight glasses of fluid a day is not scientifically supported and individual needs are likely to vary widely. However a rough guide for fluid intake is around 1–4 L a day, mainly from water, tea and coffee, and low fat dairy and soy. Alcohol has some health benefits in moderation but also considerable social and other disadvantages when over-consumed.

practice tips

PRACTICE TIPS: FLUID INTAKE

	Medical practitioner	Practice nurse
Assess	Fluid intake, not just alcohol. Whether fluids are used compulsively. The role of fluids in weight control for this patient. Dental health if using bottled water.	Fluid intake (see *Professional resources*). Habitual use of energy-rich fluids (i.e. if drunk when thirsty). Need for changes in fluid intake for this patient. Alcohol intake (see Chapter 15). Drink mixes with alcohol. Body fluid with a BIA measure if available.
Assist	Cutting back on high energy fluids. Appropriate alcohol use. Eliminating fluids such as fruit juice and choosing appropriate alternatives with artificial sweeteners if needed for tea/coffee.	Modification of fluid intake for weight control. De-conditioning of habitual drinking of sweetened fluids. By developing a strategy for putting this into action. Education about alternatives to fruit juice. Access to artificial sweetener samples. Meeting fluid needs (1–4 L/day) after determining fluid needs by patient parameters (e.g. age, sex).
Arrange	Referral to a dietitian if necessary. Referral to a practice nurse for de-conditioning and education if appropriate.	Consultation with a dietitian with knowledge of fluids. Care plan if necessary. Contact with and coordination of other health professionals.

key points

KEY POINTS FOR CLINICAL MANAGEMENT

- Do not ignore beverage energy intake when discussing weight control.
- Aim to reduce total energy intake from beverages to less than 10% of total energy.
- Discuss fluid energy requirements and the specific needs of specific patients.
- Encourage use of low energy drinks (preferably water).
- Get patients to recognise thirst as a healthy control mechanism.
- With young patients, in particular, recommend drinking water when thirsty and drinking other drinks as a treat, if necessary, but not to quench thirst.
- Teach patients how to read drink labels to recognise (and avoid) high energy-dense cut-offs.

REFERENCES

Cameron-Smith D, Egger G. (2002) *The ultimate energy guide*. Sydney: Allen and Unwin.

Cornelis MC, El-Sohemy A, Kabagambe EK et al. (2006) Coffee, CYP1A2 genotype, and risk of myocardial infarction. *JAMA* 295: 11135–41.

Gee C. (2006) Does alcohol stimulate appetite and energy intake. *Br J Community Nurs* 11(7): 298–302.

Greenberg JA, Boozer CN, Geliebter A. (2006) Coffee, diabetes and weigh control. *Am J Clin Nutr* 84: 682–93.

Jain P, Nihill P, Sobkowski J, Agustin MZ. (2007) Commercial soft drinks: pH and in vitro dissolution of enamel. *Gen Dent* 55(2): 150–54.

Kleiner SM. (1999) Water: an essential but overlooked element. *J Am Diet Assoc* 99(2): 200–06.

Lorenzen JK, Nielsen S, Holst JJ et al. (2007) Effect of dairy calcium or supplementary calcium intake on postprandial fat metabolism, appetite and subsequent energy intake. *Am J Clin Nutr* 85: 678–87.

Marques-Vidal P, Ducimetiere P, Evans A et al. (1996) Alcohol consumption and myocardial infarction: a case-control study in France and Northern Ireland. *Am J Epidem* 143: 1089–93.

Mattes RD. (2005) Alcohol, energy balance and obesity. In Mela DJ (ed) *Food, diet and obesity,* pp. 264–80. Cambridge: Woodhead Publishing Ltd.

Popkin B, Armstrong LE, Bray GM et al. (2006) A new proposed guidance system for beverage consumption in the United States. *Am J Clin Nutr* 83: 529–42.

Roglans N, Vila L, Farre M et al. (2007) Impairment of hepatic Stat-3 activation and reduction of PPAR-alpha activity in fructose-fed rats. *Hepatology* 45(3): 778–88.

Sinclair DA, Guarente L. (2006) Unlocking the secret of longevity genes. *Sci Am* 294(3): 48–51.

Tolstrup J, Jensen MK, Tjønneland A, Overvad K, Mukamal KJ, Grønbæk M. (2006) Prospective study of alcohol drinking patterns and coronary heart disease in women and men. *BMJ* 332: 1244–48.

Valtin H. (2002) 'Drink at least eight glasses of water a day.' Really? Is there scientific evidence for '8 × 8'? *Am J Physiol Regul & Integ Comp Physiol* 283: R993–R1004

Weaver C, Lupton J, King J et al. (2006) Dietary guidelines vs beverage guidance system. *Am J Clin Nutr* 84(5): 1245–46; 1246–48.

PROFESSIONAL RESOURCES: MEASURING FLUID INTAKE

Questions	Points				
	4	3	2	1	0
Alcohol					
1. How often do you drink alcohol?	every day	4–5 days a week	2–3 days a week	1–2 days a week	never
2. When you do drink alcohol, how much do you usually drink? (One standard drink is one middie of beer, one nip of spirits or one glass of wine)	more than 10 drinks	5–10 drinks	2–4 drinks	1–2 drinks	don't drink alcohol
Soft drink					
1. How often do you drink soft drinks? (Don't count diet drinks.)	every day	4–5 days a week	2–3 days a week	1–2 days a week	never
2. When you do drink soft drinks (not counting diet drinks), how much do you usually drink?	more than 10 drinks	5–10 drinks	2–4 drinks	1–2 drinks	never
Fruit juice					
1. How often do you drink fruit juices?	every day	4–5 days a week	2–3 days a week	1–2 days a week	never
2. When you do drink fruit juices, how much do you usually drink?	more than 10 drinks	5–10 drinks	2–4 drinks	1–2 drinks	don't drink fruit juices
Milk					
1. How often do you full cream milk?	every day	4–5 days a week	2–3 days a week	1–2 days a week	never
2. When you do drink full cream milk, how much do you usually drink?	more than 10 drinks	5–10 drinks	2–4 drinks	1–2 drinks	don't drink full cream milk

Scoring: Within each drink category (alcohol, soft drink, fruit juice, milk), add the score for questions 1 and 2.

Interpreting your score:

- 1 or less on any combination—drinks are not an influence on your weight
- 1–5 on any combination—drinks could be a problem
- 5+ on any combination—drinks are definitely a problem

All the drinks mentioned here can add to energy intake and hence body weight. Consequently, reducing the drink or amount drunk will help weight loss.

CHAPTER 10

Behavioural aspects of nutrition

NEIL KING, GARRY EGGER

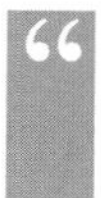

No matter how clearly one states the principles of self-help, people often misunderstand or distort them.

ELLIS AND HARPER, 1975

Introduction

In a laboratory at the University College London in 1999, health researchers fed free chocolate twice a day for two weeks to a handful of student volunteers (Gibson and Desmond, 1999), not necessarily because they liked the students, but to show that eating is not just related to biological hunger but also influenced by psychology and learning.

The researchers took a group of people identified as chocolate 'cravers' and a second group who could either 'take it or leave it'. They split the groups again and trained them by feeding them chocolate twice a day either when they were hungry (i.e. two hours after their last meal) or after they had just eaten. After two weeks, everyone was asked to rate their cravings when they were hungry or on another day, when they were full. Cravers and non-cravers who ate chocolate exclusively when hungry increased their chocolate craving post-training but, at least for the cravers, only when ratings were made while they were hungry. For those trained when they were full, chocolate craving decreased post-training, but this decrease did not depend on whether the subjects were currently hungry or full.

As complicated as this may sound, it simply suggests that cravings for chocolate or other foods may be an expression of a strong appetite or a *learned desire* for that food, elicited by hunger and acquired by repeatedly eating the craved food when hungry. In other words, eat a highly palatable and desirable food (e.g. chocolate) when you are hungry, and hunger will come to be associated (i.e. conditioned) with that food. Similarly, drinking sweetened soft drink when you are thirsty could lead to thirst being associated with a desire for sweetened soft drink, rather than water.

The implications of this are that eating and exercise behaviours are often learned or acquired. In most individuals, eating behaviour (e.g. food preference, meal pattern, eating frequency) has been established over many years and is therefore resistant to short-term changes. Of course, it is possible that they can be unlearned through such techniques as self-monitoring, stimulus control, problem solving, contingency management, cognitive re-structuring, social support and stress management (Wadden and Clark, 2005). However, it is important to recognise that eating behaviour is embedded in one's behavioural lifestyle—it will be difficult to change overnight. In this chapter, we look at the influence of learning on eating behaviour, as well as the influence of other factors such as mood states and eating context, and how these can all be managed in the clinical situation.

Hunger and appetite: are they the same?

In the scientific literature and general conversation, the terms 'hunger' and 'appetite' are often used synonymously. This is also the case in a typical medical dictionary. However, intuitively there seems to be a difference. Appetite is a generic term, which encompasses a range of factors associated with eating. Hunger is a more specific term, usually associated with the biological drive or motivation to eat; hence, it is representative of a state. As defined in the *Macquarie Dictionary*, hunger is 'the painful sensation or state of exhaustion caused by need of food' whereas appetite is 'an innate or acquired demand or propensity to satisfy a "want"'.

The distinction between *need* and *want* is important. Hunger is genuinely physiological and is based on a biological need, which cannot be willed away, which increases with the passage of time during food deprivation, and which alternative distractions cannot reduce. Only in extreme cases (e.g. anorexia nervosa, hunger strikers) is it possible to override the intense, nagging pain of hunger. Therefore, hunger is associated with homeostasis and reflects the state of energy needs (Blundell and Finlayson, 2004). 'Want' could be described more as a reflection of desire and may be uncoupled with the need to eat. More recently, the terms 'liking' and 'wanting' have been used to differentiate between the hedonic and homeostatic association with food intake (Berridge, 2004; Mela, 2006). Liking and wanting have been defined as *affective* and *motivational* factors of food intake respectively (Finlayson et al., 2007).

Hunger is of genuine concern in an environment where over-consumption can lead to energy imbalance and obesity, especially when we know that individuals eat in the absence of hunger or satiety cues (e.g. buying a pastry when passing a pleasant-smelling bakery or over-consuming at buffets). Therefore, hunger may be a *sufficient* but not a *necessary* cue for eating. The availability of food in the current environment encourages eating, particularly in the absence of hunger. Some ways of manipulating nutrient content to reduce (or delay) genuine hunger are discussed in Chapter 8. A list of these and other approaches is contained in Table 10.1.

TABLE 10.1 Possible ways of reducing/delaying biological hunger

Tactic	Process
Use a recognised meal replacement.	Replace meals or take before a main meal or before going out for a social meal.
Increase high-fibre, low energy-dense foods.	Increase food bulk while reducing calorific volume (e.g. by eating more fruit, vegetables, pasta, cereal).
Increase 'fast' protein.	Use, for example, whey from dairy, soy and, possibly seafood, to replace fat and high GI carbohydrate.
Distinguish between hunger and appetite.	Rate hunger on a virtual scale (see below); only eat when biologically hungry.
Select low fat venues when eating out.	Select generally low fat foods for social eating.
Eat more food earlier in the day.	Higher intake of low energy dense, high fibre foods in the morning reduces later intake and is 'burned off' more readily.
De-condition 'cravings'.	Separate stimulus and response through standard behavioural principles (see below).
Eat breakfast.	A low energy dense, high fibre breakfast reduces later food intake and helps 'kick-start' the metabolism.
Snack regularly.	Regular healthy (low energy-dense, high-fibre) snacks every four hours or so reduce chances of overeating through becoming too hungry.
Avoid salty foods and foods high in MSG.	Foods with added salt (e.g. peanuts, chips) tend to have less effect on satiation, meaning more can be eaten.
Increase spicy foods.	Taken as an entree or part of a main meal, these can increase metabolism and decrease total food intake.
Drink caffeine (for some people).	Caffeine may reduce hunger and food intake in some people, depending on their genetic-based reaction to caffeine.
Become 'friends' with a mild feeling of hunger.	Mild levels of hunger are innervating and stimulating. This should not be seen as something to always be avoided.
Use hunger suppressing medication.	Sibutramine and some SSRIs and SNRIs can have a genuine hunger suppressing effect. Phentermine can have short-term effects.

Genuine hunger is best determined by the use of a Likert scale (Figure 10.1).

FIGURE 10.1 Suggested hunger scale

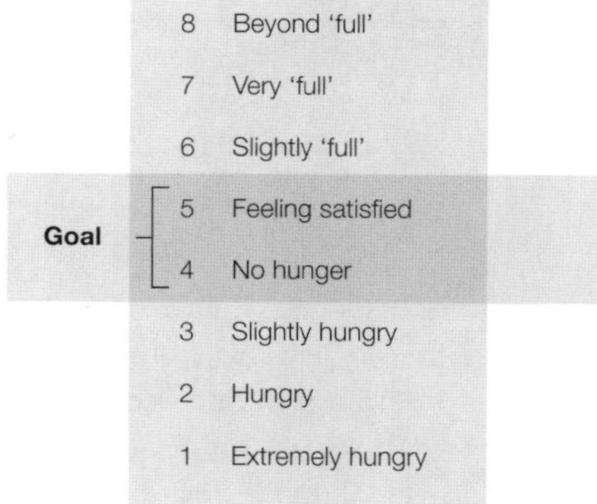

Patients should be encouraged to maintain hunger levels between three and five on the hunger scale, becoming neither too hungry nor too full. If they become too hungry, they could potentially select the wrong kinds of food to fill up on and subsequently consume more energy over the day.

Another type of drive, whether it be labelled appetite or *learned* hunger, is more psychological, is likely to diminish in intensity if one is distracted and does not necessarily increase over time. It is the identification of these two drives that enables a differentiation between the different types of drives for food and drink.

Determinants of energy intake (EI)

In animals, food seeking is primarily initiated by feelings of hunger, mediated by hormones, such as ghrelin and neuropeptide Y, originating from the gastrointestinal tract and the hypothalamus. Satiation and satiety signals also arise from the intestinal tract and, in between meals, from adipose tissue and the liver. Blundell (1990) made a clear distinction between satiation and satiety. Satiation refers to the processes involved in the termination of a meal (within meal) and satiety refers to the processes after a meal that influences the next eating episode. Satiety signals arrest the processing of food in the intestine and lead to the termination of eating. In a natural environment, hunger thus becomes a major determinant of energy intake. However, psychological factors (e.g. dietary restraint, dietary disinhibition) could also influence the onset and termination of eating episodes. The processes involved in satiation and satiety have been clearly described using the satiety cascade (Blundell, 1990). Figure 10.2 displays the various psychological and biological processes involved in satiation and satiety.

FIGURE 10.2 Satiety cascade: the temporal profile of processes involved in bringing a meal to an end (satiation) and influencing the onset of the next eating episode (satiety)

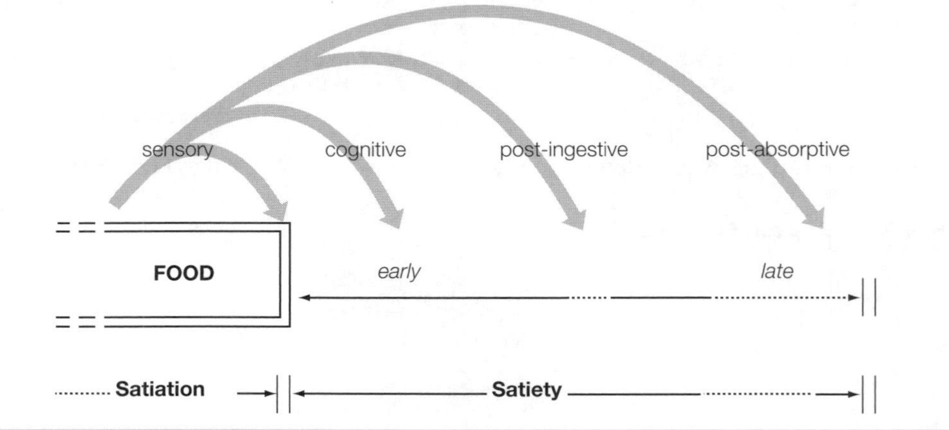

Source: Blundell, 1990

In a modern environment, hunger is just one of several factors known to be associated with EI. Some of the other factors are shown in Figure 10.3.

Some of the physical factors influencing intake shown in Figure 10.3 are discussed in Chapter 8. However, a problem with regulating food intake in the modern environment is the readily available, highly palatable and energy-dense nutrients in foods, such as sucrose and fat. This up-regulates the expression of hunger, at the same time blunting the response to satiety signals and activating the reward system, making eating as much a learned as a biological drive in the modern world. This can create habits relating to eating and drinking, some of which are due to simple conditioning (referred to here as behavioural habits) but others of which may be more complex emotionally (described here as cognitive habits).

FIGURE 10.3 Determinants of energy intake in humans

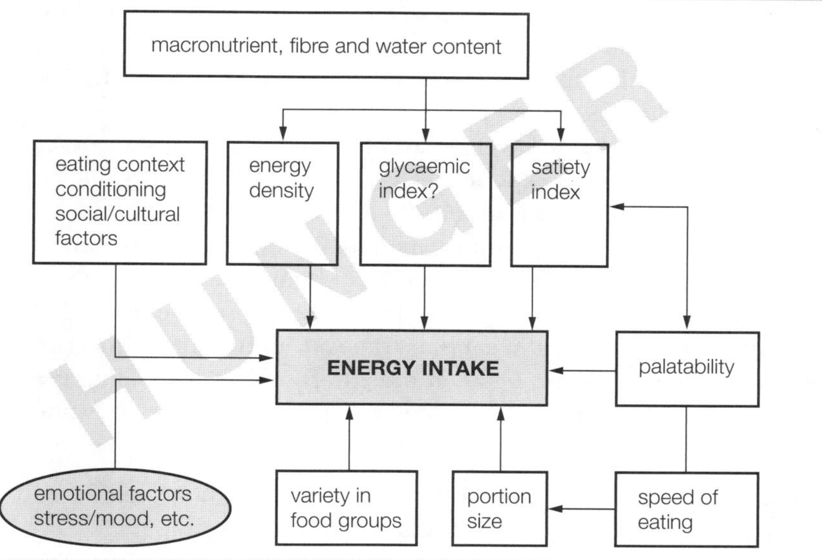

Habits

Habits are learned actions that become automatic—they are ways of responding that enable humans (and animals) to get through the day without being too distracted by repetitive actions. In the context of eating behaviours, habits can be either behavioural or cognitive. However, unlike walking, eating food (the act of putting food in the mouth) is a conscious behaviour of which individuals are usually aware. Of course, an individual may have awareness of the act of eating *per se* while remaining unaware of the mechanisms (e.g. ghrelin) that determine the expression of appetite and the pattern of eating. However, eating is a deliberate and volitional behaviour (Finlayson et al., 2007), and individuals should be made aware of this and thus control their own eating behaviours.

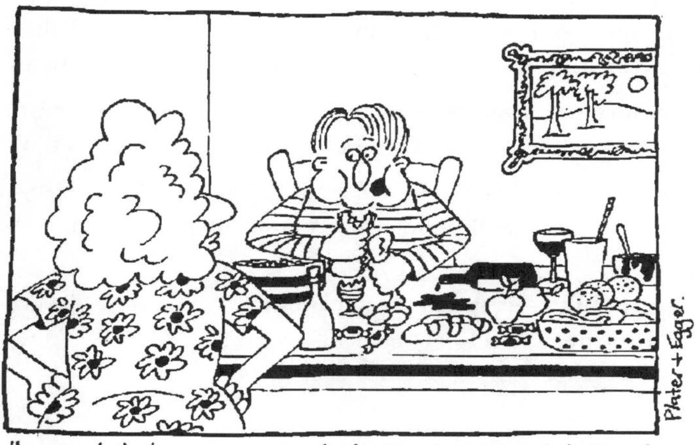

"... but this was an exception. I only ever eat this much on birthdays, public holidays, weekends and weekdays ending in a 'Y.' "

Behavioural habits

In their simplest form, habits develop as an association between a stimulus and a response. Initially, a stimulus that initiates a response is known as an unconditioned stimulus (US), resulting in an unconditioned response (UR). The stimulus is then paired with a conditioned stimulus (CS) to give a conditioned response (CR). In psychological terms this is known as classical conditioning, perhaps the best known example of which is the salivatory experiences of Pavlov's dogs, who became conditioned to the ringing of a bell (CS) such that it soon signalled food (US) and caused a salivatory response (CR) even without presentation and digestion of the meal (UR).

Similar conditioning processes can occur in human eating behaviour. An example of a typical learned response to eat in modern society, for example, would be getting up from a chair to get something to eat every time an advertisement interrupts a program on television. The association between the advertisement and eating is a surprisingly simple connection but is the kind of thing that people do every day without conscious thought. Other examples of eating behaviours that are conditioned include:

- eating at the same time every day whether hungry or not;
- reading while eating (and thus getting hungry while reading);
- always finishing everything on the plate;
- eating energy-dense, savoury snacks (e.g. peanuts, chips) with alcohol; and
- eating energy-dense, sweet snacks (e.g. cakes, biscuits) with tea or coffee.

Behavioural habits are relatively easily dealt with through behaviour modification principles. These include de-conditioning, stimulus control, self-monitoring, goal setting, cognitive restructuring and relapse prevention.

DE-CONDITIONING

This is based on the notion that eating behaviours are often conditioned by a stimulus—response connection. The first stage of recognising this is by monitoring behaviour or 'stalking the behaviour, like a hunter stalks his prey' (Tupling, 1995) through self-monitoring (see below). This can be done by keeping a diary that not only lists the foods eaten but the emotions at the time of eating. Once a conditioned behaviour (and accompanying mood states) has been identified it can then be modified by:

- **limiting exposure to the stimulus:** If having a beer leads to eating peanuts, the beer would be avoided, or limited, hence leading to 'extinction' of the response.
- **changing the response:** In the above case, an alternative response, such as eating less energy-dense foods (e.g. Japanese peas) or not eating with drinks, could be encouraged.
- **changing the stimulus—response connection:** In this case, a glass of wine might be paired with fruit to develop a new connection.

STIMULUS CONTROL

Based on the notion that environmental antecedents control behaviours, stimulus control involves changing the environments that encourage unhealthy eating. Participants in weight control programs, for example, are encouraged to increase their purchase of fruit and vegetables, wash and prepare these for easy eating, and place them prominently in the refrigerator. In contrast, unhealthy foods would be kept out of the house or in places with difficult access.

What can be done in a brief consultation

Provide a food diary to check on consequent behaviour with food/drink intake.

Check the health habits checklist provided in *Professional resources*.

Determine the importance of eating and drinking habits for particular patients.

Ask about the conditions under which special high-energy treats are consumed.

Advise not to drink sweet drinks when thirsty or eat treats when hungry.

Encourage patients to self-monitor their eating and exercise habits.

Prescribe the DAB-Q questionnaire (see Chapter 8 and www.professortrim.com/DAB-Q).

SELF-MONITORING

It is well documented that most people underestimate the amount they eat. This is even more so with the overweight (and under-reporting is also nutrient specific, that is, individuals selectively under-report the fatty foods, misrepresenting total food intake (Goris et al., 2000a). Evidence shows that even dietitians, who are trained to accurately report food intake, misreport their own food intake (Goris and Westerterp, 1999). Self-monitoring is one way of overcoming this and also providing feedback that reinforces behaviour change. This can be in the form of a diet diary, eating record or diet recall. Self-monitoring of any behaviour increases self-awareness and, in the case of unhealthy behaviours, is likely to improve that particular behaviour. This is the principle on which most commercial weight management groups work. A reduction in body weight is a likely short-term outcome of self-reporting food intake.

Because of what can be labelled the 'eye–mouth gap', there are limitations in accepting records on which to base prescription from a diet diary, given that not all foods are necessarily included. However, with the correct training and stressing the importance of compliance, self-reported food records can be a valid and reliable indicator of food intake. Indeed, evidence has shown that confronting people with their own misreported food intakes leads to improvements in the accuracy of their self-reporting (Goris and Westerterp, 2000b). Furthermore, the process of recording food intake can lead to a change in behaviour such that dietary records are not indicative of usual dietary intake. On the other hand, dietary diaries can be used to help patients ensure they are on track with their dietary intakes.

By including provision for recording mood status at the time of eating, information can also be gained about possible emotional causes of extra energy intake. An example of a self-report food diary is shown in the *Professional resources* at the end of this chapter. Generally, patients complete the date, time and detailed information about the food or drink consumed. Other methods of assessing food intake include the food frequency questionnaire, which assesses the frequency of food consumption (again, see *Professional resources*).

GOAL SETTING

Short-term, medium-term and long-term goals help provide an incentive for behaviour change. These can be process goals (such as reducing chocolate intake by one-half each week or increasing fruit to three different pieces a day) or outcome goals (such as changes in body weight or blood fats). Goals should be realistic and achievable.

COGNITIVE RESTRUCTURING

This is similar to the cognitive behaviour therapy (CBT) approaches considered in Chapter 11 and includes modifying cognitive as well as physical cues for eating, such as the sight and smell of food. Internal thoughts such as 'because I have had a bad day I deserve a treat' need to be reframed to lead to more appropriate eating behaviour. Dividing foods into good or bad, developing excuses for irrational behaviour (see below) and making comparisons with other people can all serve as negative thoughts that need to be restructured, often with the help of an experienced psychologist or counsellor.

RELAPSE PREVENTION

This involves teaching patients to anticipate the types of situations that may cause them to lapse back into poor eating habits and to plan strategies for coping with these situations. Based on principles of behaviour change, relapse should be regarded as a normal process of relearning (Marlatt and Gordon, 1985).

Some simple approaches to modifying eating behaviour are shown in Table 10.2.

TABLE 10.2 Alternative approaches to modifying eating behaviour

Cue elimination and physical environment	Manner of eating	Food choice	Alternative activities
Eat only in a designated place.	Slow the rate of eating.	Cut snacks in half.	Exercise
Eat only when sitting.	Swallow each bite before taking a second.	Measure portions.	Relaxation
Set regular eating times.	Put utensils down between bites.	Serve only the amounts pre-planned.	Meditation
Plan snacks and meals ahead.	Pause in eating.	Share desserts.	Drinking water
Rate hunger before eating.	Relax before eating.	Include favourite foods.	Imagery
Dissociate eating from other activities.	Savour foods—enjoy each bite.	Eat a variety of foods.	Tasks
Plan restaurant meals ahead.	Eat only until satisfied.	Have snacks ready.	Calling someone
Store foods in inaccessible places.	Allow time for eating.	Serve dressings 'on the side'.	Writing a letter
Store treats in opaque containers.	Leave some meal uneaten.	Use spices instead of condiments.	Re-evaluating goals
Use small plates and bowls.	Push food aside ahead of time.	Use garnishes.	Practicing assertiveness
Record food intake.	Cover food when finished.	Use low-cal substitutes.	Charting progress
Shop when not hungry.			
Use a list when shopping.			
Avoid 'problem' places and people.			
Remove plates after meal.			
Clean plates immediately.			
Write notes as reminders.			

Cognitive habits

Cognitive habits are more complex and are learned patterns of thinking, often involving emotion and including thoughts of depression, failure, worthlessness, frustration and unrealistic ideals. These can lead to cyclical ways of thinking that feed back on themselves, such as through a diet cycle as shown in Figure 10.5.

FIGURE 10.5 A vicious cycle of thinking associated with obesity

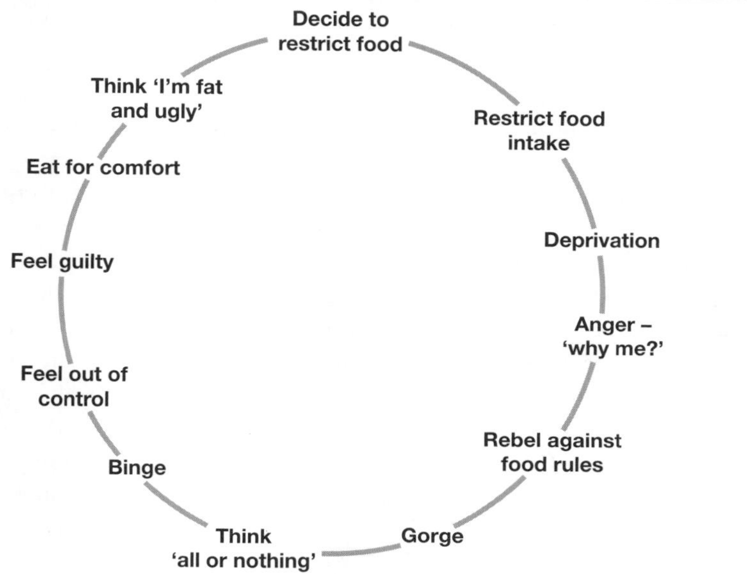

Dealing with cognitive habits often involves detailed psychological techniques, ranging from psychoanalysis to cognitive behaviour therapy, that enable the cycle of thinking shown in Figure 10.5 to be broken. Many modern psychology practitioners, however, recognise that it is *thinking* about what *may* happen as much as what *actually* has, or is about to happen, that causes many pathologies, phobias and simple unconstructive behaviours. This is not new. Indeed, there are a range of famous quotations dating back over the years to suggest this is the case (Table 10.3). Several techniques for dealing with this are covered in Chapters 12 and 13. The basics of one approach, called rational emotive therapy (RET), which forms the basis of many modern therapeutic techniques, are considered below.

TABLE 10.3 The significance of thought patterns in behaviour

We are a result of everything we have thought. Guatama Siddhartha (the Buddha, 500 BC)
People are disturbed not by things, but by the views they take of them. Epictetus, 50 AD
There's nothing either good or bad, but thinking makes it so. Shakespeare (*Hamlet*)
My life has been full of catastrophes, most of which have never happened. Mark Twain

RATIONAL EMOTIVE THERAPY (RET)

Rational emotive therapy (RET) was developed by US psychologist Albert Ellis (Ellis and Harper, 1979) to help counter the irrational beliefs that cause much minor psychopathology. RET is based around a simple format using the letters ABCD, where A = adversity, B = beliefs about that adversity (both rational and irrational), C = the consequences of beliefs about that adversity, and D = disputing of irrational beliefs about the adversity.

Ellis claimed that, 'We consciously and unconsciously choose to think and hence feel in certain self helping and self harming ways' and 'once you understand the basic irrational beliefs you create to upset yourself, you can use this understanding to explore, attack and surrender your other present and future emotional problems'. This has been picked up by others working in the area, such as Carlson (2003), who suggests that, 'being upset by your own thoughts is similar to writing yourself a nasty letter—and then being offended by that letter!'

In relation to eating behaviour, *adversity* may be a situation which breaks the pattern of healthy eating, such as a binge or overeating session. Adversity then, according to Ellis, usually takes a 'jump', leading directly to C or the consequences of this adversity. After bingeing, an overweight person might think, 'I'm useless. I can never get anything right. It could only happen to me.' However, it is the jump here from A to C that results in the form of thinking that may lead to resignation and relapse.

Weight cycling, resulting from binge eating and then dieting, is a common phenomenon with potential influences from this kind of thought process. While some degree of restrained eating to prevent weight gain may be required, there is often an irrationality of cognitive processes, instigated by unrealistic social pressures. It is the *beliefs* about this that are the real cause of much of the consequences. According to Ellis, a person's irrational beliefs are generally associated with thoughts of *musts, shoulds* and *have to's*:

- I *must* always be perfect.
- You *should* treat me well or you are an awful person.
- The world *has to* always be good to me.

Ellis also discusses ten common forms of irrational beliefs that are self-limiting in this sense and which make up the basis of RET. These, and some examples of related to weight control, are shown in Table 10.4.

TABLE 10.4 Ten common forms of irrational thinking relating to body fat maintenance

All or nothing. 'If I don't starve, I'll get fat.'
Over-generalisation. 'Things always go wrong.'
Mental filter. 'It's not the program, it's me that's wrong.'
Disqualifying the positive. 'That was just luck.'
Jumping to conclusions:
Mind reading. 'She thinks I'm useless.'
Fortune telling. 'If I did lose fat, she wouldn't like me.'
Catastrophising. 'The world will end tomorrow if I fail.'
Emotional reasoning. 'I feel so upset because I'm a failure.'
'Musturbating'. 'I must never eat anything fattening.'
Labelling. 'I'm a loser.'
The 3Ps: personal, permanent and pervasive. 'It only happens to me; I'll always be like this; It's the same with everything I do.'

Source: Egger and Swinburn, 1996

RET is a relatively simple approach to a complex problem. This, or the principles coming from it, can be applied to several aspects of behaviour, including eating and good nutrition. Psychologists skilled in this approach should be part of the referral cycle for detailed counselling on changing cognitive habits; however, other clinicians can often recognise the irrationality of beliefs relating to food and eating and their adverse effects on good nutrition.

Summary

Food and drink are not the only aspects of healthy nutrition. Much is dependent on eating behaviour. Without knowledge of this, little long-term benefit is likely to be achieved. Two significant components of eating behaviour are behavioural habits (wrong ways of doing) and cognitive habits (wrong ways of thinking). Strategies for managing eating behaviour, particularly in the presence of a plentiful food environment, are a significant component of lifestyle medicine.

PRACTICE TIPS: CHANGING EATING BEHAVIOURS

	Medical practitioner	**Practice nurse**
Assess	Whether eating behaviour is an issue. Emotional/cognitive issues involved in eating patterns. Diet record/diary. Potential eating disorders (e.g. using DAB-Q; see www.professortrim.com/DAB-Q).	Type of eating behaviour that may be an issue. Emotional/cognitive issues involved in eating patterns. Conditioned stimuli causing wrong eating. Mood factors influencing eating (from a diet diary).
Assist	Co-morbidities and treat. Understanding of eating patterns and their effect on health. In differentiating between simple habits and complex cognitive/emotional issues.	Education about eating behaviour. Development of a plan for stimulus—response control if appropriate. Patient understanding of the need for more detailed psychological help where required.
Arrange	Referral for psychological help where appropriate. Other health professionals for a care plan.	Discussion of motivational tactics with other involved health professionals. Referral to a behavioural specialist skilled in eating behaviours and/or weight control issues. Involvement with self-help groups if wanted.

key points

KEY POINTS FOR CLINICAL MANAGEMENT

- Recognise the importance of eating patterns in nutritional advice.
- Try to find and deal with the cause of emotions leading to emotional eating.
- Distinguish between wrong behavioural and wrong cognitive habits (wrong ways of acting vs. wrong ways of thinking).
- Refer to a psychologist with an understanding of eating behaviours for detailed care.
- Break stimulus—response pairing in simple conditioned eating behaviour.

references

REFERENCES

Berridge K. (2004) Motivation concepts in behavioural neuroscience. *Physiol Behav* 81: 179–209.

Blundell JE, Finlayson GS. (2004) Is susceptibility to weight gain characterised by homeostatic or hedonic risk factors for over consumption? *Physiol Behav* 82: 21–25.

Blundell JE. (1990) How culture undermines the biopsychological system of appetite control. *Appetite* 14(2): 113–15.

Carlson R. (2003) *Stop thinking. Start living 2nd edn.* London: Harper Collins.

Egger G, Swinburn B. (1996) *The fat loss leader's handbook*. Sydney: Allen and Unwin.

Ellis A, Harper RA. (1979) *A new guide to rational living*. California: Wilshire Book Company.

Finlayson GS, King NA, Blundell JE. (2007) Is it possible to dissociate 'liking' and 'wanting' for foods in humans? A novel experimental procedure. *Physiol Behav* 90: 36–42.

Finlayson GS, King NA, Blundell JE. (2007) The role of implicit wanting in relation to explicit liking and wanting for food: implications for appetite control. *Neuroscience Behav* (in press).

Gibson EL, Desmond E. (1999) Chocolate craving and hunger state: implications for the acquisition and expression of appetite and food choice. *Appetite* 32(2): 219–40.

Goris AH, Westerterp KR. (1999) Underreporting of habitual food intake is explained by undereating in highly motivated lean women. *J Nutr* 129(4): 878–82.

Goris AH, Westerterp-Plantenga MS, Westerterp KR. (2000a) Undereating and underrecording of habitual food intake in obese men: selective underreporting of fat intake. *Am J Clin Nutr* 71(1): 130–34.

Goris AH, Westerterp KR. (2000b) Improved reporting of habitual food intake after confrontation with earlier results on food reporting. *Br J Nutr* 83(4) :363–69.

Macquarie Dictionary, 3rd edn. (1997) Macquarie University: Macquarie Library Pty Ltd.

Marlatt GA, Gordon JR. (1985) *Relapse prevention: maintenance strategies in addictive behaviour change*. Guilford: NY.

Mela DJ. (2006) Eating for pleasure or just wanting to eat? Reconsidering sensory hedonic responses as a driver of obesity. *Appetite* 47: 10–17.

Tupling H. (1995) *A weight off your mind.* Sydney: Allen and Unwin.

Wadden T, Clark VL. Behavioral treatment of obesity: achievements and challenges. In Kopleman PG, Caterson ID, Dietz WH (eds). (2005) *Clinical obesity in adults and children*. Oxford: Blackwell Publishing.

PROFESSIONAL RESOURCES: MEASURING EATING BEHAVIOUR

DAB-Q for measuring food/drink intake and eating habits

See Chapter 8 *Professional resources* and www.professortrim.com/DAB-Q.

Example of a food diary

Breakfast

Time	Food/Drink	Portion/serve size	Description of cooking method

FIGURE 10.6 An example of a food frequency questionnaire

How often do you eat the following foods?	2 or more times a day	Every day	3–5 times a week	1-2 times a week	1-3 times a month	Rarely	Never
White bread	☐	☐	☐	☐	☐	☐	☐
Brown/granary bread	☐	☐	☐	☐	☐	☐	☐
Wholemeal bread	☐	☐	☐	☐	☐	☐	☐
Sweet biscuits	☐	☐	☐	☐	☐	☐	☐
Crackers/ crispbread	☐	☐	☐	☐	☐	☐	☐
Cakes, buns, pastries	☐	☐	☐	☐	☐	☐	☐
Etc.							

CHAPTER 11

Stress: its role in the S-AD phenomenon

GARRY EGGER, ROBERT REZNIK

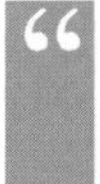

The term 'stress' has simply come to mean so much that it actually means very little in real terms.

DR ALBERT CRUM, 2000

Introduction

Although they are quite often discussed independently, there are clear links, overlaps, and confusion, between the process of *stress* and the states of *anxiety* and *depression* and their effects on human psychology and health. The connection is so close, at least in the public mind, that the urge to label them under the single acronym 'SAD' is compelling. However, we have resisted this because of the need to differentiate the distinct operational differences between these terms as they are used in lifestyle medicine. Instead, we use the broken acronym S-AD in the following three chapters. This also avoids confusion with seasonal affective disorder, associated with obesity and depression during winter.

The confusion results partly from a problem of semantics. While anxiety and depression are outcome terms, stress is more often used as a process term, reflecting a possible cause of the former (according to the *Macquarie Dictionary,* stress is 'the forces on a body which produce a deformation or strain'). In common parlance, people talk about being stressed as if it represents a medical condition, whereas the condition is actually the outcome of the stress, manifest in many different forms. According to American neuropsychiatrist Dr Albert Crum (2000), 'If we accept the dictionary definition, then stress is both a cause . . . and effect. . . The cause can be viewed as a good thing—a challenge or a push to do better—while the effect is not so good—a distress that may be felt as a momentary nervousness and free floating anxiety, or stark, paralysing fear.'

In like vein, Australian psychiatrist William Wilke (1990) suggests the term stress is increasingly misused as a synonym for distress, confusing both the response and the cause of nervous system overload. Canadian researcher Hans Selye first applied the term stress to human psychology in a 1946 journal article. Before his death in the 1990s, however, Selye admitted that he may have popularised the wrong term and that the more appropriate expression for the outcome of stress would be the engineering term *strain*. Selye suggested that stress, in itself, is not a problem. 'Stress', said Selye, 'depends not on what happens to an individual, but upon the way he reacts.' Using this, the links between stress, strain, anxiety and depression become more obvious, as shown in Figure 11.1.

FIGURE 11.1 The links between stress/strain, anxiety and depression

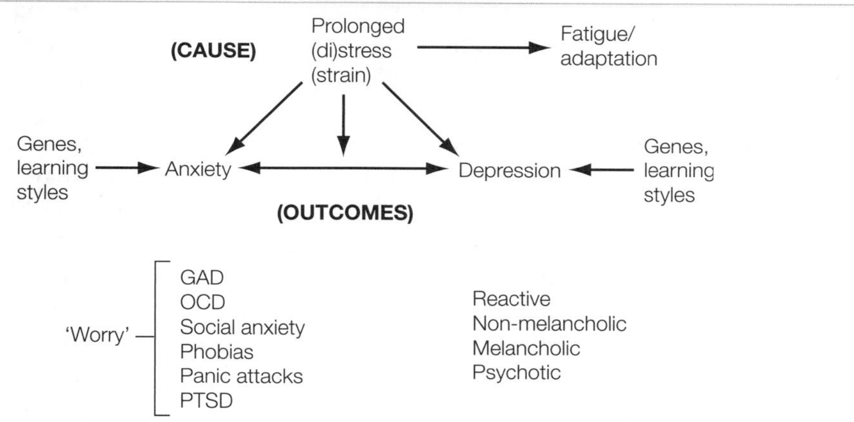

In light of this, stress would more correctly be called the 'stressed state', a 'stress reaction' or 'strain'. However, given its popular use, we will continue to use the term stress.

As we will see, not all stress is bad. However, strain—when defined as the outcome of 'distress' (in contrast to 'eustress', or the feeling of euphoria associated with the right level of stimulation), as seen in Figure 11.1—can have health-related consequences if it continues for long enough. This can lead to, or be caused by, anxiety that if maintained at a high enough level for an extended period and accompanied by a sense of loss of control can lead to depression. American psychologist Dr Martin Seligman (see Chapter 14) originally referred to this as learned helplessness (Seligman, 1972). As shown in Figure 11.1, however, anxiety and depression can also develop spontaneously within an individual, not from any obvious strain from a stressor but as a result of a genetic predisposition towards these mood states.

So, having effectively complicated the S-AD phenomena, we will attempt to alleviate the confusion by untangling the phenomenon known as stress in this chapter and discussing the idiosyncrasies of anxiety and depression separately in the following chapters. We will take a more positive approach to the clinical management of mood states by examining happiness and the move towards positive psychology in Chapter 14.

What is stress?

In a comprehensive recent review of the relationship between stress and obesity, Greek endocrinologists Ionass Kyrou and colleagues (2006) defined stress as 'a state of threatened homeostasis or disharmony caused by intrinsic or extrinsic adverse forces . . . counteracted by an intricate repertoire of physiologic and behavioural responses that aim to re-establish the challenged body composition'.

The adaptive response referred to by Kyrou et al., and earlier by Selye, refers to an elaborate physiological system involving the hypothalamic-pituitary-adrenal (HPA) axis and the central and peripheral components of the autonomic nervous system (ANS). In situations of acute stress, the response of these systems restores homeostasis through behavioural and physical adaptations, which improves the individual's chances of survival. Behavioural adaptations include increased arousal, alertness, vigilance and cognition, and suppression of hunger, feeding and sexual behaviour. Physiological adaptations involve adaptive redirection of energy through increased respiratory rate, blood pressure, heart rate, cardiovascular tone, gluconeogenesis and lipolysis. These place the body in an allostatic state, which is relieved by reactions to remove or evade the stressor. Where this does not occur, such as in a state of chronic stress, an allostatic overload results. This is caused by either a persistent stressor or a prolonged duration of the adaptive response.

Biological changes resulting from persistent changes in the HPA axis and ANS can affect a variety of physiological functions, resulting in symptoms defined as the metabolic syndrome discussed in Chapter 5, including increases in the most metabolically dangerous type of fat—visceral obesity (Bjorntorp and Rosmond, 2000). Chronic stress/strain is defined by Kryou et al. (2006) as a 'pathological state of prolonged threat to homeostasis by persistent or frequently repeated stressors . . . considered a significant contributing factor in the pathophysiology of manifestations that characterise a wide range of diseases and syndromes'.

Hence, while acute changes in homeostasis induced by a stressor can be stimulatory, chronic changes and the resultant allostatic state can have long-term health consequences. Chemical and hormonal changes that occur to assist the restoration of homeostasis through flight or flight are not corrected in the chronic state, and the body is left to 'stew in its own juices'. In readiness for flight or fight, the body prepares—the 'general adaptation syndrome'—largely through the contraction of large preparatory muscles such as the trapezius (to raise the arms for 'fight'), the abdominals (to avoid being 'winded') and the gluteals and lower back (for 'running away'). If an adaptive response occurs, the muscles are relaxed and homeostasis reigns. However, if stress is extended, these muscles remain taut and become a source of pain when palpated.

Traditionally, nature's response to the allostatic state is to 'escape' (flight or fight), either physically or mentally. This helps restore the psychological state of *perceived control,* which alleviates the stress reaction. It is these two concepts—escape and control—to which we will turn when looking at ways of dealing with stress. Before doing so, however, it is relevant to see why some people are affected more by particular stressors than other people and to examine the stages of strain through which progression can occur if stress reactions are not managed.

Genetics, resilience and hardiness

Although we talk of stress as a single concept, there are two main influencing factors: the *stressor*, or the external factor(s) causing a stress response or strain in the individual, and the internal factors within any individual leading to a stress response.

There is little doubt that some people are more resistant to the outcome of stress than others. This tends to run in families and new findings suggest that genes can actually be attributed to components such as worry. A general anxiety disorder (GAD) appears to exist in around 10% of the population and 60% of those suffering significant depression (Dolnak, 2006), and it may be that anxiety lies on a continuum, with severe phobias at one end and extreme hardiness or resilience at the other. Characteristics that appear to distinguish the hardy from the non-hardy—and which may or may not be 'hard wired'—are being empowered or having a feeling of 'control' rather than powerlessness; having the ability to see issues as a challenge rather than a threat; and having commitment as opposed to no commitment. But several other characteristics have also been identified (for further detail see Tugade et al., 2004). These provide the themes for management tips discussed here.

Learning styles can also contribute to a predisposition to develop anxiety or depression, although the extent to which this involves a genetic constituent is not known. Rumination, cyclical thinking and excessive self-based thinking, for example, can lead to a 'downhill spiral', which could result in biochemical changes that 'impress' a tendency to anxiety or depression on the brain and make this more difficult to then relieve (Dozois and Dobson, 2004).

Stages of stress/strain

The response to stress can be conceptualised as passing through a number of 'zones' and, although the transition through each may be imperceptible to the person being stressed, each zone has characteristic symptoms. These are shown in Figure 11.2.

FIGURE 11.2 The stages of stress

Stress level	Zone	Symptoms	Outcome
High	4. Danger zone	Loss of 'control' Breakdown 'Burnout'	DISTRESS ⇕
	3. Warning zone	'Brownout' Exhaustion Anxiety	
	2. Comfort zone	Excitement 'Flow' Enjoyment	EUSTRESS ⇕
Low	1. Boredom zone	Dissatisfaction Restlessness Immobilisation	DISTRESS

Distress can occur with too much or too little stress as shown in zones 1, 3 and 4 in Figure 11.2. In the case of a stimulating stressor, such strain is minimal and in fact is even sought after by the individual as a feeling of excitement, enjoyment, or 'flow'. This is the stage known as 'eustress' shown as stage 2. In the early states of distress, a stage 1 (sensory level) perception only may have been made and hence symptoms such as exhaustion and anxiety can occur with little stage 2 awareness (intellectual level) of the cause. By the time this reaches stage 4, 'burnout' becomes a common expression of symptoms, defined by the acronym DISINTEREST:

- Decreased sense of humour
- Increased physical problems (e.g. fatigue, infections)
- Social withdrawal
- Increased work load
- Not accomplishing
- Tension
- Emotional exhaustion
- Reduced sleep
- Easily taking offense
- Skipping meals and rest breaks
- Tranquilliser and/or alcohol use

According to prominent US psychologist Mihalyi Csikzentmihalyi (1992, 1975), the stages of stress and their outcomes on performance are influenced by an interaction between the severity of a stressor and the capacity of the individual being stressed (the 'stressee'), as shown in Figure 11.3.

Where a stressor is seen as insignificant by an individual capable of dealing with this (for example, a very good mountain climber on a very easy slope), boredom is the likely

FIGURE 11.3 The relationship between stressor and stressee

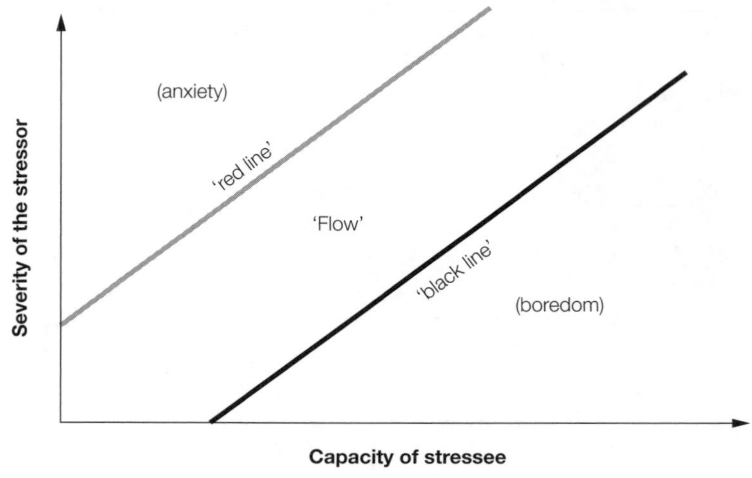

Source: Csikszentmihalyi, 1975

outcome. Where the opposite occurs (an inexperienced climber on a very hard slope), anxiety is the likely outcome. Where both are matched, a feeling of 'flow' or homeostasis is the likely outcome, putting the individual into the 'comfort zone' (or state of *eustress*). This suggests that for any given task we have a 'red line'—as seen in the top of Figure 11.3—above which the 'heat becomes too hot'. One solution is to lower the red line ('if you can't stand the heat, get out of the kitchen'). A second, 'black line' represents the level below which stimulation is insufficient and boredom results.

Stress can becomes *distress* (leading to anxiety and other problems long term, as seen in Figure 11.3) if the capacity of the stressee is genuinely overwhelmed by the severity of the stressor, or *feels* this to be the case, resulting in a feeling of loss of control. In cases of real stress, such as imminent danger, homeostasis can often only be achieved by attempting to change or eliminate the stressor. In many people, however, strain results from an inaccurate perception of stress. The classical reactions of flight or fight both lead to escape, in the broad sense of the term, either mental or physical. The concepts of control (or more correctly *perceived* control) and escape (both mental and physical) are core to the management of stress, and these can be achieved by changing the stressor and/or the stressee.

The concepts of control and escape

A feeling of loss of control, whether this is real or perceived, is what differentiates stress from distress leading to anxiety and/or depression. Some people (the more hardy or resilient) can put up with extreme stressors without difficulty, whereas others crumble at the slightest pressure. Restoring a feeling of *perceived control* is therefore a prime goal of stress reduction, whether this is by removing the individual from a stressor, reducing its potency to the stressee (by building his or her psychological immunity) or changing the stressee's reaction to the stressor. In all cases, the medium of change is encompassed in the term 'escape'.

What can be done in a standard consultation

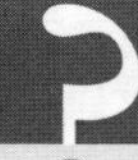

Check whether stress is a possible influencing factor on health by asking about response patterns to chronic stress (e.g. over-eating, self-medicating, passivity).

Assess the extent of any existing stress response (i.e. stress 'zone').

Explain the concepts of 'control' and 'escape' in managing stress.

Determine the patient's likely best management approach to stress: physical or mental (see *Professional resources*).

Where possible, identify and reduce the potency of stressor(s) by lowering the 'red line'.

Help restore *perceived control* within the individual.

Interestingly, the modern interest in escape as a means of coping with stress arose from research involving people who had little chance to put the real thing into practice. Sociologists Stanley Cohen and Laurie Taylor (1976) studied long-term prisoners—some of whom had life sentences—to find out about their mental processes. They found long-term inmates were no different to unconfined individuals. With no hope of physical escape the prisoners used a variety of mental escapes: fantasy, imagination, dreaming, meditation, writing, creativity and even some strange hobbies. These helped to restore the feeling of control, which is vital for the management of stress.

An approach to dealing with stress: ACE (analyse, change, evaluate)

The processes of stress management are described with a simple three-stage model ACE: analyse, change and evaluate (Figure 11.4).

FIGURE 11.4 An ACE approach to dealing with stress (analyse, change, evaluate)

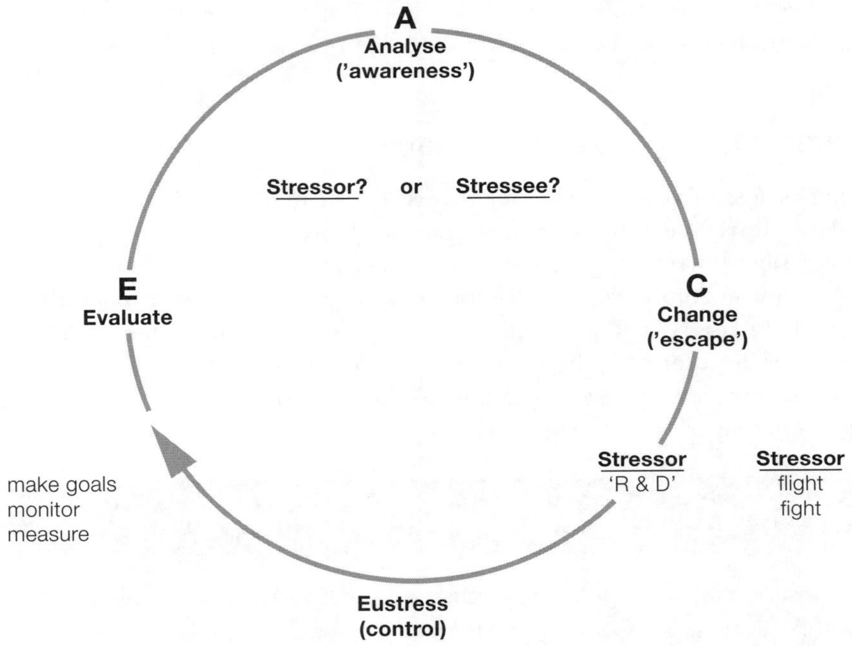

Analyse

This refers to establishing an awareness of the main source(s) of stress. As defined by Crum (2000), it involves moving from a stage 1 (sensory) to a stage 2 (intellectual) perception of the problem and the effects of stress are the results of particular external stressors or the individual's own coping mechanisms. Where a stress reaction is manifest with a less specific stressor or one that changes over time, a general anxiety disorder, or a higher order anxiety may be suspected. Where a stressor can be identified, and the stress reaction would be reduced or eliminated if this was made to disappear or reduced in potency, the obvious solution is to work on changing the stressor. Where removal of this would not reduce the reaction, it is more important to build immunity in the stressee. The exact situation determines the operational procedures of the next stage.

Change (escape)

CHANGING THE SRESSOR

Where an obvious stressor can be identified and is easily modified, changing the stressor is the obvious way to deal with the problem. A simple formula for this is the 'R & D' method:

• Reduce it	Do it
• Remove it	Delegate it
• Replace it	Delay it
• Rethink it	Discuss it
• Reframe it	Drop it

However, because the causes of most stress reside in the home, work or financial environments, and because these are situations that are often difficult to change, dealing with the stressor or the underlying cause of the problem is often not an option. As the prayer goes, 'God grant me the serenity to accept the things I cannot change, the courage to change the things I can, and the wisdom to know the difference'. Once a stressor is identified, these options can be considered. Most stress, however, comes from the individual's reaction and calls for changing the stressee.

CHANGING THE STRESSEE

As discussed above, all methods of dealing with stress can be considered as involving some form of escape. Escapes can be either maladaptive (e.g. drug abuse, violence, blame, displacement) or adaptive. Maladaptive approaches work only in the short term; they do not solve a chronic problem and may even lead to its worsening. Alcohol and stimulant drugs such as caffeine, for example, may even lead to panic attacks (see Chapter 12). Medication can help patients change the situation but needs to be seen as an adjunct to a greater understanding and management of the problem, rather than treatment as such.

The adaptive approaches involve the classic two reactions—flight or fight. These still form the basis of modern stress management solutions. In the past, flight may have meant running away, but it is clear that escape can be either mental or physical (or both). This can mean removing oneself physically from a stressor (a holiday, quitting a stressful job, exercise) or using techniques of mental 'escape'. Similarly, tackling the situation head on physically through fight is now not always possible or advisable. However, other options, both physical and mental, are available and examples of these (as well as the flight options, divided into physical and mental approaches) are shown in Table 11.5. The examples shown are not meant to be exhaustive but to provide examples of the wide range of options available, depending on individual interests and capacity. The range is vast, and individual preferences probably explain why no one theory of stress management fits all.

In general, it can be said that some people escape best physically (by running long distances, sport, going to the gym, paddling a canoe, riding a bike). Recent research provides evidence for positive physiological effects of exercise on central functions related to stress and depression in the brain (Tsatsoulis and

TABLE 11.1 Somatic (physical) and cognitive (mental) escapes

FLIGHT		FLIGHT	
Physical	**Mental**	**Physical**	**Mental**
Exercise	meditation	confrontation	cognitive
Sport	muscle relaxation	challenge	restructuring
warm baths	pause/prayer	preparation	rational emotive
holidays	concentration	social engineering	therapy
mini breaks	counting to ten	nutrition	assertiveness
hobbies	art	direct action	psychotherapy
games	mind games	expression	planning
yoga	music	talking	mind control
tai chi	creativity	meeting	financial control
breathing	reading		positive self-talk
massage	trance		rehearsal
sex	biofeedback		thought stopping
sleep	mind mapping		brainstorming

Fountoulakis, 2006). Others do it best mentally (by meditation, cognitive behaviour therapy, prayer, tai chi, yoga, meditation, distractions such as reading or watching movies). A third group uses a combination of techniques. A brief test shown in the *Professional resources* is one way of assessing the most appropriate approach for an individual.

Evaluate

Once change has been effected through some form of appropriate escape, setting stress-reduction goals and monitoring the patient's homeostatic state through standard measures such as blood pressure, blood glucose and other biochemical measures, as well as through simple stress questionnaires, can test the outcome. If an appropriate outcome is not achieved, the process outlined in Figure 11.4 may need to be instituted again, until a measure of control, and homeostasis, is restored.

Summary

The term stress is often confused with the outcome of a chronic period of allostatic overload (strain), which can cause a variety of disorders—metabolic, physical and psychological—often leading to more overt disease. There are major differences in hardiness (representing individual responses to a stressor), much of which seems to be genetically based and which, at one extreme, can lead to a range of phobic responses and even general anxiety disorder (GAD). Stress management provides a range of mental or physical escapes appropriate to the individual which help restore a sense of perceived control over the situation or one's life.

PRACTICE TIPS: MANAGING STRESS

	Medical practitioner	Practice nurse
Assess	Whether stress is an issue likely to cause health problems. Effects of stress on health behaviours (e.g. eating, obesity). Whether stress is a cause of greater morbidity (e.g. anxiety, depression).	Stress as a factor in disease states. Stress levels with questionnaires (baseline and during monitoring). Stress type (see *Professional resources*). Cardiovascular risk factors.
Assist	Patient to identify stressors where possible. By identifying goals. By providing (short-term) medication if needed. By explaining the control and escape concepts for stress management. Identification of 'escapes'. Review. By using templates as appropriate.	General education about stress management, including suggesting or providing good literature.
Arrange	Referral for stress management if appropriate. List of other health professionals for a care plan.	Discussion of stress management tactics with other allied health professionals. Input from a psychologist or psychiatrist. Contact with self-help groups if desired.

KEY POINTS FOR CLINICAL MANAGEMENT

- Differentiate between stress and the outcome of chronic strain.
- Consider stress as a cause of other morbidities (e.g. anxiety, depression), not an outcome in itself.
- Offer techniques for reducing stress independent of treating other outcomes.
- Use medication as a window of opportunity for dealing with the lifestyle basis of the problem.
- Aim to empower the patient by restoring perceived control.
- Target the stressor or stressee according to where the problem lies.

REFERENCES

Bjorntorp P, Rosmond R. (2000) The metabolic syndrome—a neuroendocrine disorder? *Br J Nutr* 83(Suppl 1): S49–S57.

Cohen S, Taylor L. (1976) *Escape attempts*. London: Allen Lane.

Crum A. (2000) *The 10-step method of stress relief: decoding the meaning and significance of stress*. CRC Boca Raton Fa: Press.

Csikszentmihalyi M. (1975) *Beyond boredom and anxiety*. San Francisco: Jossey Bass.

Csikszentmihalyi M. (1991) *Flow: the psychology of optimal experience*. NY: Harper and Rowe.

Dozois DJA, Dobson KS (eds). (2004) *The prevention of anxiety and depression: theory, research, and practice*. American Psychological Association: Washington, D.C.

Dolnak DR. (2006) Treating patients for comorbid depression, anxiety disorders and somatic illnesses. *J Am Osteopath Ass* 106(Suppl): S9–S14.

Kyrou J, Chrousos GP, Tsigos C. (2006) Stress, visceral obesity and metabolic complications. *Ann NY Acad Sci* 1083: 77–110.

Macquarie Dictionary. Third edition. (1997) Macquarie Library Pty Ltd: Macquarie University.

Seligman M. (1972) *Learned helplessness*. Random House: NY.

Selye H. (1946) The general adaptation syndrome. *J Clin Endocrinology* 6:177.

Tsatsoulis T, Fountoulakis S. (2006) The protective role of exercise on stress system dusregulation and comorbidities. *Ann NY Acad Sci* 1083: 196–213.

Tugade MM, Fredrickson BL, Barrett LF. (2004) Psychological resilience and positive emotional granularity: Examining the benefits of positive emotions on coping and health. *J Personality* 72(6): 1161–90.

Wilke W. (1990) *Understanding stress breakdown*. ANZEA Books: Sydney.

professional resources

PROFESSIONAL RESOURCES: A STRESS-TYPE TEST

Patient instructions: Rate the degree to which you generally or typically experience each of the following symptoms when you feel anxious or stressed.

	Not at all				Very much
A. I have difficulty concentrating because of uncontrollable thoughts.	1	2	3	4	5
B. My heart beats faster.	1	2	3	4	5
C. I worry too much over something that doesn't really matter.	1	2	3	4	5
D. I imagine terrifying scenes.	1	2	3	4	5
E. I feel jittery in my body.	1	2	3	4	5
F. I get diarrhoea.	1	2	3	4	5
G. I can't keep anxiety-provoking pictures out of my mind.	1	2	3	4	5
H. I feel tense in the stomach.	1	2	3	4	5
I. Unimportant things bother me.	1	2	3	4	5
J. I feel like I am losing out because I can't make up my mind quickly.	1	2	3	4	5
K. I nervously pace.	1	2	3	4	5
L. I become immobilised.	1	2	3	4	5
M.I perspire.	1	2	3	4	5
N. I can't keep anxiety-provoking thoughts out of my mind.	1	2	3	4	5

Scoring:

Add scores in the following way

1. Physically oriented = B + E + F + H + K + L + M = TOTAL SCORE
2. Cognitively oriented = A + C + D + G + I + J + N = TOTAL SCORE

The results can indicate whether a respondent is best suited to a somatic (physical) or cognitive (mental) approach to managing stress.

CHAPTER 12

Dealing with worry and anxiety

ANDREW BINNS, GARRY EGGER, ROBERT REZNIK

> *Anxiety is a thin stream of fear trickling through the mind. If encouraged, it cuts a channel into which all other thoughts are drained.*
>
> ARTHUR SOMERS ROCHE

Introduction

If depression is 'learned helplessness', anxiety could be thought of as 'feared helplessness'. Unlike depression, where the sufferer has all but 'given up', the anxiety sufferer is still trying to cope, albeit in the presence of 'a very unpleasant feeling of impending doom or disaster, a feeling that there is something wrong somewhere, which is associated with body symptoms of jumpiness and tenseness' (Wilke, 1990). The fear is recognised by individuals as being out of proportion to the event or situation but nevertheless they feel unable to control this. Psychodynamically, the anxiety and its associated signs and symptoms are often the displacement of conscious and unconscious stresses that are unresolved or seemingly insoluble.

Anxiety disorders follow a chronic course, often with relapse and remission, and although there is a significant genetic component involved in causality, lifestyle factors such as alcohol and drug use, caffeine, poor nutrition, smoking and obesity can cause a significant exacerbation, or indeed initiate the symptoms (Blashki et al., 2007).

Health effects of anxiety

While excessive and prolonged anxiety itself can be debilitating, excessive anxiety can lead to an allostatic state of disequilibrium, which, over time, can result in a range of metabolic disorders up to and including heart disease (Yusuf et al., 2004). Pathologies can also include somatoform disorders—such as body dysmorphic syndrome, irritable bowel, hypochondriasis and variants of fibromyalgia—where the focus of the anxiety becomes the body functioning. Recently, worry (as a sub-component of anxiety) has also been shown to affect long-term memory and the risk of Alzheimers disease.

Types of anxiety disorders

There are a number of separate classifications within the general category of anxiety disorders, ranging from generalised anxiety disorder (GAD), obsessive compulsive disorder (OCD), social anxiety disorder (SAD), panic disorder (PD), and specific phobias through to posttraumatic stress disorder (PTSD). However, these can be co-morbid with each other and with depression (Aina and Susman, 2006). For example, more than 50% of patients with GAD and 30% of those with SAD also meet criteria for major depressive disorder (van Ameringen et al., 1991; Yonkers et al., 1996).

Typically, an anxiety disorder will precede the development of depression (Kessler et al., 2003), although not all anxiety sufferers will progress to depression and not all depressive patients will suffer anxiety (Aina and Susman, 2006). Also, although each disorder has its own primary manifestation, symptoms of other disorders can be experienced in conjunction with the principal disorder. Indeed, the most common disorder of all (still not accepted as a disorder by DSM, although it contains research criteria) is a mixed anxiety/depression disorder (Dozois and Dobson, 2004).

The extent of the problem

Anxiety disorders exist in up to 10% of the population at any one time but usually do not begin until the late teens. Studies have shown that up to 18% of over 18-year-olds may have an anxiety disorder in any one year. Over a lifetime, however, more than one in four adults will experience at least one anxiety disorder (Kessler et al., 2005). One study of almost 1 000 patients at fifteen US primary care centres showed that 19.5% had at least one anxiety disorder, 8.6% had PTSD, 7.6% had GAD, 6.8% had a PD and 6.2% had SAD (Kroenke et al., 2007)—and yet fewer than two in three sufferers reported receiving any treatment for their disorder. It has been estimated that anxiety accounts for around 30% of the total expenditure for mental illness (equivalent to about one-third the cost for heart disease) and that over half of this is accounted for by anxiety drug therapy (Kessler et al., 2005).

GAD is the most common of the anxiety disorders and makes up about 60% of anxiety cases. This is a pervasive problem, where patients have chronic daily anxiety that can interfere with their daily functioning and may require medication use. PD, on the other hand, produces discrete symptom attacks that arise suddenly, escalate over ten to fifteen minutes, then subside. We will look here only at the moderate end of the scale of anxiety, leaving severe panic attacks, PTSD and OCD for specific attention from the appropriate allied health professionals. However, some of the treatment approaches discussed will be appropriate for a range of anxiety disorders.

Various websites, such as www.beyondblue.org, give easy-to-follow descriptions of the symptoms of the different forms of anxiety disorder as well as brief self-tests for signs, symptoms and potential risk factors. This and other websites quoted below also discuss treatment options and give details of where patients can get personalised help.

The role of lifestyle

While anxiety in its various forms has undoubtedly been with humans from time immemorial, certain modern lifestyle factors may have exacerbated the problem, and anxiety management needs to include a close analysis of lifestyle and thought patterns followed by appropriate modification.

Decreases in sleep time and quality, for example, can cause nervous system changes favouring increased parasympathetic arousal. This can be augmented by excessive caffeine, alcohol, and recreational drugs such as marijuana, cocaine and amphetamines. Caffeine use can also raise anxiety levels in those predisposed individuals, particularly patients with GAD (Telch et al., 1996).

Inactivity, which fails to produce the standard modulatory hormonal effect on the sensory nervous system, is likely to have a similar effect (Tsatsoulis and Fountoulakis, 2006). Modern levels of obesity may increase anxiety as a result of social discrimination, workplace disadvantage, decreased sexual potence, and the resultant negative self-images that these create.

Diagnosis

Unlike depression, anxiety may not be openly declared to a clinician. It can be picked up in a screening questionnaire such as the Hamilton Anxiety Scale (HAMA) or through questions about mood states (e.g. anxious mood, tension, difficulty getting to sleep, fears, worries, compulsions).

Somatic pain is often a presenting symptom, as with depression. Although anxiety may be co-morbid with depression, the two symptoms have different internal mood states. Depression is characterised by feelings of helplessness, worthlessness, despair and anger that reduces the patient's energy to carry out the activities of daily living. Anxiety, on the other hand, is an excess of energy generated by intense fear and panic, coupled with excessive worry. Anxiety sufferers typically have difficulty getting to sleep, whereas depressives typically have early morning wakening with excess sleeping at other times (however, the increased arousal associated with the depressed state can lead to a pervasive sense of exhaustion for the sufferer).

Diagnoses that may need to be ruled out include: thyroid disorders; other, less common medical disorders; use of a variety of medications including over-the-counter preparations and herbal remedies; substance abuse; and extreme over-use of caffeine, especially in those easily influenced by the effects of caffeine (such as the person who becomes jittery and hyperaroused after only one or two cups of strongly brewed coffee). It is also worth remembering that many substances contain caffeine, including all the so-called energy drinks, many diet drinks and, especially, green tea. Care should also be taken to distinguish anxiety from bipolar disorder.

Aspects of each of the individual anxiety disorders are covered in detail in several specific texts (e.g. Barlow, 2002; Blashki et al., 2007) and popular publications (e.g. Fox, 1994; Wilke, 1990).

Worry as a ubiquitous characteristic of anxiety

Worry, in some form, is an underlying feature in all anxiety disorders (Shearer and Gordon, 2006). It also manifests as hypochondriasis in about 1% of the population (where displaced anxiety manifests as changes in somatic states that are interpreted by the person as a marker of significant or indeed catastrophic medical conditions) and up to 5% of those in primary care (Barsky and Ahern, 2004). Worry is a short-term response to uncertainty that can become self-perpetuating, with adverse long-term consequences.

However, worry differs in the forms it takes in different anxiety disorders. In PD, for example, worry is often specific to the cause, whereas those with GAD generally report a pervasive sense of worry about everything and almost any new stress is assumed to result in a negative outcome (Roemer et al., 1997). Scores on worry tests correlate with the frequency of statements related to personal inadequacy, suggesting that this may be a characteristic of individuals who worry excessively (Davey and Levy, 1998). Older people (>65) worry more than the young, and the nature of the worry is usually different; over half the worries of older people are health related, whereas those of the young are more about psychological wellbeing and social evaluation (Barlow, 2002).

Following evolutionary principles, worry (like anxiety) serves a purpose by diverting an individual's energies away from possible future life-threatening situations. People who worry chronically often believe that their worry serves positive functions. This is because the low probability of occurrence of feared events can often reward worry, shaping beliefs that this somehow has prevented bad things from happening. The reinforcement of the worried state can then, in extreme circumstances, be extended to 'worrying about worrying' (meta-worry), taking the problem full circle (Barlow, 2002).

> *Ain't no use worryin 'bout things you can't control, 'cause you can't control them. And ain't no use worryin' bout things you can control, 'cos you can control them. So just ain't no use worryin'.*
>
> Ed Moses (Olympic gold medallist 400 m hurdles 1976, 1984)

Management of excessive worry is covered in the general principles discussed below and primarily includes pharmacotherapy and cognitive behaviour therapy. Somatic and mental approaches such as relaxation training and meditation are likely to be less than fully effective because they do not specifically target the source of worry. Nevertheless, they do allow the person to develop a generalised lower level of arousal and to experience thoughts coming and going (with attendant tension and worry increasing and then dissipating). This process enhances the individual's sense of self-efficacy (i.e. control), a critical element for achieving proper homeostasis. Thought-stopping techniques are now out of favour, because, just as with telling someone not to think of white elephants, the deliberate effort to suppress some types of thought often just serves to promote these. Use of a 'worry outcome diary' has been suggested (Borkovec et al., 1999) to help de-condition worry with a lack of reinforcement. This involves recording specific negative predictions (worries), then going back and assessing whether the outcomes justified such worry. It provides a form of extinction when positive reinforcement of the worry state is not forthcoming.

What can be done in a standard consultation

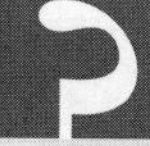

Ask about ongoing worry if anxiety is suspected as a cause of ill-health (see *Professional resources*).

If necessary, administer a worry scale to quantify this (see *Professional resources*).

Suggest a worry outcome diary to be checked in retrospect to de-condition worry.

Ask diagnostic questions to check on specific anxiety disorders (see *Professional resources*).

Offer pharmacotherapy if appropriate.

Offer or refer for cognitive behavioural and other psychological treatments.

Management

Dealing with the extreme anxiety disorders generally requires a specialised psychologist or psychiatrist, but many of the principles of treatment are common and are discussed in summary here (Dolnak, 2006). There are three main categories of treatment: pharmacotherapy, psychological processes and self-help, including nutrition and exercise management and supplementation (see Table 12.1)

TABLE 12.1 Management of anxiety

	Pharmacotherapy	**Psychological treatment**	**Self-help**
General anxiety/ all anxiety disorders	SSRIs/SNRIs	CBT and other psychological processes RET education	reduced caffeine/stimulants support groups
GAD/excessive worry	anxiolytics TCAs	positive psychology EMDR	kava exercise relaxation relaxation massage yoga support groups
Social anxiety/ panic disorder	anxiolytics	positive psychology systematic desensitisation interpersonal therapy EMDR	bibliotherapy public speaking training kava 'safe place' training
OCD	TCAs	exposure and response prevention psychotherapy	bibliotherapy

CONTINUED OVERLEAF

Management of anxiety (Continued)

PTSD	propranolol anxiolytics	counselling psychotherapy	support groups
Phobias	anxiolytics	exposure/flooding psychotherapy	support groups bibliotherapy

bibliotherapy = researching the problem; EMDR = eye movement desensitisation and reprocessing; GAD = general anxiety disorder; kava is a soporific drink used by Pacific Islanders and is available as anxiolytic in Europe; OCD = obsessive compulsive disorder; PTSD = posttraumatic stress disorder; RET = rational emotive therapy; selective serotonin reuptake inhibitor/selective noradrenaline reuptake inhibitor; TCA = tricyclic antidepressant

Source: Adapted from Shearer and Gordon, 2006

Pharmacotherapy

This consists largely of the selective serotonin reuptake inhibitors (SSRIs) or serotonin and noradrenaline reuptake inhibitors (SSNRIs) as the first-line treatment (for a detailed list of specific medications see Shearer and Gordon, 2006 and Parker, 2002). Tricyclic and bupropion antidepressants can also help in GAD and OCD. In some cases (GAD, SAD, PD, specific phobias), anxiolytics may also be indicated and a beta-blocker such as propranolol has been found to be effective in treating PTSD. Where a patient is accepting of this, pharmacotherapy is most effective when combined with psychological and self-help practices.

Psychological processes

These are generally based around cognitive behaviour therapy (CBT), education and other psychological processes, with specific counselling focusing on accepting uncertainty, curtailing reassurance seeking, thought stopping, rational emotional therapy, behavioural strategies (e.g. worry periods, worry recording) and mindfulness meditation. Psychological processes including CBT usually involve some means of changing internal thought processes.

An exception is eye movement desensitisation and reprocessing (EMDR). This involves focusing on a moving object while concentrating on the source of anxiety for a set period, followed by a period of relaxation or meditation. Meta-analyses show the effectiveness of this technique in many cases (i.e. PTSD), although the mechanisms of action are not known (Parnell, 2007; Shapiro, 2005).

Education and counselling that challenges thought processes (see Shearer and Gordon, 2006, for a list of strategies) are also effective in dealing wih anxiety and form the mainstay of cognitive therapy (combined with the behavioural strategy of exposure leading to adaptation). For PTSD, websites such as www.acpmh.unimelb.edu.au and www.beyondblue.org provide some levels of self-help.

Self-help practices

These begin with the elimination of stimulant foods and drinks from the diet, including those containing caffeine (e.g. coffee, tea, chocolate, cocoa) and the inclusion of exercise sessions, particularly endurance or extended exercise to reduce somatic tension. Exercise is effective because anxiety is associated with increased sympathetic activity and vagal tone and exercise tends to dampen this down through muscular contractions (Tsatsoulis and Fountoulakis, 2006). Morning exercise may be expected to be best

(although there is little current research on this) because it can have a somatic effect that lasts through the day and because it is more likely to prevent the build up of anxiety. The most appropriate types of exercise are extended aerobic activities or resistance training. Progressive resistance training can be especially useful in the frail and elderly because it increases insulin sensitivity as well as decreasing anxiety and depression.

Self-help psychological processes such as developing a highly specific 'safe place' in the mind for retreat and escape will help. For anxiety-provoking situations such as public speaking, training through groups such as Toastmasters will build confidence and allow for the mind's adaptive capacity to reduce anxiety with exposure. Progressive muscular relaxation techniques can also help some patients who are willing to put in effort for treatment. Relaxation training, however, is less effective for inveterate worriers and thought stopping techniques, as mentioned above, are no longer recommended for this group (Shearer and Gordon, 2006).

A review of self-help and complementary treatments has shown kava, the soporific drink (or tablet) used by Pacific Islanders, to have the best evidence for management of GAD (Jorn et al., 2004). However, although this is available as an anxiolytic in tablet form in Europe, it is not available (nor probably appropriate) in Australia. Other evidence-based self-help treatments are relaxation training and bibliotherapy (researching the problem). Common treatments with only limited evidence are acupuncture, music, inositol (a B vitamin derivative), and alcohol avoidance. Support groups and other self-help resources (see below) can also assist in management of the milder anxiety disorders.

Simple approaches for self-management of anxiety

Choose your battles wisely.

Be aware of the snowball effect of thinking.

Ask yourself, 'Will this matter a year from now?'

Become aware of your moods—and don't be fooled by the low ones.

Practice random acts of kindness.

Do one thing at a time.

Think of what you have—not what you want.

Think of problems as potential teachers.

If someone throws you the ball, you don't have to catch it.

Keep asking the question, 'What is really important?'

Be open to 'what is', not 'what should be'.

Ask yourself 'What do I lose by not doing what I fear?' if the consequence you fear is highly unlikely or far into the future.

Source: Carlson, 1997

When to refer

Referral to a psychiatrist, psychologist or anxiety specialist should occur if:

- the patient fails to respond to simple treatments;
- medical problems, such as medication use, complicate treatment or have not been ruled out as possible causes;
- side effects occur from standard treatments; or
- the problem is escalating.

Summary

At least one in four people have a lifetime risk of an anxiety disorder. This can range from a simple general anxiety disorder (GAD) to posttraumatic stress disorder (PTSD), panic attacks or extreme phobia. Worry is a ubiquitous characteristic of all anxiety disorders and often needs to be managed with pharmacotherapy or cognitive behavioural techniques. The three methods of management of anxiety include pharmacotherapy, psychological techniques and self-help processes, including relaxation therapy. Anxiety is a chronic condition with frequent recurrences, and a significant proportion of cases (around 50%) can progress to depression.

practice tips

PRACTICE TIPS: DEALING WITH ANXIETY

	Medical practitioner	**Practice nurse**
Assess	Worry as a health risk. Possible types of anxiety disorder. Physical effects of anxiety/worry.	Worry/anxiety (see *Professional resources* for tests).
Assist	By offering medication if appropriate. By discussing relaxation/meditation practices. By suggesting a worry outcome diary if appropriate.	General education about worry/anxiety. By providing good literature. By monitoring cardiovascular risk factors. Monitoring anxiety levels.
Arrange	Referral for CBT if appropriate. List of other health professionals for a care plan. Access to self-help websites.	Discussion of anxiety management tactics with other allied health professionals. Referral to a psychologist/psychiatrist. Contact with self-help groups.

key points

KEY POINTS FOR CLINICAL MANAGEMENT

- Be aware of anxiety as an underlying cause of somatic problems.
- Consider specific aspects of 'worry' in anxiety.
- Classify anxiety within accepted disorders.
- Use anxiolytic medication (such as a benzodiazepine, e.g. diazepam or alprazolam) only as a short-term option for GAD.
- Aim to empower the patient by restoring perceived control.

references

REFERENCES

Aina Y, Susman JL. (2006) Understanding comorbidity with depression and anxiety disorders. *J Am Osteopath Assoc* 106 (Suppl 2): S9–S14.

Barlow DH. (2002) *Anxiety and its disorders: the nature and treatment of anxiety and panic,* 2nd edn. New York: Guilford.

Barsky AJ, Ahern DK. (2004) Cognitive behavior therapy for hypochondriasis: a randomized control trial. *JAMA* 291: 1464–70.

Borkovec TD, Hazlett-Stevens H, Diaz ML. (1999) The role of positive beliefs about worry in generalized anxiety disorder and its treatment. *Clin Psychol & Psychotherapy* 6: 126–38.

Blashki G, Judd F, Piterman L. (2007) *General practice psychiatry*. Sydney: McGraw–Hill.

Carlson R. (1997) *Don't sweat the small stuff.* NY: Hyperion.

Davey GCL, Levy S. (1998) Catastrophic worrying: personal inadequacy and a perseverative iterative style as features of the catastrophizing process. *J Abnom Psych* 107: 576–86.

Dozois DJA, Dobson KS (eds). (2004) *The prevention of anxiety and depression: theory, research, and practice*. Washington: American Psychological Association.

Dolnak DR. (2006) Treating patients for comorbid depression, anxiety disorders and somatic illnesses. *J Am Osteopath Ass* 106(Suppl): S9–S14.

Fox B. (1994) *Anxiety attack: don't panic*! Melbourne: Longman Cheshire.

Fricchione G. (2004) Clinical practice. Generalised anxiety disorder. *N Eng J Med* 351: 675–82.

Jorn AF, Christensen H, Griffiths KM et al. (2004) Effectiveness of complementary and self help treatments for anxiety disorders. *Med J Aust* 181(7): S29–S46.

Kessler RC, Berglund P, Demler O et al. (2003) The epidemiology of major depressive disorder: results from the National Co-morbidity Survey Replication (NCS-R). *JAMA* 289: 3095–105.

Kessler RC, Berglund P, Demler O et al. (2005) Lifetime prevalence and age-of-onset distributions of DSM-IV disorders in the National Comorbidity Survey Replication. *Arch Gen Psychiatry* 62: 593–602.

Kroenke K, Spitzer RL, Williams JBW et al. (2007) Anxiety disorders in primary care: prevalence, impairment, comorbidity, and detection. *Ann Int Med* 146(5): 317–25.

Parker G. (2002) *Dealing with depression: a commonsense guide to mood disorders*. Allen and Unwin: Sydney.

Parnell L. (2007) *A therapist's guide to EMDR*. WW Norton and Co.: NY.

Roemer L, Milina S, Borkovec TD. (1997) An investigation of worry content among generally anxious individuals. *J Nerv Ment Dis* 185(5): 314–19.

Shapiro R (ed). (2005) *EMDR solutions: pathways to healing*. NY: WW Norton and Co.

Shearer S, Gordon L. (2006) The patient with excessive worry. *Am Fam Phys* 73(6): 1049–56.

Telch MJ, Silverman A, Schmidt NB. (1996) Effects of anxiety sensitivity and perceived control on emotional responding to caffeine challenge. *J Anx Disord* 10: 21–35.

Tsatsoulis A, Fountoulakis S. (2006) The protective role of exercise on stress system dysregulation and comorbidities. *Ann NY Acad Sci* 1083: 196–213.

Tugade MM, Fredrickson BL, Barrett LF. (2004) Psychological resilience and positive emotional granularity: examining the benefits of positive emotions on coping and health. *J Personality* 72(6): 1161–90.

Van Ameringen M, Mancini C, Styan G et al. (1991) Relationship of social phobias with other psychiatric illness. *J Affect Disord* 21(2): 93–99.

Wilke W. (1990) *Understanding stress breakdown*. Sydney: ANZEA Books.

Yonkers KA, Warshaw MG, Massion AO et al. (1996) Phenomenology and course of generalized anxiety disorder. *Br J Psychiatr* 168: 308–13.

Yusuf S, Hawken S, Ounpuu S et al. Interheart Study Investigators. (2004) Effect of potentially modifiable risk factors associated with myocardial infarction in 52 countries (the INTERHEART study). *Lancet* 364(9438): 937–52.

PROFESSIONAL RESOURCES: MEASURING ANXIETY

Clinical question

Approximately 90% of people with GAD will answer positively to the following question (Fricchione, 2004): *During the past four weeks, have you been bothered by feeling worried, tense or anxious most of the time?*

Penn State Worry Questionnaire

Patient instructions: Enter the number that best describes how typical or characteristic each item is of you.

	Not at all typical		Somewhat typical		Very typical
1. If I don't have enough time to do everything, I don't worry about it.	1	2	3	4	5
2. My worries overwhelm me.	1	2	3	4	5
3. I don't tend to worry about things.	1	2	3	4	5
4. Many situations make me worry.	1	2	3	4	5
5. I know I should not worry about things, but I just cannot help it.	1	2	3	4	5
6. When I am under pressure I worry a lot.	1	2	3	4	5
7. I am always worrying about something.	1	2	3	4	5
8. I find it easy to dismiss worrisome thoughts.	1	2	3	4	5
9. As soon as I finish one task, I start to worry about everything else I have to do.	1	2	3	4	5
10. I never worry about anything.	1	2	3	4	5
11. When there is nothing more I can do about a concern, I do not worry about it any more.	1	2	3	4	5
12. I have been a worrier all my life.	1	2	3	4	5
13. I notice that I have been worrying about things.	1	2	3	4	5
14. Once I start worrying, I cannot stop.	1	2	3	4	5
15. I worry all the time.	1	2	3	4	5
16. I worry about projects until they are all done	1	2	3	4	5

Practitioner instructions: Reverse score items 1, 3, 8, 10 and 11, then sum all 16 items. Possible scores range from 16 to 80. Means for groups with generalised anxiety disorder range from 60 to 68.

Signs and symptoms of anxiety disorders

For checklists for common types of anxiety disorders, see www.beyondblue.org.

CHAPTER 13

Depression

ROBERT REZNIK, ANDREW BINNS, GARRY EGGER

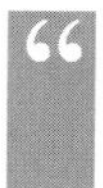

He who has a why to live for can bear with almost any how.

NIETZCHE

Introduction

Aldous Huxley in his 1932 novel *Brave New World* predicted a future of people 'high' on mood-enhancing drugs. That future, it seems, is now. Antidepressants are among the most popularly prescribed medications in western cultures. Up to one in five Australians *admit* to suffering from anxiety and/or depression, and depression is predicted to become the second most common form of morbidity in western societies in the next twenty years (WHO, 2007). Is this a real phenomenon or just an artefact of modern living?

Indications from surveys carried out up to fifty years ago suggest that there has been a genuine tenfold increase in levels of depression over time (Seligman, 2006). Why this is so is a source of conjecture, but most analysts associate it with the advances in technology discussed in Chapter 2. While leading to improvements in living standards, these have resulted in a loss of the 'meaning' gained from earlier struggles for survival. A more recent and interesting theory links inactivity, obesity and depression through neural changes in the brain (Ernst et al., 2006; Pereira et al., 2007), and this may explain the well-proven benefits of exercise in treating depression (discussed below).

In this chapter we look at the theory of, and management techniques for, depression. It specifically covers the less severe end of the scale. While reference is given to bipolar disorder and major depressive disorder, these require more detailed treatment than they are given here. In Chapter 14, a more positive slant is given to the management of mild mood disorders through a developing discipline known as 'positive psychology'.

What is depression?

Depression has been defined as 'the common cold of psychopathology' (Tan and Ortberg, 1995). It is further defined as 'an abnormal state characterised by exaggerated feelings of sadness, melancholy, dejection, worthlessness, emptiness and hopelessness that are inappropriate and out of proportion to reality'. Up to 25% of women and 17% of men admit to suffering depression at any one time—although men are less likely to admit it (Kessler et al., 2003). Those who have suffered one episode of depression have a 50% chance of a second episode if untreated (15% if treated); two episodes carries a 70% chance of relapse; and three episodes, a 100% chance (Parker, 2004).

Although it seems to be a useless emotion, Maguire (1997) suggests that depression has an evolutionary function as the adaptive response to a loss of status or social holding power in a community. Depression reduces conflict and allows the social group to reach out and help the injured party and thus help maintain social cohesion within the group. According to Maguire, this is seen in many primate colonies following is a successful coup of an alpha male, where serotonin levels reflect alpha male status.

Depression and health

Although depression has its own pathological sequelae, including suicide (about 10% of depressed patients will attempt suicide; Kessler et al., 1999), it is also associated with a range of other metabolic problems (Kessler et al., 2005). Depression can both follow and precede heart disease, type 2 diabetes (T2DM), and possibly other chronic diseases, suggesting a sound basis for screening and treating those with recent disease for depression. Recently, depression has also been identified as an independent risk factor both for heart disease and T2DM (Lustman et al., 2000; Yusef et al., 2004). The risk of further infarction after an initial myocardial infarct can be increased up to four times by depression. Somatic complaints are also higher in those with depression. In a study of almost 17 000 patients in Washington, somatic symptoms of four common medical disorders (diabetes, pulmonary disease, heart disease, arthritis) were at least as strongly associated with depression and anxiety as were objective physiologic measures (Katon et al., 2007). Improvement in depression outcome was associated with decreased somatic symptoms without improvement in physiologic measures.

Depressive disorders

As with anxiety, there are a number of depressive disorders, and these have been classified in a number of ways. The classification shown in Table 13.1, based on that by Professor Gordon Parker (2004) of the Black Dog Institute, is typical of most.

Reactive depression is a normal response to a major life event and does not usually last for more than about two weeks. Depressive disorders of concern here are those that last for at least two weeks and affect daily functioning. Patients with 'mild' depression probably vary most in the initial presentation, while those with major depression vary least.

TABLE 13.1 Classification of depressive disorders

Minor depressive disorders
reactive (non-clinical) depression
non-melancholic depression
Major depressive disorders
melancholic depression
psychotic depression/melancholia (including bipolar disorder)

Source: Parker, 2004

Non-melancholic depression lacks the psychomotor dysfunction of the more severe depressive categories, and sufferers usually have brief periods of cheerfulness with fewer lapses in concentration and memory. Often it is spontaneously remitting and different treatments—drugs, counselling or psychotherapy—have similar effects.

Melancholic depression is more severe than its non-melancholic counterpart. It is often described as more endogenous or biologically based and includes psychomotor disorders. This level of depression generally requires medication as the first-line therapy because non-medical treatments are less effective.

Psychotic melancholia lies at the severe end of the scale and usually involves psychotic phenomena such as hallucinations and delusions. It includes bipolar disorder and responds only to medical treatments.

Postnatal depression is well described in new mothers, with increasing attention now being paid to early recognition and treatment. However, less has been reported on *antenatal depression*, which may occur in up to 20% of pregnant women (Bowen and Muhajarine, 2006) but which may be less well acknowledged because of the focus on maternal and fetal wellbeing and the attribution of complaints to the physical and hormonal changes associated with pregnancy. Moreover, many who suffer from postnatal depression will, on retrospective questioning, give a history of antenatal depression. Antidepressant medications are less advisable here, but lifestyle-based therapies including exercise, adequate nutrition and adequate sleep are recommended (Bowen and Muhajarine, 2006). For more severe cases, clinical judgment must balance the reluctance of the mother to take medication against the dangers of inadequate treatment of her depression. The clinician must remember that maternal bonding (a critical phase in the development of the newborn) cannot be adequately provided by a depressed mother and poor bonding may lead to an increased risk of depression for the child in later life.

Risk factors

The important signs to look for when screening for depression are a family history of depression and a previous episode. Some chronic illnesses—including stroke, Parkinson's disease, dementia, cancers and heart attack, as well as adverse life events in susceptible people—are risk factors for depression. Personality types such as the less hardy or resilient (see Chapter 11) or the pessimistic are at increased risk.

Risk factors for antenatal depression include a history of depression, lack of a partner, marital difficulties, lack of social support, poverty, family violence, increased life stress, substance abuse, history of previous abortions, unplanned pregnancy, ambivalence toward the pregnancy, and anxiety about the fetus (Bowen and Muhajarine, 2006).

It is now clear that depression has a biological as well as a psychological component, affecting neural connections and transmitters in different parts of the brain. A possible way in which the biological—psychological link works in minor depression is shown in Figure 13.1, which suggests that continuation of adverse life events in susceptible people can lead to more severe depression through biological changes that require physical rather than psychological treatments (i.e. medication).

FIGURE 13.1 Suggested biological–psychological links in depression

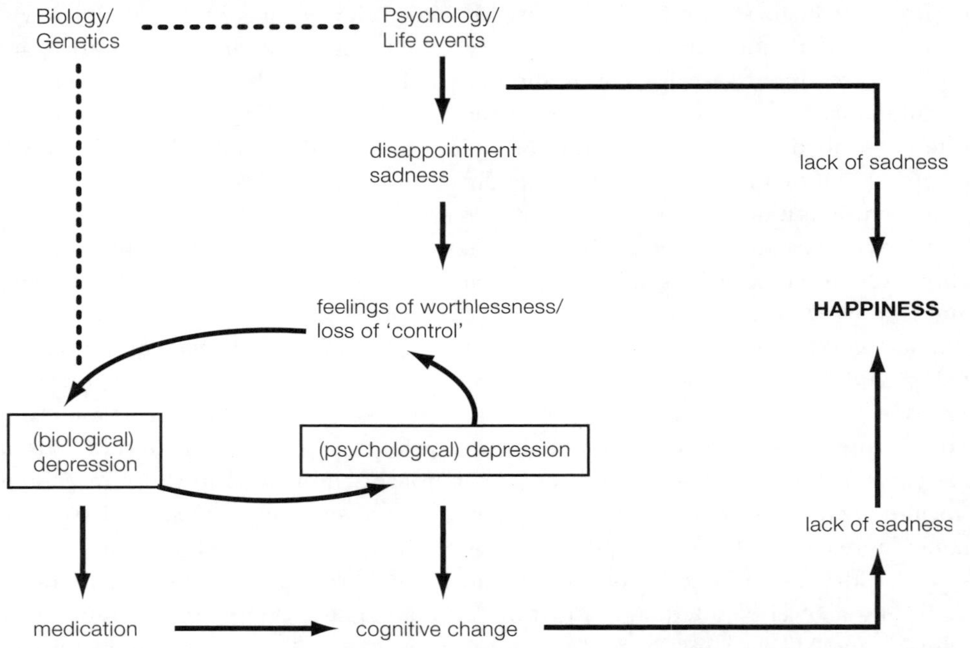

Diagnosis

Several publications and websites provide lists of symptoms for diagnosing depression; however, some simple questions appear to have high validity in diagnosis (see *Professional resources*). Symptoms can vary widely, but the acronym SIGECAPS (Mahendron and Yap, 2005) lists the defined DSM-V symptoms:

Sleep increase/decrease

Interest in formerly compelling or pleasurable activities diminished

Guilt, low self-esteem

Energy low

Concentration poor

Appetite increase/decrease

Psychomotor agitation/retardation

Suicidal thoughts

Aaron Beck, the leading cognitive behaviour therapist, says there is a typical 'thinking' triad in the depressed client (Beck, 1987). This involves:

- a negative view of the self;
- a tendency to interpret all external events as negative; and
- a pattern of viewing the future as negative.

The Beck Depression Inventory (Beck et al.,1996) is a licensed test for measuring depression, and it and the Hamilton Rating Scales for Depression (HAM-D) can be used for detailed screening for depression as well as general anxiety disorder. Other measurement instruments are listed and discussed in Tolman (2001).

Management

There are significant crossovers between treatments for anxiety and depression, with perhaps a greater emphasis on physical treatments (drugs) at the extremes of major depressive disorders. Table 13.2 lists possible options and indications for treatment.

TABLE 13.2 Treatment options for depression

Disorder	Pharmacotherapy	Psychological treatment	Non-pharmacotherapy (self help)
General/all disorders	SSRIs/SNRIs	CBT	exercise
	TCAs	education	support groups
	MAOs	counselling	bibliotherapy
Mild depressive	St John's wort	psychological	positive psychology
disorder	SAMe	'immunisation'	
Non-melancholic	SSRIs/SNRIs	psychological	positive psychology
depression	St John's wort	'immunisation'	
	SAMe		
Melancholic	SSRIs/SNRIs	psychotherapy	light therapy for SAD
depression	TCAs	interpersonal	
	MAOs	therapy	
Psychotic depression	antipsychotics	psychotherapy	
		interpersonal therapy	

CBT = cognitive behaviour therapy; MAO = monamine oxidase inhibitor; SAD = seasonal affective disorder; SAMe = S-adenosyl-L-methionine; SSRI/SNRIs = selective serotonin reuptake inhibitor/selective noradrenaline reuptake inhibitors; TCA = tricyclic antidepressants

Source: Adapted from Parker, 2004

Pharmacological treatments

First-line pharmacological therapy today involves third-generation antidepressants known as SSRIs or SNRIs. These appear to have less side effects than earlier generation monoamine oxidase inhibitors (MAOs) or tricyclic or tetracyclic antidepressants (TCAs) and better long-term outcomes. However, side effects such as sexual dysfunction remain a problem, particularly in some middle-aged men. One of the more common side effects is a reduction in sensitivity of the glans penis and, in those more seriously affected, anorgasmia. The upside is less premature ejaculation, and for this reason antidepressants are commonly prescribed by sex therapists for men with this problem. Side effects must be balanced against clinical improvement and the patient's preferences. For many, minor discomfort from side effects may be far outweighed by the benefits.

Importantly, when one medication fails to give a good clinical response, a change in medication may be beneficial; consequently, a number of different medications may need to trialled. A useful point to remember is that if a medication is going to work, 80% of responders will report an improvement (with up to a 50% decrease in depression) within two weeks. It is also worth stressing that, although patients may reach a good clinical response within 6–8 weeks of treatment with SSRIs, the improvement will continue, albeit at a reduced rate, for weeks and months later. A summary of the appropriate use of antidepressant medications for depression is given in Parker (2004, pp. 76, 82) and Tolman (2001, pp. 62–66) and by www.beyondblue.org. Possible limiting side effects of some of the major antidepressants medications are discussed in Chapter 21.

There are links between depression and obesity, which are complicated by some depression medications. Obesity can cause depression in some people, for obvious reasons. Seasonal affective disorder (SAD), although more common in high latitude countries with limited winter sunlight, is an increased negative energy balance and depression occurring in some individuals in winter. Depression, on the other hand, can also lead to obesity because of increased inertia, decreased physical activity and increased comfort eating. Some SSRIs are obesogenic. People who eat more when depressed (typically women) may lose weight following treatment with antidepressants that do not cause weight gain, for example, fluoxetine or sertraline. People who eat less when depressed (typically men, who eat less but drink more) may eat more and gain weight following treatment.

Psychological treatments

Psychological treatments are extensive and range from the simple 'immunisation' and self-help approaches discussed above to detailed psychodynamic approaches. A summary of the main approaches is shown in Table 13.3. More detail is obtainable from Tolman (2001, pp. 33–58).

There is a good evidence base for treatments such as cognitive behaviour therapy (CBT) and its components, cognitive therapy and behaviour therapy. Interpersonal therapy and psychodynamic approaches have also been shown to be effective under certain circumstances, including in combination with pharmacotherapy. There is less evidence base for processes such as hypnosis, but these may have positive benefits in select individuals.

Other treatments

As with anxiety, effective non-pharmacological interventions—such as exercise, relaxation training, meditation, research (bibliotherapy) and education—can have positive effects in some cases. Support groups, both in person and via the internet, can also be effective (see *Professional resources*). Exercise, even without weight loss, is particularly effective in reducing

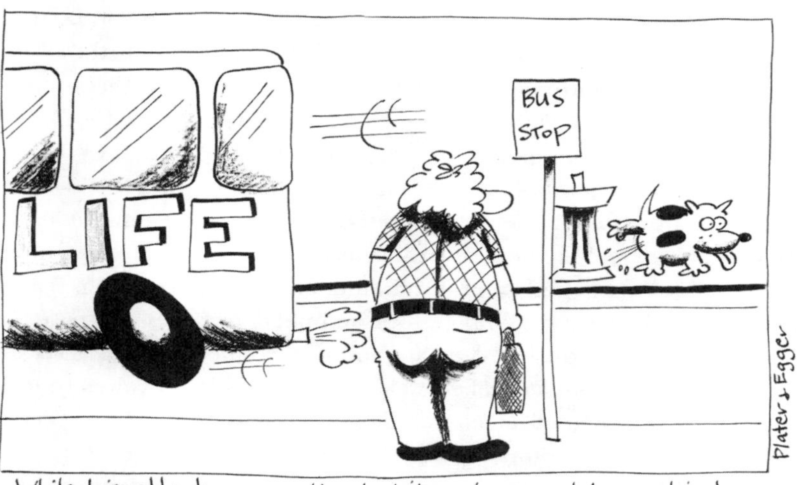

While his attention was diverted it just seemed to pass him by.

TABLE 13.3 The main psychological treatments for depression

	Description	Indications
Cognitive behaviour therapy	Focuses on changing irrational and ruminative thoughts and images that affect patterns of behaviour and social reinforcement. Includes awareness of thought distortion, rational emotive therapy, thought stopping, hypothesis testing, 'homework' and behavioural techniques.	Internalising, 'ruminating' thinkers
Behaviour therapy	Based on learning principles of reinforcement. Involves self-monitoring, tracking moods, assertiveness training, problem solving, role playing, and behavioural rehearsal and relaxation.	Externalisers Habit-influenced patients
Interpersonal therapy	Proposes that current functions are influenced by past relations. Designed to relieve relationship issues. Uses problem solving to resolve issues, improve communication, and form healthier relationships.	Where relationship difficulties are an obvious cause
Psychodynamics	Uses a range of psychoanalytic processes. Generally requires experienced psychotherapy training.	Complex early experience issues

depression (Craig et al., 2006). This is not only because it fulfils one of the main recommendations for depression (to 'just do it') but because it may promote the release of 'feel good' neurotransmitters and help re-form neural links in parts of the brain associated with depression (Ernst et al., 2006). As with anxiety, morning exercise is likely to be the most effective way to maintain mood throughout the day. It also reduces the problem of early wakening and the negative effects of rumination that can arise from lying awake.

In those who have suffered a depressive episode, psychological immunisation and cognitive exercises can help prevent or reduce the severity of a recurrence (Dozois and Dobson, 2004). Self-help books (e.g. Carlson, 2003; Tanner and Ball, 1991) and research (bibliotherapy) often have the most profound effects on mild depressives who have tried everything else. Because depression and sleep are positively connected (and sleep and activity negatively connected), a process called wake therapy—which involves reducing sleep hours—has also been promoted, albeit with limited supporting evidence (Giedke, 2002).

Although many over-the-counter (OTC) medications, such as ginseng, veridian and lemon balm, are promoted for depression relief, only two formulations have reasonable supporting evidence. These are the herbal substance St John's wort (Jorm et al., 2002) and SAMe (S-denosyl-L-methionine), which is a naturally occurring amino acid and part of the natural dopamine–serotonin biochemical cycle associated with feelings of well being (Bressa, 1994; Papakostas et al., 2003). One problem with herbal mixes such as St John's wort is the dose of active ingredient, which may vary between manufacturer and tablets. There is little supporting evidence for other alternative therapies, such as massage, folate or yoga, although some forms of meditation do appear to be more helpful for depression than for anxiety, where concentration is particularly difficult.

Although electroconvulsive therapy (ECT) has received bad press, it can be a highly effective form of therapy—life saving in some cases. Kitty Dukakis is the wife of Michael Dukakis, the former Democratic presidential opponent to George Bush, Senior. She has suffered from severe lifelong depression and found ECT to be the only thing that has helped her live a normal life. She regularly travels the United States speaking of its virtues and has written a book and developed a DVD for the public use to dispel myths and mistruths about this form of therapy.

What can be done in a standard consultation

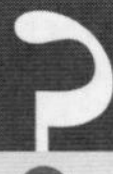

Check for anxiety (see Chapter 12).

Check for a family history of depression, anxiety and/or suicide.

Determine the degree of depression and refer where appropriate.

Check depression risk in pregnancy.

Question life stages and events as triggers (e.g. heart problems, illness).

Try to remove or reduce chronic stressor(s) that are obvious progenitors.

Address the use of alcohol and psychoactive substances.

Begin with simple steps (e.g. increased activity, activity planner) and add psychological and pharmacological treatments if required.

When to refer

While suicidal thoughts are not necessarily likely to lead to completion of the act, obsessive and continual thoughts may require experienced help or referral to a psychologist or psychiatrist. Psychotic depression, including bipolar disorder, may be managed by the GP but also require ongoing care and advanced psychological input from a qualified therapist.

Summary

Depression is a common and serious cause of misery for many people. It is important for the clinician and patient to recognise that this can be treated by a variety of methods. Whatever method is chosen, an objective measure such as a questionnaire or symptom check list provides a useful baseline to enable both parties to evaluate treatment. Trying to remove or resolve a chronic stressor is a first line of attack; if this is not possible, consider reducing its significance. Education is critical, as is forming a partnership between the sufferer and clinical helper. As with most psychological problems, the earlier treatment is initiated, the better the outcome. Treatment begins with simple steps—such as increased activity levels or an activity planner—and, depending upon response, the addition of one of the forms of psychological treatment outlined above, with or without medication. However, no treatment for depression will succeed if co-morbidity or other medical issues are not addressed, especially the use of psychoactive substances such as alcohol or illicit substances such as cocaine, amphetamines or cannabis.

practice tips

PRACTICE TIPS: MANAGING DEPRESSION

	General practitioner	Practice nurse
Assess	Depression, particularly in heart/diabetes patients. Possible co-morbidities. Somatic problems. Suicidal ideation. The nature of any depressive disorder. Interest in self-help groups.	Depression: use depression scales on heart/diabetes patients if indicated. Co-morbidity risk factors. The nature of any depressive disorder Stressors and how these might be removed.
Assist	Understanding differences between anxiety and depression. By prescribing medication if indicated. By discussing other options for treatment. By referring to self-help books. By providing handouts. By developing prevention strategies with the patient. By providing ongoing support.	By offering alternative strategies for treatment/accompanying medication. By teaching management techniques (if able). With self-help treatments. By referring to self-help books. By providing handouts. By referring to self-help groups/internet sites. By providing ongoing support.

Arrange	List of other health professionals for a care plan. Referral to psychological/psychiatric care where appropriate. Referral for suicide counselling if appropriate.	Care plan. Contact with and coordination of other health professionals. Discussion of options with other professionals.

KEY POINTS FOR CLINICAL MANAGEMENT

- Identify the level of depression and extent of treatment required.
- Consider the role of worry and anxiety.
- Aim to reduce stressors where these are an obvious cause of concern.
- Use medication as a window of opportunity rather than a lifetime treatment (if possible).
- Encourage involvement in self-help and self-seeking.
- Make use of modern resources such as self-help websites (see *Professional resources*).

REFERENCES

Beck AT. (1987) Cognitive models of depression. *J Cog Psychother* 1: 5–37.

Beck AT, Steer RA, Brown GK. (1996) *Beck depression inventory, 2nd edn*. San Antonio, TX: Psychological Corp.

Bowen A, Muhajarine N. (2006) Antenatal depression. *Can Nurse* 102(9): 26–30.

Bressa GM. (1994) S-adenosyl-L-methionine (SAMe) as antidepressant: meta-analysis of clinical studies. *Acta Neur Scand Suppl* 154: 7–14.

Carlson R. (2003) *Stop thinking and start living*. London: Harper Collins.

Craig CL, Bauman A, Phongsavan P et al. (2006) Fit and fat: Should we be singing the 'Santa Too Fat Blues'? *CMAJ* 175(12): 1563–66.

Dozois DJA, Dobson KS (eds). (2004) *The prevention of anxiety and depression: theory, research, and practice*. Washington, D.C: American Psychological Association.

Ernst C, Olson AK, John PJ et al. (2006) Antidepressant effects of exercise: Evidence for an adult-neurogenesis hypothesis? *Rev Pyschiat Neurosci* 31(2): 84–91.

Giedke H. (2002) Therapeutic use of sleep deprivation in depression. *Sleep Med Rev* 6(5): 361–77.

Jorm AF, Christensen H, Griffiths KM et al. (2002) Effectiveness of complimentary and self-help treatments for depression. *Med J Aust* 176(10 Suppl): S84–S96.

Katon W, Lin EH, Kroenke K. (2007) The association of depression and anxiety with medical symptom burden in patients with chronic medical illness. *Gen Hosp Psychiatry* 9(2): 147–55.

Kessler RC, Berglund P, Demler O et al. (2003) The epidemiology of major depressive disorder: results from the National Co-morbidity Survey Replication (NCS-R). *JAMA* 289: 3095–105.

Kessler RC, Berglund P, Demler O et al. (2005) Lifetime prevalence and age-of-onset distributions of DSM-IV disorders in the National Comorbidity Survey Replication. *Arch Gen Psychiatry* 62: 593–602.

Kessler RC, Borges G, Walters EE. (1999) Prevalence of risk factors for lifetime suicide attempts in the National Comorbidity Survey. *Arch Gen Psychiatry* 56: 617–26.

Lovibond SH, Lovibond PF. (1995) *Manual for the depression anxiety stress scales,* 2nd edn. Sydney: Psychology Foundation.

Lustman P, Anderson RJ, Freedland KE et al. (2000) Depression and poor glyaemic control: a meta-analytic review of the literature. *Diab Care* 23: 934–42.

Mahendran R, Yap HL. (2005) Clinical practice guidelines for depression. *Singapore Med J* 46(11): 610–15.

Mcguire MT. (1997) *Darwinian psychiatry*. Cambridge, Ma: Harvard University Press.

Papakostas GI, Alpert JE, Fava M. (2003) S-adenosyl-methionine in depression: a comprehensive review of the literature. *Curr Psychiatry Rep* 5(6): 460–66.

Parker G. (2004) *Dealing with depression, 2nd edn.* Sydney: Allen and Unwin.

Pereira AC, Huddleston DE, Brickman AM et al. (2007) An in vivo correlate of exercise-induced neurogenesis in the adult dentate gyrus. *PNAS* 104: 5638–43.

Seligman M. (2006) Paper presented to Australian Psychological Society Meeting, Sydney, August 2006.

Tan SY, Ortberg J. (1995) *Coping with depression: the common cold of the emotional life.* Grand Rapids, MI: Baker Pub Group.

Tanner S, Ball J. (1991) *Beating the blues: a self help approach to overcoming depression.* Sydney: Southwood Press.

Tolman AO. (2001) *Depression in adults*. Kansas City, Mo: Compact Clinicals.

WHO (World Health Organization). *World health statistics 2007.* Geneva: WHO.

Yusuf S, Hawken S, Ounpuu S et al. Interheart Study Investigators. (2004) Effect of potentially modifiable risk factors associated with myocardial infarction in 52 countries (the INTERHEART study): case-control study. *Lancet* 364(9438): 937–52.

professional resources

PROFESSIONAL RESOURCES: MEASURING DEPRESSION

Clinical questions

During the past month have you often been bothered by feeling down, depressed or hopeless?

During the past month have you often had little interest or pleasure in doing things?

The DASS$_{21}$ (Depression, Anxiety and Stress Scale—short version)

This is a valid Australian single test measuring stress, anxiety and depression. It was developed by Lovibond and Lovibond (1995). It can be downloaded from www.psy.unsw.edu.au/groups/dass and a manual purchased if desired.

Patient instructions

Please read each statement and circle a number 0, 1, 2 or 3 to indicate how much the statement applied to you over the past week. There are no right or wrong answers. Do not spend too much time on any statement.

The applicability rating scale:

0 Did not apply to me at all

1 Applied to me to some degree or some of the time

2 Applied to me to a considerable degree or a good part of time
3 Applied to me very much or most of the time

1.	I found it hard to wind down.	0	1	2	3	**S**
2.	I was aware of dryness of my mouth.	0	1	2	3	**A**
3.	I couldn't seem to experience any positive feeling at all.	0	1	2	3	**D**
4.	I experienced breathing difficulty (e.g. excessively rapid breathing, breathlessness in the absence of physical exertion).	0	1	2	3	**A**
5.	I found it difficult to work up the initiative to do things.	0	1	2	3	**D**
6.	I tended to overreact to situations.	0	1	2	3	**S**
7.	I experienced trembling (e.g. in the hands).	0	1	2	3	**A**
8.	I felt that I was using a lot of nervous energy.	0	1	2	3	**S**
9.	I was worried about situations in which I might panic and make a fool of myself.	0	1	2	3	**A**
10.	I felt that I had nothing to look forward to.	0	1	2	3	**D**
11.	I found myself getting agitated.	0	1	2	3	**S**
12.	I found it difficult to relax.	0	1	2	3	**S**
13.	I felt downhearted and blue.	0	1	2	3	**D**
14.	I was intolerant of anything that kept me from getting on with what I was doing.	0	1	2	3	**S**
15.	I felt I was close to panic.	0	1	2	3	**A**
16.	I was unable to become enthusiastic about anything.	0	1	2	3	**D**
17.	I felt I wasn't worth much as a person.	0	1	2	3	**D**
18.	I felt that I was rather touchy.	0	1	2	3	**S**
19.	I was aware of the action of my heart in the absence of physical exertion (e.g. sense of heart rate increase, heart missing a beat).	0	1	2	3	**A**
20.	I felt scared without any good reason.	0	1	2	3	**A**
21.	I felt that life was meaningless.	0	1	2	3	**D**

Practitioner instructions

Apply the template to both sides of the sheet and sum the scores for each scale. For the short (twenty-one item) version, multiply the sum by two. Bolded letters should be printed on a plastic template for scoring: S = stress, A= anxiety, D = depression. The total score for each of the four subscales is evaluated using the severity-rating index given in Table 13.4. Normative data are available on a number of samples. From a sample of 2 914 adults the means (and standard deviations) were 6.34 (6.97), 4.7 (4.91) and 10.11 (7.91) for the depression, anxiety and stress scales, respectively. A clinical sample reported means (and standard deviations) of 10.65 (9.3), 10.90 (8.12) and 21.1 (11.15) for the three measures.

TABLE 13.4 Severity-rating index for the $DASS_{21}$

	Depression	Anxiety	Stress
Normal	0–9	0–7	0–14
Mild	10–13	8–9	15–18
Moderate	14–20	10–14	19–25
Severe	21–27	15–19	26–33
Extremely severe	28+	20+	34+

OTHER RESOURCES

www.adaa.org

Anxiety Disorders Association of America; has excellent self-tests for different anxiety disorders.

www.anxieties.com

Free self help for anxiety sufferers; includes a good free newsletter.

www.beyondblue.org

Australian site with a range of excellent information, free advice, and referrals for anxiety and depression.

www.blackdoginstitute.com.au

Australian site concentrating on the management of different levels of depression.

CHAPTER 14

Happiness and mental health: the flip side of S-AD

ROB DONOVAN, GARRY EGGER

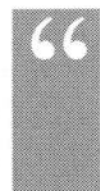

Hans Selye is wrong; it is not stress that kills us. It is effective adaptation to stress that permits us to live.

GEORGE VAILLANT, 1996

Introduction

Psychiatrist George Vallaint was three years old when the long-term prospective study of Harvard alumni commenced. He was in the third decade of his life when he joined the study and began to forge his career based on a detailed understanding of how humans use ego mechanisms of defence to adapt, with varying degrees of success, to life's trials and tribulations.

Vaillant's message, based on five decades of observation of growth to maturity, is a simple one: 'soundness is a way of reacting to problems, not an absence of them'. Of all the 287 men studied, none had only 'clear sailing through life'. What interested Vaillant was the adaptation mechanisms used to cope with the inevitable conflicts that occurred. Vaillant and his team identified four main types of defence mechanisms, from psychotic (in people typically managing least effectively in their adaptation to life) to mature (those who manage most effectively). The levels are shown in Table 14.1.

The Harvard findings represent an early awareness of mental 'health' in contrast to mental illness. This has since been adopted by the 'positive psychology' movement which has developed practices for capitalising on this to promote, if not happiness, then a form of positive affect with potential benefits for health.

Depression and happiness

It goes without saying that nobody likes to be 'bitten by the black dog' of depression. But it seems as though more people than ever before are suffering from depression

TABLE 14.1 Adaptive mechanisms of (ego) defence

Level	Mechanisms
Level 1: psychotic mechanisms (common in psychosis, dreams and childhood)	denial (of external reality) distortion delusional projection
Level 2: immature mechanisms (common in severe depression, personality disorders and adolescents)	fantasy projection hypochondriasis passive-aggressive behaviour (e.g. masochism, turning against the self)
Level 3: neurotic mechanisms (common in everyone)	intellectualisation (isolation, obsessive behaviour, rationalisation) repression reaction formation displacement (conversion, phobias) dissociation (neurotic denial)
Level 4: mature mechanisms (common in 'healthy' adults)	sublimation altruism suppression anticipation humour

Source: Vaillant, 1996

and anxiety disorders. True depression is undoubtedly a serious and apparently growing problem in modern societies, as we saw in Chapter 13. But does feeling unhappy from time to time justify reaching for the latest soma pill? Are there other ways of dealing with mood fluctuations? Can we use George Vallaint's mechanisms of defence or develop other more positive ways of preventing mental illnesses (which Vaillant describes as a continuum, rather than a discrete entity) or lessening their severity or duration when they do strike? The answer lies in an understanding of what is good mental health, other than simply the absence of disease.

What is (good) mental health?

Mental health has been defined by the World Health Organization (WHO) as 'a state of wellbeing in which the individual realises his or her own abilities, can cope with the normal stresses of life, can work productively and fruitfully, and is able to make a contribution to his or her community' (WHO, 2001). In lay terms, being mentally healthy means being alert, socially competent, emotionally stable, enthusiastic and energetic (Donovan et al., 2003).

In this chapter we look at these positive aspects of mental health, with a view to encouraging patients to take up activities that build and maintain good mental health. Because most people associate mental illness with the term mental health, it is suggested that during consultations, mental health issues be discussed in a context of 'keeping mentally healthy'. Being mentally healthy—or having good mental health—has positive health connotations and is generally described by lay people as being content with who they are and what they have; being in control of their lives; being mentally competent and emotionally stable; generally feeling happy most of the time; being able to cope with problems and crises in life; and being interested and involved in things in their lives (Donovan et al., 2003).

Defining happiness

It has been said that the search for happiness is one of the main sources of unhappiness in the world. Defining happiness, on the other hand, is like trying to describe a colour or wrestle with a column of smoke. Happiness has been variously defined as:

- an activity of the soul expressing virtue (Aristotle);
- the absence of desire (Epicurus);
- unity with one's nature (John F. Schumaker);
- a way station between too little and to much (Channing Pollock); and
- a way of travel, not a destination (Roy M. Goodman).

Contemporary society tends to focus on the affective nature of happiness and on overall enjoyment with one's life as a whole: 'feeling good—enjoying life and wanting that feeling to be maintained' (John Layard). Of most importance to our discussion here, is that happiness is more than just the absence of feeling sad.

Mental health and happiness

While the study of (good) mental health has been and continues to be neglected, the study of *happiness* has a long history. The volume of research has increased exponentially in the past decade. In one sense, this is a good thing because many of the factors that predict good mental health also predict happiness. In some cases, the terms happiness and psychological health are used interchangeably (e.g. Belliotti, 2004), especially when talking about happiness as measured by ratings of wellbeing and in a positive psychology context. Overall, happiness researchers tend to be individually and affective focused, whereas mental health researchers tend to be more population and determinant focused and thus place more emphasis on environmental influences.

There is little agreement among psychologists and philosophers on what does or should constitute happiness (Belliotti, 2004; Eckersley, 2004) and confusion about the terms wellbeing, contentment and life satisfaction. Nevertheless, agreement has been reached on a number of factors influencing happiness and good mental health.

The left column of Table 14.2 summarises the factors that appear to predict higher levels of happiness, wellbeing or life satisfaction; the right column looks at factors that negatively impact on wellbeing and mental health (see Donovan et al., 2003; Eckersley 2004; Layard, 2005). Interestingly, these factors, obtained from multivariate analyses of large databases, are strikingly similar to those listed by Aristotle (and others) almost 2500 years ago (i.e. wealth, plenty of friends, good friends, good health, athletic powers, good children and resources) (McMahon, 2006).

TABLE 14.2 Factors affecting mental health/happiness/wellbeing

Positive factors	Negative factors
family relationships (marriage)	child abuse and neglect
leisure activities	coercive treatment by those in authority
money/financial situation	discrimination/racism
physical health and disability/mobility	drug and alcohol abuse
personal freedom (from government control)	violence (family, intimate partner, civil war/terrorism, sexual assault)
personal values and religion	approaches to mental health
social networks, community and friends (social capital—trust in others)	
work situation (job security, job satisfaction)	

Warr (1994) listed nine environmental factors (Table 14.3) that underlie good mental health. Although Warr considered these in an occupational environment, they also apply across family, school, recreational, sporting and institutional environments.

TABLE 14.3 Environmental factors that contribute to good mental health

Factor	Examples
opportunity for control	opportunities for decision making and personal control
opportunity for skill use	opportunities to apply learning and feel that these applications are valued
externally generated goals	having structured routines set by others
variety	having varied roles and responsibilities changes in routine
environmental clarity	feedback about consequences of actions; being able to foresee a stable and secure future; having clear knowledge of expectations and role requirements
availability of money	sufficient resources for food, clothing, shelter, entertainment and education relative to wider society
physical security	feeling safe at home; feeling safe in public places; workplace safety
opportunity for interpersonal contact	quantity and quality (especially) of interactions; good communication emotional and instrumental support
valued social position	respect from others; self-respect; self-esteem

Source: Warr, 1994

There are a number of overlapping areas of interest in the promotion of good mental health. One stream, called positive psychology, grew out of mainstream psychology and hence tends to focus on the individual. Positive psychology is differentiated from traditional clinical psychology by its emphasis on individual strengths rather than weaknesses and by putting equal emphasis on building mental health and happiness in the absence of pathology.

A second stream is more concerned with the factors that contribute to or detract from wellbeing or satisfaction with life, as measured by structured items in large-scale population surveys (Eckersley, 2004; Headey and Wearing, 1992). Where positive psychologists are concerned with individual applications of their principles, wellbeing researchers see their data as also applicable at the population level.

The third stream looks at mental health from a more comprehensive and proactive view. While drawing on both of the above, it takes a broader view of the factors that lead to poor mental health, provide resilience to stressors and strengthen mental health. This approach is concerned more with the neglected area of mental health *promotion*: increasing proactivity about the positive sides of mental health (Donovan et al., 2006).

Positive psychology

Dr Martin Seligman, a former head of the American Psychological Society, became famous in the 1970s for 'shocking the living daylights' out of rats. This was not because he was a sadist, but rather to prove a point. Seligman found that if the rats were warned by a light that they were going to be shocked through the iron grills of a cage floor, and were able to learn a task to avoid that shock, they stayed happy and healthy—in rat terms, of course. However, if the ability to escape was taken away from them, they gradually became agitated, then catatonic, then just gave up trying until they eventually died. Seligman called this 'learned helplessness', and this was the title of his seminal book (Seligman, 1976). His thesis was that stress per se is not such a bad thing—in fact, it can even be invigorating. It is an organism's ability to react to that stressor which is important.

Fast forward to the 1990s and Dr Seligman has a road to Damascus moment. He realises that rats and people are different. He also appreciates that studying helplessness, anxiety and depression only helps one relieve these symptoms—it does not do the more positive things that make people happy. Hence, he was converted (along with many other psychologists of the time) to *positive psychology*, or the study of human happiness.

Seligman's Positive Psychology Centre (www.ppc.sas.upenn.edu) defines positive psychology as 'the scientific study of the strengths and virtues that enable individuals and communities to thrive'. Positive psychology focuses on positive affect (contentment with the past; happiness in the present; hope for the future) and individual strengths and virtues such as the capacity for love and work, courage, compassion, creativity, curiosity, resilience and integrity. It also aims to create positive families, communities, schools and other social institutions.

Positive psychology has three main characteristics that distinguish it from other forms of psychopathology:

- it works on an individual's underlying strengths and virtues, rather than concentrating on weaknesses;
- it is aimed mainly at untroubled or mildly troubled people, not the pathological; and
- it works on making people happy, not just on making them less miserable.

There are a number of practical applications involved in doing this (see www.authentichappiness.com). These include:

- **Finding and working on signature strengths** A questionnaire, designed to identify signature strengths and based on the *Handbook of signature strengths* (Pearson and Seligman, 2004), offers a short cut to identifying an individual's five most prominent strengths. Strengths include such things as the ability to find humour, summon enthusiasm, appreciate beauty, be curious and love learning. The idea of the exercise is that using one's 'signature' strengths may be a way to become engaged in satisfying activities. One or more strengths is then applied each day in a different way.

- **Counting blessings** At the end of each day, patients are advised to think of three good things that have happened that day and analyse why they have occurred. This enables them to focus on the good things that happen, which might otherwise be forgotten because of daily disappointments.

- **Expressing appreciation** Patients are advised to find someone who has done something helpful at some stage, and for whom proper appreciation was never given, and to thank them for this. This increases attention to good relationships and the good things that have happened in life, in contrast to the bad.

Other practical techniques include:

- savouring the pleasing things in life, such as a warm shower or a good breakfast;
- writing down what one may want to be remembered for, to help bring daily activities in line with what is really important;
- regularly practicing acts of kindness for strangers; and
- thinking about the happiest day in one's life over and over again, without analysing it.

The general idea is to improve self-image and promote good interactions with others. Participants who perform a variety of acts, rather than repeating the same ones, have been shown in published research to have an increase in happiness, even a month after the experiment ended. Those who kept on doing the acts on their own did better than those who did not.

Lives led

Positive psychology assumes that there are different levels of life that can be led on the road to happiness.

- **The pleasant life** Seligman defines this as the superficially happy life espoused by modern celebrity worship, which is generally artificial and based around material possessions.

- **The engaged life (interest and involvement)** This involves more engagement in activities that include a feeling of belonging and interest, such as joining a sports or interest group.

- **The meaningful life (giving/commitment)** At this level, a sense of purpose and meaning in what has been committed to provides an inner satisfaction. This may or may not involve religious belief and can include such things as political, social or environmental action or commitment.

As discussed below, Seligman's lives led can be transposed into action at a public health as well as a clinical level.

Is positive psychology the way for everybody?

Most psychologists working in the area of mental health acknowledge the organic nature of much mental illness. At the extreme ends, this requires pharmacological as well as psychological intervention. However, much of the so-called normal population is burdened with what have been called neuroses, often encouraged by a happiness-fixated media, resulting in an inability to thrive and achieve full potential. As pointed out by Schock (2006), 'somewhere between Plato and Prozac, happiness stopped being a lofty achievement and became an entitlement'. Positive psychology aims to assist people in achieving a level of happiness by focusing on core strengths and de-emphasising neurotic failings.

Mental health promotion

Mental health promotion is any action taken to maximise mental health and human well-being that focuses on improving the environments that affect mental health and the coping capacity of communities and individuals. *Prevention* refers to interventions that prevent the development of a disorder by targeting known risk factors. *Early intervention* involves actions that specifically target people displaying the early signs and symptoms of a mental disorder (Australian Government Department of Health and Aged Care, 2000). In this chapter, we are concerned mainly with mental health promotion and prevention, although the activities suggested below are equally applicable as part of an early intervention process.

While there are a number of school and worksite interventions aimed at building positive mental health, most community-wide campaigns have been aimed at early detection and treatment of mental problems and de-stigmatisation of mental illness (Saxena and Garrison, 2004). The Western Australia 'Act-Belong-Commit' campaign is one of the few positive community-wide mental health promotion campaigns in the world. The principles behind it are as applicable to use in one-to-one clinical practice as they are for public health.

The Act-Belong-Commit (ABC) approach to mental health promotion

The *Act-Belong-Commit Mentally Healthy WA* campaign is a community-wide intervention, developed from qualitative and quantitative research, that encourages individuals to be proactive about their mental health. The public health aspect of the campaign also targets appropriate 'partner' organisations to promote their activities as beneficial to mental health. The ABC message provides a simple mnemonic of concepts that are relevant at the clinical and public health levels.

The primary objective for the ABC campaign is to reframe individual perceptions of mental health away from simply the *absence* of mental *illness* to the belief that an individual can (and should) act proactively to protect and strengthen his or her mental health.

Participants in formative research identified a number of factors that impact on mental health, ranging from economic and sociocultural factors to individual personality and lifestyle factors. These include: unemployment or job insecurity; early childhood experiences and coercive parenting; exposure to violence, alcohol and drug abuse; and being subject to discrimination (on the basis of race, age, gender, sexual orientation or disability).

A number of factors were seen to increase resilience and ability to cope with stressors, including: positive parenting; educational and workplace practices; having access to good support networks; good self-esteem; and feelings of self-efficacy. There was near-universal agreement that keeping oneself active (physically, socially and mentally), having good friends, being a member of various groups in the community, and feeling in control of one's circumstances were necessary for good mental health.

There was also widespread agreement that having opportunities for achievable challenges—at home, school or work, or in hobbies, sports or the arts—were important for a positive sense of self.

Helping others (e.g. volunteering, coaching, mentoring) was also frequently mentioned as a source of satisfaction, as well as providing a source of activity and involvement with others. These factors are similar to those identified by experts and listed in Tables 14.2 and 14.3.

The *Mentally Healthy WA* campaign has two themes, one encouraging individuals to be more proactive about their own mental health and one helping individuals in authority over others to be more aware of their impact on mental health. The former encourages individuals to engage in activities that would enhance their mental health (e.g. social, arts and sporting organisation membership; community involvement; physical and mental activities; family socialising; hobbies) and simultaneously encourages community organisations offering such activities to promote their activities under a mental health benefit message. The latter focuses on interactions between those in authority and those under their charge or care (e.g. supervisors and their workers; parents and their children; teachers and their students; coaches and their trainees; service personnel and customers), with the aim of replacing coercive, negative styles with encouraging, positive styles.

The ABC slogan is a simple message. The three verbs 'act', 'belong' and 'commit' were chosen not only because they provide an ABC but because they represent three major domains of factors that both the research literature and people in general consider contribute to good mental health (Donovan et al. 2003; Donovan et al., 2007). A summary of suitable actions is shown in Table 14.4.

TABLE 14.4 The ABC for good mental health

ACT	Maintain or increase levels of physical activity (e.g. walk, garden, dance), cognitive activity (e.g. read, do crossword puzzles, study) and social activity (e.g. say hello to neighbours, chat to shopkeepers, maintain contacts with friends).
BELONG	Maintain or increase level of participation in groups if already a member or join a group. Maintain or increase participation in community events and with family and friends.
COMMIT	Take up a cause or challenge (e.g. volunteer for a good cause, learn a new and challenging skill).

For example, a person can ACT by reading a book; BELONG by joining a book club; and COMMIT by becoming the secretary/organiser for the book club or by occasionally reading challenging books rather than just 'pulp fiction'.

These three domains may also be viewed as a hierarchy of increasing contribution to an individual's sense of self and mental health.

Act

'Act' suggests that individuals strive to keep themselves physically, socially and cognitively active. This is supported by evidence from a variety of sources indicating that individuals with higher levels of physical, cognitive and/or social activity have higher levels of wellbeing and mental health and that such activities can alleviate mental problems such as anxiety and depression (Dunn et al., 2005; Saxena et al., 2005). At the basic physical and cognitive levels, individuals can be encouraged to take a walk, read a book, do a crossword puzzle, garden, take a correspondence course, visit a museum, and so on. At a basic social level, individuals are encouraged to interact with salespeople while shopping, talk to their neighbours, and maintain contact with family and friends. Actions at this level are encompassed under Seligman's pleasant life. They can improve an individual's mental coping capacity but alone are unlikely to lead to 'bliss point' satisfaction.

Belong

'Belong' refers to being a member of a group or organisation (whether face to face, formal or informal) in order to strengthen an individual's connectedness with the community and sense of identity. Many activities can be done alone or as a member of a group (e.g. reading a book vs. joining a book club; going for a walk alone or joining a walking group; playing solitaire or playing bridge). In some cases, there are synergistic effects: belonging to a book club not only adds a connectedness dimension but is likely to expand the cognitive activity involved; joining a walking group can expand the physical activity while adding a social dimension.

Regular involvement in social activities, whether via hobby groups, professional interest groups, family or friends, is likely to result in a strong personal support group, one of the most important factors for maintaining mental (and physical) health (Kawachi and Berkman, 2001). Involvement in local community activities and organisations builds social cohesion (or social capital), which is also important for individual mental health (Fullilove, 1998; Ziersch, 2005). Overall, the more an individual is active within the context of connectedness, the greater the contribution to mental health and the greater the availability of assistance in coping with the vicissitudes of life and threats to mental health (WHO, 2004).

Belonging implies the engaged life proposed by Seligman.

Commit

'Commit' refers to the extent to which an individual becomes involved with (or commits to) some activity or organisation. Commitment provides a sense of purpose and meaning to one's life, which some researchers claim is the single most important factor contributing to life satisfaction/wellbeing (Headey and Wearing, 1992). Commitment can be to a cause or organisation that benefits the group or wider community or can be to the achievement of some personal goal.

Meeting challenges provides a sense of accomplishment, feelings of efficacy and a stronger sense of self (Csikszentmihalyi, 1990). Religious belief is an obvious form of commitment, but meaning can be obtained from short-term as well as long-term commitment to an ideal, as pointed out by Victor Frankl in developing 'Logotherapy' while incarcerated in a Nazi concentration camp. The WA health promotion ad *Feeling Blue? Act Green* (Figure 14.1), aimed at increasing interest in nature, captures the notion of joint rewards from physical activity.

Volunteering and undertaking activities to benefit the community at large, especially where these involve the disadvantaged, have special returns for feeling good about oneself and overall mental health benefits, particularly in the retired elderly (Vaananen et al., 2005). Volunteering and greater participation in community activities and organisations also have substantial implications for community cohesion and social capital and hence quality of life (ESRC, 2004).

FIGURE 14.1 Feeling blue? Act green!

Feeling **blue?** Act **green!**

It seems that watching wildlife shows, exploring parks and gardens, looking at fabulous mountain and ocean views, and getting away from it all to the bush and Pacific island beaches are not only pleasurable, but are actually good for us!

Eminent biologists, psychologists and health professionals are showing that contact with nature – whether through parks, natural bush, pets or farm animals – helps us recover from stress and mental fatigue, helps us relax and puts us in a good frame of mind.

Of course, most of us know this intuitively and it's probably why we are drawn to nature instinctively. We all know that a walk on the beach, down a bush track or in a park is good to clear the head when we feel a little tired or stressed.

So, next time you are feeling like a lift, 'act green': do some gardening, pet the cat or dog, take a walk around the park or head down to the water for some time out.

Better still, don't wait until you're tired or feeling flat. Act green more often. Being in touch with nature makes us feel good, builds good mental health and helps beat the blues. And it's as easy as A-B-C

Act – do some gardening; take a walk around the local park; watch a wildlife documentary; take time to watch the sun set; spend time with pets ...

Belong – get a group together for a picnic in a natural setting; visit a wildlife sanctuary with friends; join a hiking group ...

Commit – become a 'civic environmentalist'; join a tree planting group; volunteer to keep your local parks & gardens clean; take up orienteering; learn more about ecology; offer to take a home-bound person out to a park ...

Being active, having a sense of belonging, and having a purpose in life all contribute to happiness and good mental health.

If you want to know more, visit www.mentallyhealthywa.org.au Phone Professor Rob Donovan on 9266 4598 or email r.donovan@curtin.edu.au

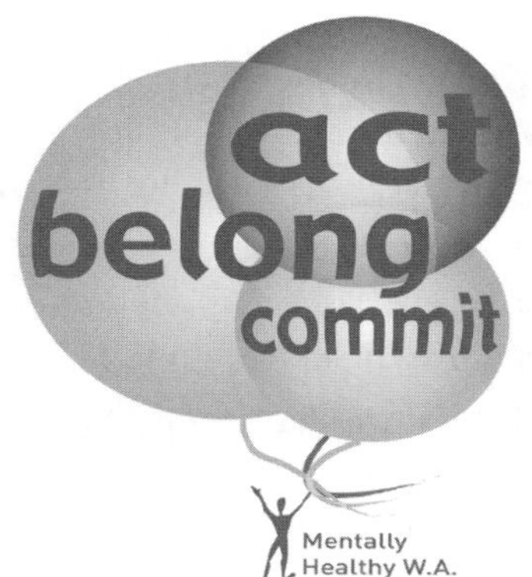

www.mentallyhealthywa.org.au

Health professional goals

The health professional's main aims should be to:

- increase patients' understanding that maintaining good mental health is just as important as maintaining good physical health;
- increase patients' salience that there are things that they can and should do to build and maintain good mental health (summarised under the ABC framework); and
- encourage patients to take up ABC activities where they appear to lack 'sufficient' participation.

While there are no agreed levels for what is considered sufficient, our view is that areas of deficiency would be clearly noticeable and provide clear indications for areas of increase.

What can be done in a standard consultation

Explain the ABC acronym.

Go through each in detail (see *Professional resources*).

Check on hobbies, interests and commitments and suggest possibilities.

Get patients to check signature strengths and other procedures from the website www.authentichappiness.com.

Suggest 'happiness' reading material.

Other indications would be provided by a patient's symptoms. For example, the following kinds of patients could benefit from the various elements within the ABC framework: those showing signs of mild to moderate depression or diffuse anxiety; those expressing feelings of excess stress or an inability to relax; those feeling bored or expressing a lack of energy or enthusiasm for general activities; and those lacking social support. However, all patients can benefit from an increased awareness of how they can strengthen and maintain good mental health.

Applying the procedure involves three steps:

1. Establishing to what extent the patient is physically, mentally and socially active (more severe cases may need to be referred or managed more intensively). This may involve the exhortation to 'just do it'.
2. Establishing to what extent the patient is an active member of groups and actively participates in community activities or events, and discussing possibilities for doing this where this may be appropriate.
3. Establishing to what extent the patient engages in activities, hobbies or interests that provide purpose and meaning in his or her life. Considering an individual's interests and philosophical bent can help in providing assistance in this direction.

The questioning style outlined in Table 14.5 is a useful starting point.

TABLE 14.5 A useful questioning style

Act	How often do you do something physically active that requires some effort, such as walking, gardening, dancing, golfing or playing other sports? How often do you do something requiring some mental activity, such as reading, learning something new, doing crosswords or playing card games that require you to concentrate? How often do you have contact with other people where you stop for a chat or talk on the phone?
Belong	Do you belong to any groups, clubs or organisations, formal or informal? How often do you meet or interact with other group members? Do you hold any office or position in any of those groups? What does that involve?
Commit	Are you a volunteer for any charitable organisation or cause? What does that involve? How often do you do that? When was the last time you took on a challenge in which you had to work hard to achieve and you felt a great sense of satisfaction by doing what you did? Are you doing anything challenging at the moment? (Some indication of commitment may have already been identified through membership and office holding under 'Belong' and via challenging activities under 'Act'.)

Analysing and identifying activities

Some patients may have 'social overload' through their jobs or family commitments but still not get enough physical or mental activity; others may get plenty of mental stimulation but make little time for socialising or physical activity; still others may be active individually but appear socially isolated; and some may have few or no real commitments to causes or challenges.

If an individual is lacking in all three areas, the aim would be to get him or her to join some group activity that involves physical and/or mental activity along with the group membership. The first step would be to establish the activities he or she might like doing and then provide a contact name (preferably) or organisation providing such activities. Uncovering past hobbies, activities and interests is a step to identifying possible interests. If the patient is too shy to personally make contact, try to provide a contact name.

Similar principles apply to increasing levels for ABC involvements where they are deemed deficient. An important step is to identify activities he or she may be interested in and capable of doing. Older people are quite receptive to the mental and physical benefits of increasing their levels of mental and physical activity and appreciate the sense of satisfaction from volunteering. Younger persons may be more interested in participating in activities requiring some challenge and learning new things. For the 'Commit' component, depending on time and other commitments, people can be encouraged to look at their local TAFE or other skills providers, whether for a qualification certificate or simply personal development. This can provide cognitive and social activity as well as building self-esteem through achievements.

Minimal social activity can be maintained by something as simple as encouraging patients to say hello to neighbours and shopping/service personnel and by maintaining contacts with friends and family, whether in person (preferably) or via telephone or email.

Most local governments have listings of community sporting, recreational and service organisations that can be given to patients. There is a wide variety of activities that can be done alone or as a member of a group, and there are many groups that can benefit from people with time on their hands.

The Act-Belong-Commit website has additional information and resources (www.actbelongcommit.org.au).

practice tips

PRACTICE TIPS: ENCOURAGING HAPPINESS

	Medical practitioner	**Practice nurse**
Assess	Presence of mild depression. Level of ABC. Physical and mental activities. Social contacts. Your own 'happiness' status.	Details of ABC. Belonging to 'causes'. Time available and commitment (overload or underload). Your own 'happiness' status.
Assist	By providing medication for risk if appropriate. By providing a website for checking on signature strengths. By discussing actions from signature strengths. By suggesting appropriate reading materials.	By providing a list of available organisations. By checking places for volunteering. By suggesting options for daily actions (e.g. counting blessings). By providing reading materials.
Arrange	Contact with psychologists who work in positive psychology. Access to self-help websites.	A relationship with a psychologist to enhance happiness. Contact with self-help groups.

key points

KEY POINTS FOR CLINICAL MANAGEMENT

- Consider mental health and not just mental illness.
- Regard everyone as a potential target for good mental health.
- Practice good personal mental health tactics.
- Encourage the patient to do personal research (reading, searching websites).

references

REFERENCES

Australian Government Department of Health and Aged Care. (2000) *Promotion, prevention and early intervention for mental health—a monograph.* Canberra: Mental Health and Special Programs Branch, Department of Health and Aged Care.

Belliotti R. (2004) *Happiness is overrated.* Maryland: Rowman and Littlefield Publishers Inc.

Csikszentmihalyi M. (1990) *Flow: the psychology of optimal experience.* NY: Harper Perennial.

Donovan R, Henley, N, Jalleh, G et al. (2007). People's beliefs about factors contributing to mental health: implications for mental health promotion. *Health Promotion Journal of Australia* 18(1): 50–56.

Donovan RJ, James R, Jalleh G et al. (2006) Implementing mental health promotion: the 'Act-Belong-Commit' Mentally Healthy WA campaign in Western Australia. *International Journal of Mental Health Promotion* 8(1): 29–38.

Donovan RJ, Watson N, Henley N et al. (2003) *Report to Healthway: mental health promotion scoping project.* Curtin University, Centre for Developmental Health: Perth, WA.

Dunn AL, Trivedi MH, Kampert JB et al. (2005) Exercise treatment for depression: efficacy and dose response. *American Journal of Preventive Medicine* 28(1): 1–8.

Eckersley R. (2004) *Well & good.* The Text Publishing Company: Melbourne.

ESRC (Economic Research Council). (2004) *The art of happiness . . . is volunteering the blueprint for bliss?* ESRC Press Release. Available from www.esrc.ac.uk/esrccontent/news/september04-2.asp.

Fullilove MT. (1998) Promoting social cohesion to improve health. *Journal of American Medical Women's Association* 53(2): 72–76.

Heady B, Wearing A. (1992) *Understanding happiness: a theory of subjective well-being.* Longman Cheshire: Melbourne.

Heady B, Wooden M. (2004) The effects of wealth and income on subjective well-being and ill-being. *Economic Record* 80: S24–33.

Kawachi I, Berkman LF. (2001) Social ties and mental health. *Journal of Urban Health: Bulletin of the New York Academy of Medicine* 78(3): 458–67.

Layard R. (2005) *Happiness: lessons from a new science.* London: Penguin.

McMahon DM. (2006) *Happiness: a history.* NY: Grove Press.

Pearson C, Seligman M. (2004) *Character strengths and virtues.* USA: Oxford University Press.

Saxena S, Garrison PJ. (2004) *Mental health promotion: case studies from countries.* Geneva: World Health Organization and World Federation for Mental Health.

Saxena S, Ommeren MV, Tang KC et al. (2005) Mental health benefits of physical activity. *Journal of Mental Health* 14(5): 445–51.

Schock R. (2006) *The secrets of happiness.* London: Profile Books.

Seligman M. (1976) *Learned helplessness*.

Vaananen A, Buunk BP, Kivimaki M et al. (2005) When it is better to give than to receive: long-term health effects of perceived reciprocity in support exchange. *Journal of Personality and Social Psychlogy* 89(2): 176–93.

Vaillant, G. (1996) *Adaptation to life,* 2nd edn. London: Harvard University Press.

Warr P. (1994) A conceptual framework for the study of work and mental health. *Work and Stress* 8(2): 84–97.

——. (2004) *Prevention of mental disorders: effective interventions and policy options*. *A report of the WHO and the Prevention Research Centre, Universities of Nijmegen and Maastricht.* Geneva: WHO.

World Health Organization. (2001) *Strengthening mental health promotion.* World Health Organization (Fact Sheet no. 220). Geneva: WHO.

Ziersch AM. (2005) Health implications of access to social capital: findings from an Australian study. *Social Science & Medicine* 6(1): 2119–31.

CHAPTER 15

Understanding addictions: tackling smoking and hazardous drinking

JOHN LITT, GARRY EGGER

> *Addiction must be viewed at the outset as a personal problem rather than a chemical problem. To discuss the alcohol problem, the heroin problem or the marijuana problem makes as much sense as discussing suicide as the hanging problem, the wrist slashing problem and the bridge jumping problem.*
>
> UNKNOWN

Introduction to smoking

Smoking is the largest single preventable cause of death and disease in Australia, with an estimated 19 000 deaths and 142 500 hospital admissions per year.

In developed countries, smoking is estimated to cause 87% of lung cancer deaths, 82% of emphysema deaths, 40% of heart disease deaths among people under 65 years old, 21% of all heart attack deaths, 33% of all cancers and 10% of all infant deaths. No other single avoidable factor accounts for such a high proportion of deaths, hospital admissions or GP consultations.

Lifelong smokers have a 50–60% chance of dying from a tobacco-related disease and more than half of these deaths will occur in middle age (25–54 years) (Fagerstrom, 2002). The non-voluntary and social costs of smoking are vast, totalling at least $AUD21 billion in Australia in 1998–99. While the Australian government collects

$5.2 billion in tobacco excise, a net deficit of $15.8 billion remains (the health effects of smoking and the benefits of quitting are summarised in a poster developed for primary care workers, available from www.quitsa.org.au/cms_resources/documents/resource_ doctorsposter.pdf.)

Despite the enormous impact of smoking on ill health and disease, in the early 1990s one in four men and one in five women continued to smoke. The prevalence of smoking in Australia has nearly halved in the last twenty years from 35% to approximately 19% of the population (AIHW, 2002). This mirrors a similar trend in other western countries. Significant declines in Australian smoking rates have been seen for males but less so for females. In the 15–29 age group, a third of women and 40% of men smoke. In the subsequent ten years, the prevalence decline to 25% in men and women 18–24 years and 29% in men and 24% in women 25–34 years (AIHW, 2005).

Just over half the people who smoke are seriously thinking about quitting in the next six months and nearly half of all smokers have made a quit attempt in the last twelve months. However, only a minority of these will achieve permanent abstinence: the majority will cycle through periods of relapse and remission. Quitting smoking is associated with immediate and long-term health benefits.

Introduction to alcohol

Hazardous alcohol consumption is associated with considerable morbidity and mortality. An estimated 31 132 Australians (23 431 or 75% males; 7 703 or 25% females) died from risky and high-risk alcohol use in the ten-year period 1992–2001. The leading cause of death was alcohol-related liver disease, followed by road crash injury, cancer and suicide. These types of deaths reflect a pattern of drinking to intoxication, with more people dying from the acute rather than the chronic effects of alcohol. Deaths from acute effects of alcohol were more common among younger age people (15–29 years) whereas, perhaps not unexpectedly, deaths from chronic effects of alcohol were more common among older people (45 years and over) (AIHW, 2004).

Alcohol is a major contributor to the global burden of disease. Apart from cardiovascular disease, morbidity shows a dose–response relationship with the amount of alcohol consumed. Up to 10% of cancers, 20% of intentional injuries and 7% of all deaths can be attributed to alcohol. Heavy drinking increases the risk of high blood pressure, stroke, unintentional injuries and cancer. It is also implicated in a significant number of hospital admissions and imposes a significant cost burden on society. While moderate consumption of alcohol has been associated with some benefits, especially a lower incidence of cardiovascular events and cardiac-related deaths and (in some studies) reduced all-cause mortality, heavier consumption has been consistently associated with poorer quality of life and increased mortality. The effects of high-risk drinking on the body are shown in Figure 15.1.

Hazardous drinking contributes substantially to social morbidity, where it is associated with many criminal activities, accidents and violence (Ezzati et al., 2002). In Australia, the estimated direct and indirect costs of this alcohol-related morbidity is $8.18 billion each year, which is consistent with estimated costs for other developed countries. A recent review found that offering evidence-based treatment to people with alcohol use disorders would produce a significant population health gain.

FIGURE 15.1 Effects of high-risk drinking on the body

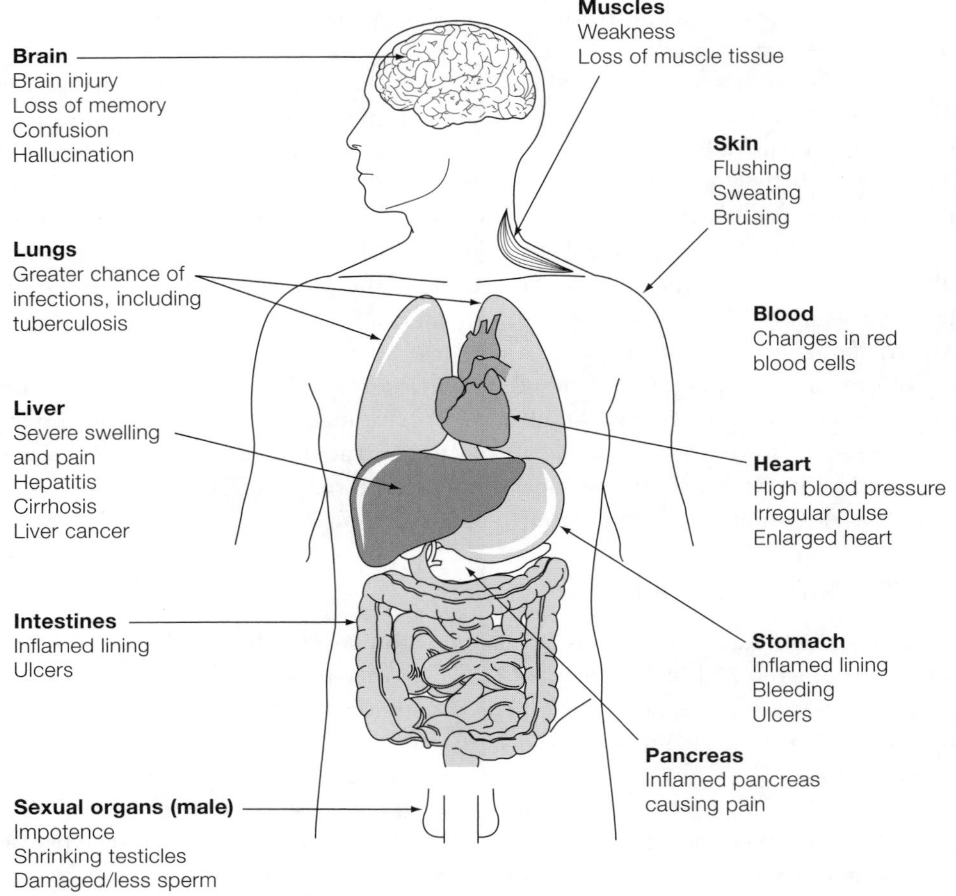

Source: Babor et al., 2001; Australian Government Department of Veterans' Affairs (available from www.dva.gov.au/health/menshealth/images/10_pills_potions_alco.gif)

Although the likelihood of adverse consequences and the risk to health is directly related to the level of alcohol consumption, it is the large number of binge drinkers and moderate to heavy drinkers that accounts for most of the morbidity and mortality. This so-called prevention paradox strengthens the case for addressing consumption in the general population and not just in those with more advanced alcohol-related problems.

Levels of hazardous drinking vary with the definition. In many populations, there is also a considerable opportunity for intervention because hazardous use is common (10–15%) in the population and people with hazardous levels of consumption make more frequent visits to the GP. In a typical United Kingdom general practice, at least 5% of patients will be drinking at a harmful level, 2% will have an alcohol-related problem and nearly 1% will be dependent upon alcohol (Paton et al., 1982). Others studies have found similar patterns in two different Australian general practice settings (Murtagh, 1987; Redman et al., 1987).

Why is addressing smoking and drinking so difficult?

There are a number of reasons why addressing smoking and drinking in the consultation room can be difficult, including factors specific to the patient, barriers for the clinician and aspects of the practice setting.

Patient factors

Both smoking and drinking are social activities that provide both enjoyment and a way for many people to reduce stress and put them at ease. These are potent influences on maintaining both habits.

MANY ARE NOT ASKED ABOUT THEIR DRINKING

Less than a third of patients in general practice are asked about their drinking (Litt, 2007). Men are more likely to be asked about their drinking than women.

LACK OF KNOWLEDGE OF THE HEALTH EFFECTS FROM AND BENEFITS OF TREATMENT

Most studies report that patients are aware of the main risks of smoking to their health. Nevertheless, according to Yong et al. (2005) smokers, when contrasted with ex-smokers, are more likely to:

- have less health-related knowledge about the effects of smoking;
- express less concern about the health effects of smoking;
- downplay the health-related risks of smoking;
- report greater potential for harm from nicotine medications than nicotine in cigarettes;
- be less aware of effective treatment strategies for quitting; and
- be overly optimistic about their ability to quit at any time.

Lack of awareness of the effectiveness of a number of treatments is also a barrier for both smokers and hazardous drinkers.

LACK OF CONCERN

Many heavy drinkers view their consumption as moderate and not harmful. This may contribute to the mixed perceptions that individuals have about both the role and effectiveness of GPs in assisting them to cut down on their drinking. Prevention activities or health-related behaviours are also influenced by patients' perceptions of their susceptibility to or risk of contracting a lifestyle-related disease and whether they believe that the behaviour in question is harmful to their health (Cunningham et al., 2005). In a US national household survey, only 8% of women with untreated alcohol dependence perceived a need for treatment (Wu and Ringwalt, 2004). In the National Survey of Mental Health and Well-being in Australia, only 9.2% of men and 16.2% of women with alcohol dependence sought treatment in a twelve-month period (Teeson et al., 2006).

SENSITIVITY OF THE TOPIC

Many patients find discussing their smoking or drinking habits a sensitive issue. The negative stereotyping associated with a health-related behaviour or illness can affect the likelihood that patients seek help or assistance.

UNDERESTIMATING THE DIFFICULTY ASSOCIATED WITH CHANGING BEHAVIOUR

For smokers and hazardous drinkers, a significant barrier to making changes is the perception that they may be able to sort the problem out themselves without seeking help, if they really wish to.

Many health-related behaviours are difficult to change. For smokers, there are a large number of barriers that make it difficult to quit. Barriers to quitting smoking also influence patients' preparedness to seek help. These include:

- addiction to nicotine;
- perceived difficulty of quitting;
- fear of weight gain;
- concerns about dealing with stress;
- lack of support; and
- presence of other smokers in the household.

RELUCTANCE TO SEEK HELP

Less than a third of smokers ask their GP to help them quit and a minority of smokers call the National Tobacco Campaign's Quitline. Hazardous drinkers, similarly, find it difficult to cut back. The barriers to doing this include:

- physical dependence on alcohol;
- lack of support;
- difficulty coping with stress and using alcohol as a coping strategy;
- stigmatisation associated with the label of problem drinker;
- reluctance to seek help, especially from medical sources; and
- lack of self-efficacy.

A number of smokers report a sense of fatalism or a feeling that it is too late to do something. Nevertheless, most smokers are interested in quitting and up to 70% of smokers have made at least one attempt to quit.

Clinician barriers

Table 15.1 highlights the perceived advantages and disadvantages associated with the individual versus the practice population approach to delivering preventive care, including lifestyle assessment and counselling.

KNOWLEDGE

Clinicians' knowledge of the guidelines for low-risk levels of drinking is variable. Similarly, there is a wide spectrum of clinician awareness of effective behavioural interventions for unhealthy lifestyles.

ATTITUDES AND BELIEFS

Many clinicians are pessimistic about their effectiveness in facilitating behaviour change in patients who smoke or who drink at hazardous levels, despite good evidence to the contrary.

TABLE 15.1 GP-reported perceived advantages and disadvantages to the individual patient with the practice population approach

	Potential benefits and advantages	Costs
Systematic practice population approach	improved provision of effective preventive care (e.g. smoking) improved quality of care improved health outcomes promotes equity and reduces disadvantage additional clinical income from increased provision of preventive services improved patient safety	additional work and responsibility variable perceptions about effectiveness not enough time not rewarded financially patients may be offended/not interested extra expectations and work not worthwhile/not valued by peers
Haphazard approach (status quo)	'if it ain't broke, don't fix it'—a prevailing culture that is both familiar and personal perceived effectiveness perceived efficiency (i.e. providing care to those who need it) individual, patient focused	variable effectiveness of delivery ranging from good (e.g. BP) to poor (e.g. asking about drinking habits, adult immunisation) poorer health outcomes ad hoc networks, variable communication channels, referrals and collaboration reactive care often fails to identify those who either need or want prevention

SKILLS AND PRACTICES

Research has shown that GPs less frequently than desired:

- refer smokers to a Quitline service;
- arrange a follow-up visit to review patient progress with quitting; or
- prescribe some form of nicotine replacement therapy.

All three strategies are associated with higher quit rates. Similarly, GPs under-utilise effective strategies with hazardous drinkers, including routine enquiry and brief non-judgmental advice. GPs' own health practices can also influence their likelihood of providing lifestyle counselling. GPs who smoke, do little exercise, or eat a less healthy diet are less likely to counsel about these areas.

Practice setting

LACK OF TIME

Lack of time is a major barrier to the effective delivery of prevention. Most prevention activities, including counselling, is provided opportunistically. The disposable time available to tackle issues on the clinician's agenda, after dealing with the reasons that the patient has come to the doctor, is generally 60–90 seconds. This limits the nature and extent of the counselling that can be provided. It has also stimulated the move to think about how this limited time can be used more effectively and efficiently (Litt, 2005; RACGP, 2006).

LACK OF ORGANISATIONAL INFRASTRUCTURE

The most successful lifestyle implementation strategies use the skills of the entire healthcare team and the practice infrastructure to provide timely, pertinent information during a medical visit and subsequently (RACGP, 2006).

A supportive organisational infrastructure includes:

- practice policies (e.g. standing orders, protocols and procedures);
- clarification of roles and responsibilities;
- accessible, evidence-based guidelines;
- availability and use of appropriate resources (e.g. practice nurses);
- multifaceted delivery options (e.g. delegation to a practice nurse, use of multidisciplinary clinics and group sessions, appropriate referral to groups or agencies);
- information management and information technology systems (e.g. practice registers of age, sex and disease; recall and reminder systems; health summaries);
- waiting room materials (e.g. posters and pamphlets with patient education and information material);
- screening and information gathering materials and strategies (e.g. patient questionnaires, inventory of practice prevention, clinical audit); and
- consultation materials (e.g. decision aids, computer decision support systems, patient education and information material).

The barriers discussed above contribute to the reluctance of clinicians to be involved both in screening for alcohol consumption and associated risks and problems and in providing brief intervention.

What works?

Smoking cessation guidelines

Smoking status should be assessed for every patient over ten years of age. Patients who smoke, regardless of the amount they smoke, should be offered regular brief advice to stop smoking (Zwar et al., 2004).

Alcohol guidelines

All patients from fourteen years of age should be asked about the quantity and frequency of alcohol intake and number of alcohol-free days each week. Those with at-risk patterns of alcohol consumption should be offered brief advice to reduce their intake (RACGP, 2004; Whitlock et al., 2004). The risk of harm associated with drinking in the short term is shown in Table 15.2.

TABLE 15.2 Australian alcohol guidelines for short-term drinking and the level of risk to health for males and females of average or larger body size (e.g. over 160 cm in height and 50 kg in women, 60 kg for men)

	Risk of harm in the short term		
	low risk (standard drinks)	**risky (standard drinks)**	**high risk (standard drinks)**
males	≤6 on any one day, no more than three days per week	7–10 on any one day	≥11 on any one day
females	≤4 on any one day, no more than three days per week	5–6 on any one day	≥7 on any one day

A standard drink contains 10 g of alcohol, which is the equivalent of 12.5 mL of alcohol
Source: NHMRC, 2001

An acronym for treatment: the five A's

GPs are a credible, authoritative, effective and cost-effective source of smoking cessation advice. The key components of brief interventions for smoking cessation and assisting hazardous drinkers are the five A's: ask, assess, advise, assist and arrange (or, for better recall, the three A's used throughout this book: assess, assist and arrange). Table 15.3 outlines the key components of this approach for drinking (more detail for smoking is given in *Professional resources*). This brief intervention takes into account the time available for counselling and takes only five minutes.

TABLE 15.3 The three A's and alcohol: a brief alcohol intervention

Ask	About current patterns of consumption (e.g. waiting room checklist).
Assess	Stage of change (see Chapter 3) and level of risk (e.g. AUDIT; see *Professional resources*).
Assist	By assessing the pros and cons of current patterns of use. By using motivational interviewing techniques. By considering referral. By considering drug treatment for cravings or dependence (e.g. acamprosate).
Advise	On safe drinking guidelines and ways to cut down. By giving feedback on current level of drinking. By discussing barriers to cutting down. By negotiating and setting realistic goals.
Arrange	Follow up in 2–4 weeks.

Source: National Centre for Education and Training on Addiction (NCETA) Consortium, 2004; RACGP, 2004

The first step is to adopt a systematic approach to the identification of patients who drink hazardously or who smoke. Patient surveys in the waiting room can help to identify these groups (RACGP, 2006).

Raising the issue

The next step is to raise the issue of patients' smoking or drinking in a sensitive manner. Practical tips from Litt (2005) for minimising the likelihood of confrontation and aggravation include:

- normalising the enquiry (ask all your patients and provide a context for asking);
- avoiding making a judgment prematurely. Premature advice or attempting to 'close the loop' too soon is likely to be met with resistance.
- providing the patient with time and space to work through the consequences of the information. Seeing a connection between a behaviour and health consequences is a necessary first step in the change process. Just because the doctor regards it as a problem does not mean the patient does. Acceptance and preparedness to change takes time.
- understanding the patients' perspective. Ask how they feel about their behaviour. What do they get out of it? What are the benefits? Acknowledge that changing behaviour is difficult.

- maintaining rapport/therapeutic alliance by working with the patient. Ensuring agreement on what the problem is and respecting the patient's autonomy both facilitates the communication process and improves the likelihood of success.
- leaving the door open. Patients see their GP five to six times a year. The next consultation could provide an opportunity to follow up where you left off.
- assessing the patient's interest and confidence in changing (e.g. quitting smoking, cutting down on drinking), using motivational interviewing techniques (Litt, 2005; Rollnick et al., 1999). Explore the patient's perceptions of any costs and the perceived benefits of cutting down on drinking or quitting smoking.
- assessing dependence on nicotine or alcohol. Time to first cigarette (less than one hour) and smoking more than fifteen cigarettes a day are associated with nicotine dependence. Alcohol dependence can be assessed using AUDIT or the CAGE questionnaire (see *Professional resources*).CAGE should be used after assessing consumption, not as a substitute for it. AUDIT is considered the instrument of choice.

Assess whether the patient's alcohol intake is risky. A useful acronym to highlight the areas of enquiry is LIMPED:

Legal problems (e.g. driving under the influence of alcohol, assaults)

Injury (e.g. any trauma or motor vehicle accidents). Alcohol contributes to:

- 20% of all injuries
- 33% of falls and drownings
- 30% of MVAs
- 12.5% of suicides

Medical problems. Patients drinking more than the NHMRC recommended levels long term are more likely to have a range of medical problems. These include a range of cancers (lip, mouth, throat, oesophagus, stomach, pancreas, liver); fatty change (hepatic steatosis) and inflammation (steatohepatitis) of the liver; cirrhosis of the liver; brain insult/injury, including cognitive problems, dementia and Wernicke-Korsakoff syndrome; increased risk of cardiovascular diseases (hypertension, haemorrhagic stroke, ischaemic stroke, heart failure, cardiomyopathy); peripheral neuropathy (limb muscle weakness); and male sexual impotence.

Psychological and psychiatric problems (e.g. anxiety, depression, sleeping difficulties). Heavy drinking can also aggravate symptoms in people with milder degrees of anxiety and depression. While alcohol consumption may bring some short-term relief from anxiety or stress, it tends to worsen mood in the longer term, especially at higher levels of consumption.

Employment problems (e.g. fall off in work performance, accidents). Alcohol contributes to 10% of industrial accidents; 13% of all employees on sick leave have alcohol problems.

Domestic problems (e.g. relationship difficulties, violence, financial worries). Forty to fifty per cent of all incidents involving aggression occur while under the influence of alcohol.

If patients acknowledge that any of these issues may be relevant, ask about whether they (or others) have concerns about this. It is also useful to assess the barriers to change and high-risk situations. Many of these are listed above.

Making changes

Providing clear, actionable advice with an explanation of the mechanisms of cause can help. Table 15.4 provides some examples.

TABLE 15.4 Clear, actionable advice and explanations for people wanting to change their alcohol or cigarette use

For drinking	The level of alcohol you are consuming is probably contributing to your stomach pain. Alcohol increases the production of acid in the stomach and helps to weaken the protective layer of mucus lining the stomach. Both these effects are contributing to your gastritis.
For smoking	When you smoke around your children, the tobacco smoke tends to weaken the cilia in the respiratory tract. The cilia are like little vacuum cleaners that help to mop up dust and infective agents (bacteria and viruses) and remove them from the respiratory tract. Children exposed to environmental tobacco smoke are more prone to respiratory infections and meningococcal meningitis (they are for to six times more likely to get it) and have more episodes of asthma.

The goals for change should be both incremental and realistic. This is more challenging for smoking, where quitting is the only option. Cutting down is often associated with a change in the patient's inhalation pattern to redress the declining nicotine levels. For many hazardous drinkers, cutting down is a reasonable end-point. Abstinence is more appropriate if there is evidence of alcohol dependence or other physical or mental impairment from alcohol use.

Behavioural self-management training can be used to foster self-management strategies in the patient who is drinking heavily. Strategies include: self-monitoring (e.g. using a drink diary); setting drinking limits; controlling rates of drinking; identifying high-risk drinking situations; and identifying rewards for limiting drinking.

Pharmacotherapy

Pharmacotherapy is useful for patients who are dependent upon either nicotine or alcohol. Nicotine replacement therapies (NRT) are very effective when there is nicotine dependence. Remember that most of the NRTs contain less nicotine than the patient generally smokes. Occasional patients may need two forms of NRT, for example, a nicotine patch to provide basal levels of nicotine and a nicotine lozenge to deal with early morning cravings.

For patients dependent on alcohol, acamprosate (which blocks glutamate receptors and activates GABA receptors) and naltrexone (an opioid receptor antagonist) are useful agents. Both can be used to reduce cravings and increase the likelihood of the patient remaining abstinent. Acamprosate also reduces relapse rates, has no significant drug interactions and has fewer side effects than naltrexone. Naltrexone has the advantage of once daily dosing and a fairly rapid onset. The disadvantages are the blocking of opioid analgesia and the numerous drug interactions. Unfortunately, patient adherence with both medications is relatively low.

All patients who receive some assistance with quitting or cutting down should be followed up. Follow-up significantly increases the likelihood of a patient quitting or cutting down on their drinking.

What stimulates change?

The most commonly given reasons for change are concerns about health, money and relationships (Cunningham et al., 2005). For smokers, health-related concerns top the list of factors that stimulate the need to quit (McCaul et al., 2006; Yong et al., 2005).

While patient motivation is a strong predictor of treatment outcomes in patients who drink at hazardous levels, many hazardous drinkers express little interest in cutting down and some are only prepared to cut down when they hit 'rock bottom'.

practice tips

PRACTICE TIPS: QUITTING SMOKING, DECREASING ALCOHOL

	Medical practitioner	**Practice nurse**
Assess	Smoking and drinking, in a sensitive manner. Possible health effects from smoking/drinking. Alcohol dependence. Whether alcohol intake is risky (e.g. with LIMPED).	Smoking and drinking: provide *Lifescripts* questionnaires in waiting room; administer AUDIT or CAGE questionnaires (see *Professional resources*).
Assist	By providing clear, non-judgmental advice. By providing feedback on the impact of a patient's drinking or smoking and explaining the mechanisms. By setting realistic and incremental goals. By offering pharmacotherapy where appropriate.	By providing written information about drinking or smoking (e.g. *Lifescripts* information).
Arrange	Referral for behavioural self-management training. Follow-up. Other health professionals for a care plan (e.g. psychologist). Referral to existing programs (e.g. QUIT, AA).	Care plan. Contact with and coordination of other health professionals.

KEY POINTS FOR CLINICAL MANAGEMENT

- Initiate opportunistic discussions of smoking and drinking.
- Be aware of the sensitive nature of enquiries about smoking and alcohol.
- Develop a 'one minute' routine that you can use regularly with most patients.
- Sensitive enquiry about drug and alcohol use coupled with practical and clear advice is very effective and generally improves patient satisfaction.

REFERENCES

Australian Government Department of Veterans; Affairs. (2004) Alcohol Screen. Available at URL: www.therightmix.gov.au/pdfs/AlcoholScreen.pdf.

AIHW (Australian Institute of Health and Welfare). (2005) *2004 National Drug Strategy Household Survey. First results.* Canberra: AIHW.

——. (2004) *A guide to Australian alcohol data.* Canberra: AIHW. Available from www.aihw.gov.au/publications / phe/gaad/gaad.pdf.

——. (2002) *Australia's health 2002.* Canberra: AIHW.

Babor T, Higgins-Biddle J, Saunders J et al. (2001) *AUDIT: the alcohol use disorders identification test, guidelines for use in primary care.* Geneva: WHO.

Cunningham JA, Blomqvist J, Koski-Jannes A et al. (2005) Current heavy drinkers' reasons for considering change: results from a natural history general population survey. *Addict Behav* 30: 581–84.

Ezzati M, Lopez A, Rodgers A et al. (2002) Comparative Risk Assessment Collaborating Group. Selected major risk factors and global and regional burden of disease. *Lancet* 360: 1347–60.

Fagerstrom K. (2002) The epidemiology of smoking. Health consequences and benefits of cessation. *Drugs* 62: 1–9.

Litt J. (2005) Smoking and GPs: time to cough up: successful interventions in general practice. *Aust Fam Physician* 34: 425–29.

Litt JC. (2007) *Exploration of the delivery of prevention in the general practice setting.* PhD thesis. Department of General Practice, Flinders University, Adelaide.

McCaul KD, Hockemeyer JR, Johnson RJ et al. (2006) Motivation to quit using cigarettes: a review. *Addict Behav* 31: 42–56.

NCETA (National Centre for Education and Training on Addiction). Consortium. (2004) *Alcohol and other drugs: a handbook for health professionals.* Canberra: AIHW.

Murtagh J. (1987) Alcohol abuse in an Australian community. *Australian Family Physician* 16: 20–24.

NHMRC (National Health and Medical Research Council). (2001) *Australian alcohol guidelines: health risks and benefits.* Canberra: NHMRC.

Paton A, Potter J, Lewis K. (1982) *Detection in general practice. Alcohol problems.* London: BMJ Publications.

RACGP (Royal Australian College of General Practitioners). (2006) *Putting prevention into practice. Guidelines for the implementation of prevention in the general practice setting.* Melbourne: RACGP.

——. (2004) *SNAP (smoking, nutrition, alcohol and physical activity). A population health guide to behavioural risk factors in general practice.* Melbourne: RACGP.

Redman S, Cockburn J, Reid A et al. (1987) Alcohol consumption and alcohol related problems: prevalence amongst a general practice population. *Aust Drug and Alcohol Rev* 6: 245–52.

Rollnick S, Mason P, Butler C. (1999) *Health behavior change.* Edinburgh: Churchill Livingstone.

Teesson M, Baillie A, Lynskey M et al. (2006) Substance use, dependence and treatment seeking in the United States and Australia: a cross-national comparison. *Drug Alcohol Depend* 81: 149–55.

Whitlock E, Polen M, Green C et al. (2004) Behavioral counseling interventions in primary care to reduce risky/harmful alcohol use by adults: a summary of the evidence for the US Preventive Services Taskforce. *Ann Int Med* 140: 557–68.

Wu L, Ringwalt CL. (2004) Alcohol dependence and use of treatment services among women in the community. *Am J Psychiatry* 161: 1790–97.

Yong H, Borland R, Siahpush M. (2005) Quitting-related beliefs, intentions, and motivations of older smokers in four countries: findings from the International Tobacco Control Policy Evaluation Survey. *Addict Behav* 30: 777–88.

Zwar N, Richmond R, Borland R et al. (2004) *Smoking cessation guidelines for Australian general practice.* Canberra: DoHA.

professional resources

PROFESSIONAL RESOURCE: MEASURING ADDICTION

CAGE questionnaire

In the last 12 months, have you ever felt you **ought** to cut down on your drinking?

- [ ] yes
- [ ] no

In the last 12 months, have people annoyed you by criticising your drinking?

- [ ] yes
- [ ] no

In the last 12 months, have you ever **felt guilty** about your drinking?

- [ ] yes
- [ ] no

In the last 12 months, have you ever **had a drink first thing in the morning** to steady your nerves or to get rid of a hangover?

- [ ] yes
- [ ] no

FIGURE 15.2 Alcohol screen (AUDIT)

Australian Government
Department of Veterans' Affairs

Alcohol Screen (AUDIT)

Light Beer 425ml 2.9% Alcohol	Full Strength Beer 285ml 4.9% Alcohol	Wine 100ml 12% Alcohol	Fortified Wine 60ml 20% Alcohol	Spirits 30ml 40% Alcohol	Full Strength Can or Stubbie 375ml 4.9% Alcohol

The guide above contains examples of ***one standard drink****.* A full strength can or stubbie contains ***one and a half standard drinks****.*

Introduction

Because alcohol use can affect health and interfere with certain medications and treatments, it is important that we ask you some questions about your use of alcohol. Your answers will remain confidential, so please be as accurate as possible. Try to answer the questions in terms of **'standard drinks'**. Please ask for clarification if required.

AUDIT Questions Please tick the response that best fits your drinking.

Question						Score	Sub totals
	Never	*Monthly or less*	*2 - 4 times a month*	*2 - 3 times a week*	*4 or more times a week*		
1. How often do you have a drink containing alcohol?	☐ Go to Qs 9 & 10	☐	☐	☐	☐	☐	
	1 or 2	*3 or 4*	*5 or 6*	*7 to 9*	*10 or more*		
2. How many standard drinks do you have on a typical day when you are drinking?	☐	☐	☐	☐	☐	☐	
	Never	*Less than monthly*	*Monthly*	*Weekly*	*Daily or almost daily*		
3. How often do you have six or more standard drinks on one occasion ?	☐	☐	☐	☐	☐	☐	☐
4. How often during the last year have you found that you were not able to stop drinking once you had started?	☐	☐	☐	☐	☐	☐	
5. How often during the last year have you failed to do what was normally expected of you because of drinking?	☐	☐	☐	☐	☐	☐	
6. How often during the last year have you needed a first drink in the morning to get yourself going after a heavy drinking session?	☐	☐	☐	☐	☐	☐	☐
7. How often during the last year have you had a feeling of guilt or remorse after drinking?	☐	☐	☐	☐	☐	☐	
8. How often during the last year have you been unable to remember what happened the night before because you had been drinking?	☐	☐	☐	☐	☐	☐	
	No		*Yes, but not in the last year*		*Yes, during the last year*		
9. Have you or someone else been injured because of your drinking?	☐		☐		☐	☐	
10. Has a relative, friend, doctor, or other health care worker been concerned about your drinking or suggested you cut down?	☐		☐		☐	☐	☐
						TOTAL ☐	

Supplementary Questions	*No*	*Probably Not*	*Unsure*	*Possibly*	*Definitely*
Do you think you presently have a problem with drinking?	☐	☐	☐	☐	☐
	Very easy	*Fairly easy*	*Neither difficult nor easy*	*Fairly difficult*	*Very difficult*
In the next 3 months, how difficult would you find it to cut down or stop drinking?	☐	☐	☐	☐	☐

The World Health Organization's Alcohol Use Disorders Identification Test (AUDIT) is a very reliable and simple screening tool which is sensitive to early detection of risky and high risk (or hazardous and harmful) drinking. It has three questions on alcohol consumption (**1 to 3**), three questions on drinking behaviour and dependence (**4 to 6**) and four questions on the consequences or problems related to drinking (**7 to 10**).

The **Supplementary Questions** do not belong to the AUDIT and are **not** scored. They provide useful clinical information associated with the client's perception of whether they have an alcohol problem and their confidence that change is possible in the short-term. They act as an indication of the degree of intervention required and provide a link to counselling or brief intervention following feedback of the AUDIT score to the client.

Scoring the AUDIT

- The columns in the AUDIT are scored from left to right.
- **Questions 1 to 8** are scored on a five-point scale from **0, 1, 2, 3,** and **4**.
- **Questions 9 & 10** are scored on a three -point scale from **0, 2** and **4**.
- Record the score for each question in the **"score"** column on the right, including a zero for questions **2 to 8** if 'skipped'.
- Record a total score in the **"TOTAL"** box at the bottom of the column. The maximum score is 40.

Consumption score

Add up **questions 1 to 3** and place this sub-score in the adjacent single box in the far right column (maximum score possible = 12). A score of 6 or 7 may indicate a risk of alcohol-related harm, even if this is also the total score for the AUDIT (e.g. consumption could be over the recommended weekly intake of 28 for men and 14 for females in the absence of scoring on any other questions). Drinking may also take place in dangerous situations (e.g. driving, fishing/boating). Scores of 6 to 7 may also indicate potential harm for those groups more susceptible to the effects of alcohol, such as young people, women, the elderly, people with mental health problems and people on medication. Further inquiry may reveal the necessity for harm reduction advice.

Dependence score

Add up **questions 4 to 6** and place this sub-score in the adjacent single box in the far right column (maximum score possible = 12). In addition to the total AUDIT score, a secondary 'dependence' score of 4 or more as a subtotal of questions 4 to 6, suggests the possibility of alcohol dependence (and therefore the need for more intensive intervention if further assessment confirms dependence).

Alcohol-related problems score

Any scoring on **questions 7 to 10** warrants further investigation to determine whether the problem is of current concern and requires intervention.

AUDIT Total score	*Dependence score*	*Risk level*	*Possible Interventions*
0 - 7	below 4	**Low-risk**	• Use 'Right Mix' materials to reinforce low-risk drinking, particularly for those who previously had alcohol problems or whose circumstances may change. • Harm reduction advice may be appropriate for those in susceptible groups (see 'Consumption Score' above).
8 - 15	below 4	**Risky** or **hazardous level.** Moderate risk of harm. May include some clients currently experiencing harm (especially those who have minimised their reported intake and problems).	• Brief Intervention - feedback of AUDIT and harm reduction advice may be sufficient Ideally also: - setting goals and limits - a motivational interview - self-monitoring of drinking - use of "The Right Mix" self-help guide
	4 or more	Assess for dependency	• Counselling may be required.
16 - 19	below 4	**High-risk** or **harmful level.** Drinking that will eventually result in harm, if not already doing so. May be dependent.	• Brief Intervention (all components) is a minimum requirement. • Assessment for more intensive intervention. • Counselling using CBT principles and motivational interviewing in individual sessions and/or in groups. • Follow-up and referral where necessary.
	4 or more	Assess for dependence	
20 or more	below 4	**High-risk** Definite harm, also likely to be alcohol dependent. Assess for dependence.	• Further assessement preferably including family and significant others. • More intensive counselling and/or group program. • Consider referral to medical or specialist services for withdrawal management.
	4 or more	**Almost certainly dependent.** Assess for dependency.	• Pharmacotherapy to manage cravings. • Relapse prevention, longer-term follow-up and support.

Source: Australian Government Department of Veterans' Affairs, 2004.

The five A's

The five A's is an evidence-based framework which has been developed and evaluated for smoking cessation in healthcare settings.

Ask	**Identify and document smoking status routinely and review at least every twelve months**	Current, ex- or never smoker
Assess	**Interest in quitting**	How interested in quitting are you? How important is smoking in your life?
	Identify barriers to quitting	For example, what would be the hardest thing about quitting?
	Level of nicotine dependence	Time to first cigarette in the morning (<60 minutes) Number smoked per day (>15 cigarettes) Previous symptoms of withdrawal
	Explore motivation and confidence	On a scale of 1 to 10 (where 10 = very motivated to quit) how would you rate your motivation to quit? On a scale of 1 to 10 (where 10 = very confident to quit) how would you rate your confidence?
	Explore barriers to quitting	Ask about dealing with stress, weight, peer pressure, social aspects.
	Quitting history	For example, what worked? What didn't work? What tipped you back?
	High-risk situations	Which cigarette would be the hardest to give up? When might 'slips' occur? Even one puff greatly increases the risk of relapse.
Advise	**Provide brief, clear, personalised and non-judgmental advice to quit.**	As your doctor, I think it is very important for your health that you quit smoking.
	Set quit date.	
	Address the three main domains.	Dependence (e.g. withdrawal symptoms, craving) Habit (e.g. triggers) Dealing with negative emotions.
	Brainstorm solutions.	For example, provide options; explore what is likely to support their ability to quit.
	Negotiate/advise on how to deal with high-risk situations.	
Assist	**Offer a Quitbook and give the Quitline number 131 848.**	
	Negotiate a separate smoking cessation-oriented consultation.	It would be very useful for us to spend some time on helping you quit (e.g. exploring the barriers and possible strategies to deal with them, looking at medications to counter withdrawal symptoms).
	Enrol in Quit twelve-week active call back program.	Quit provide proactive support over the first three months through phone calls at times convenient to you.
	Discuss/offer pharmacotherapy.	
	Develop a plan to deal with nicotine withdrawal, habit, negative moods, weight gain, stress and high-risk situations.	

Arrange	**Follow-up (ideally in the first seven days).**	
	Recruit support (e.g. partner, family).	Having your partner quit at the same time doubles your chances of success.

Bolded items can each be completed in <1 minutes; other aspects can each be covered in 1–5 minutes.

Remember: The unsupported quit rate is about 3%. This can be improved eight-fold with 2–3 visits of 10–15 minutes.

Source: Adapted from DATIS Clinical Support Service, GASP; Quit

CHAPTER 16

To sleep, perchance . . . to get everything else right

CAROLINE WEST WARNE, GARRY EGGER

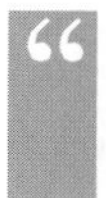

Sleep touches on nearly every aspect of our physiology and psychology, of our interaction with the world and with others.

WILLIAM C. DEMENT, 1999

Introduction

Sleep research, such as was carried out by some of the pioneers in the area in the 1960s and, '70s, might in a different setting have been classified as torture. Researchers kept subjects awake for extended periods and, just when they tended to nod off, would wake them every minute or so throughout an entire night. They then evaluated their alertness the next day. Not surprisingly, this was found to be less than optimal. But the important thing was how and why daytime functioning was affected by sleep deprivation and what this tells us about the functions of—and reasons for—sleep.

Humans, like most mammals, sleep for about a third of their lives. Anyone living to the current average age (for women) of eighty-two will have slept for a staggering twenty-seven years. Yet, given the amount of time invested in sleep, it is surprising how little time is spent prioritising it—until something goes wrong. In many ways, healthy sleep is the anchor for a healthy life. Healthy sleep not only helps boost mood and IQ and improve memory and concentration, it also decreases the risks of heart disease, diabetes, depression and even obesity (Alvarez and Ayas, 2004).

Sleep disorders are also on the rise. As many as 80% of people will suffer from a sleep problem at some stage in their life (Dement, 1999), ranging from mild intransient insomnia to severe and crippling narcolepsy. The burden is even heavier in lower socioeconomic groups, where obesity, sleep-disordered breathing and cardiovascular risk are all greater (See et al., 2006). At any given time as many as 30–50% of people will have difficulty sleeping.

Modern lifestyles are often in direct competition with sleep, so much so that it could be argued that the majority of modern sleep problems have a basis in lifestyle choices. Inactivity, poor nutrition, anxiety, depression and stress—all by-products of modernity—have an impact on sleep. Obesity, another by-product of modernity, has been linked both with too little and too much sleep (Carmelli et al., 2000). The good news, however, is that sleep can often be dramatically improved with a healthy approach to lifestyle and a simple, structured approach to sleeping patterns. While we will consider the best ways of achieving this here, this is not intended to be an in-depth discussion of medically related sleep problems. Our main concerns are those sleep issues that are related to, and can be modified by, lifestyle factors and the lifestyle changes that can make sleep more functional for ongoing wellbeing.

The reasons for sleep

Ironically, despite the importance of sleep in human lives and functioning, there is still no agreed understanding of why it is necessary. The notion of giving the brain and/or body a 'rest' seems facile in light of the fact that body organs such as the heart, liver and kidneys function twenty-four hours a day. Other suggestions are that sleep serves an energy conservation function, a body tissue restitution function, or a temperature down-regulation function.

Regardless of the reason(s), it is clear that sleep plays an important role in human health and wellbeing. The fact that the world record for avoiding sleep is only a matter of days in a lifespan that lasts scores of years suggests that the psycho-physiological rationale of sleep, albeit illusive, is undoubtedly significant.

How much sleep do we need?

Humans have large variations in their individual needs for sleep, ranging from 1–2 to 12–14 hours a day. Variations occur with age, life stages, health conditions, lifestyle patterns and other conditions. On average, most adults need 7–8 hours a night to wake refreshed and function well during the day, and individuals reporting both an increased (>8 hours/day) or reduced (<7 hours/day) sleep duration are at moderately increased risk of all-cause mortality, cardiovascular disease and symptomatic diabetes (Spiegel et al., 2005). Unfortunately, though, the number of hours slept per day appears to be decreasing, with increasingly busy lifestyles. The average of 8–9 hours in previous years has now dropped to about seven hours per night, according to the National Sleep Foundation (2002). The proportion of young adults getting less than seven hours sleep per night has more than doubled from 15.6% in 1960 to 37.1% in 2002.

What are the consequences? Is sleep deprivation really a problem, or can humans simply be conditioned to sleep less? Accumulating evidence suggests that sleeping less than five hours a night over an extended period can significantly raise the risks of all those health problems referred to above. There is also evidence that chronic sleep deprivation of as little as an hour or more a day can lead to a situation of sleep debt (Dement, 1999). This can have an enormous impact on the risk of fatigue-related accidents (Taylor and Dorn, 2006). In other words, if sleep is not taken seriously, there is a price to pay.

Sleep cycles

Prior to the invention of the EEG in 1929 by Hans Berger, very little was known about sleep. Up until that point, sleep was often considered to be a blank state, an unconscious wasteland. However, the EEG revealed that sleep was dynamic, varied and complex. It was soon discovered that sleep could be divided into five stages, each with its own distinct brain-wave patterns. And sleep was far from a linear journey. While on average each cycle or journey of sleep lasts around ninety minutes, each can be slightly different. For example, later in the evening, people may drift from the deep sleep of stage 4 back to the light sleep of stage 2 before going into stage 5 REM (rapid eye movement) or dream sleep.

The sleep cycle: stages of sleep

Stage 1 Very light sleep, theta brain waves. During this phase we may experience fleeting visual images called 'hypnagogic hallucinations'.

Stage 2 Light/transitional sleep characterised by theta waves with K complex waves and sleep spindles.

Stage 3 Deep sleep with a combination of theta and delta waves.

Stage 4 Deepest sleep, theta waves disappear and there are only delta waves.

Stage 5 REM (dream) sleep.

Individuals usually have about five sleep cycles per night. The earlier part of the night may be characterised by more time spent in deep sleep, and often as the night progresses more time is spent in REM sleep. We know that REM/dream sleep is important for preparing the mind for peak daytime performance and improving memory retention and recall (Dujardin et al., 1990). Too little sleep can certainly come at a cost. Missing out on the longer periods of REM sleep that come near morning can also have serious consequences for thinking, memory and daytime performance.

The concept of sleep debt

One of the most accepted axioms among sleep researchers is the concept of 'sleep debt'. Sleep debt accumulates during periods of wakefulness. In fact, according to many sleep researchers all periods of wakefulness are sleep deprivation and add to sleep debt (Dement, 1999). This is usually paid back after a good night's sleep. However, if this does not occur, and the debt is left unpaid, it accumulates progressively until eventually it has to be paid off in another form, for example, with sickness, mood change or ongoing fatigue (Haack and Mullington, 2005). According to McEwen (2006), sleep deprivation is a chronic stressor that causes cognitive problems, which can exacerbate pathways that lead to disease. Researchers who woke sleepers regularly found that while one-minute sleep periods followed by forced awakenings (leading to sleep deprivation) caused major deficits in alertness the next day, longer periods of sleep (10–15 minutes) had much less of an effect. This suggests that there are minimal units of restorative sleep.

As Dement (1999) put it, 'It's as if the bank that keeps track of sleep debt doesn't accept small deposits'. Siestas, and naps, on the other hand, seem to play a significant role in restoring debt. Heart disease rates are lower in countries where siestas are part of daily life (Naska et al., 2007). Paradoxically, short daytime naps (<30 mins) also appear to be more effective than longer naps in maintaining alertness (Dhand and Sohal, 2006).

In terms of performance, vigilance, alertness, decision making and reaction times, sleep loss can been compared to the effects of blood alcohol. This has particular relevance for shift workers (and indeed hospital doctors), who are at risk of fatigue-related accidents and mistakes. Dawson and Reid (1997) showed that seventeen hours of wakefulness had an equivalent effect on performance to a blood alcohol level (BAL) of 0.05%; twenty-four hours without sleep was the equivalent of a BAL of 0.1%.

While accountants deal with monetary debts and bankers call in bad loans, the body deals with sleep debt, and clinicians are left to deal with the unpaid loans by treating sleep-related disorders.

Fatigue and excessive daytime sleepiness (EDS)

As might be expected, poor or inadequate sleep can lead to fatigue (tiredness without increased sleep propensity) and excessive daytime sleepiness (EDS), the latter of which has been found to be quite common (about 10% of the population; Bixler et al., 2005). This is often attributed to periods of wakefulness caused by obstructive sleep apnoea, which in turn is causally related to obesity. A recent review, however, has shown that obese individuals without sleep apnoea can suffer EDS and fatigue and those with sleep apnoea may not (Vgontas et al., 2006). This has led to the suggestion that other factors—such as depression, diabetes and inactivity in the obese—may be risk factors for daytime fatigue and EDS, independent of night-time sleep quality. In turn, fatigue and EDS may themselves cause disease via a link to cytokines and the stress system. Vgontas et al. (2006) suggest that fatigue is associated more with psychological distress and EDS with metabolic factors such as insulin resistance and diabetes. This suggests the need to distinguish between both conditions in treating the problem. Apnoea should also not be discounted as a cause.

Risk factors associated with poor sleep

As well as the common disorders that occur in sleep (see below), there is a range of pathological conditions associated with inadequate or poor quality sleep. These include:

- depression/anxiety
- obesity
- heart disease
- decreased cognition/performance/memory
- impaired decision making
- impaired immunity

- fatigue and work-related accidents
- car accidents
- substance abuse
- suicide risk

Poor sleep can also include too much sleep. Although this is controversial, some researchers suggest that sleeping for prolonged periods may adversely affect health, although perhaps not nearly to the same extent as short sleeping (Youngstedt and Kripke, 2004). The deleterious effects of sleep duration less than eight hours a day appear to be related to depression and low socioeconomic status (Patel et al., 2006). Hence, it could be argued that the ideal amount of sleep (as with many lifestyle issues) may be like a U-curve, with too little or too much placing an individual at risk of health problems.

Sleep and lifestyle interactions

As with most topics discussed in this book, there are significant interactions between other components of lifestyle, sleep and disease. The process is often cyclical, with lifestyle-related problems causing poor sleep patterns, which then make the initial problems worse. Treating lifestyles behaviour is therefore necessary to break this cycle and reduce the chances of further ill health. Research suggests there are two-way interactions between sleep problems and a range of health problems that include obesity, alcohol misuse and diabetes, for example.

Sleep and obesity

The findings on sleep and body weight are interesting and challenging. On the one hand, a lack of sleep may be an important trigger for obesity (Spiegel et al., 2005). Sleep deprivation can lead to a surge in appetite. According to recent research, people who sleep only four hours a night are 73% more likely to be obese, and those sleeping five hours have a 50% higher risk of obesity (Gangwisch and Heymsfield, 2005). Even those who sleep six hours a night (about one hour less than the current seven hour average) are 23% more likely to be very overweight. In one systematic meta-analysis of studies from 1996–2006, short sleepers had a two-fold rate of obesity (Cappuccio et al., 2007).

The reasons for this may be complex. There may be a mechanism humans have evolved to protect themselves against famine in winter, when food is in shorter supply. Sleeping less could act as a trigger to eat more. Sleep deprivation also affects hormone levels associated with appetite and satiation. Leptin is decreased (making it harder to sense satiety) and grehlin, the stomach hormone related to hunger, is increased. Cortisol levels are also increased with sleep deprivation, and this can encourage weight gain (Spiegel et al., 2005).

Quality and length of sleep may also play an important role in childhood obesity. Researchers from the U.K. found that a short duration of sleep can adversely influence weight in children (Reilly et al., 2005).

Obesity also decreases sleep quality by increasing the risk of sleep apnoea and snoring (see below). For these reasons, a sleep review is vital when managing other lifestyle-related health conditions, such as overweight or obesity. Improving sleep quality can help prevent weight gain while adding benefit to other weight loss initiatives.

What can be done in a standard consultation

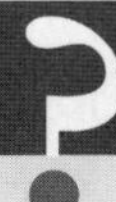

Ask about sleep quality, as well as daytime fatigue and excessive daytime sleepiness (EDS).

Ask if patients have ever been told they snore.

Test for diabetes in cases of unexplained fatigue.

Consider psychological factors as a cause of fatigue and insulin resistance as a cause of EDS.

If a sleep problem is suspected, get the patient to complete a sleep diary (see *Professional resources*).

Explain the link between obesity, inactivity, depression, anxiety and sleep.

Order a home sleep study if apnoea is suspected.

Sleep and alcohol

Alcohol and sleep are not the best bedfellows. Although a nightcap is often seen as a relaxant that will help with sleep, the reality is that alcohol (along with caffeine and nicotine) is a sleep thief. While alcohol may help you get off to sleep a little faster (reducing sleep latency), it has a definite downside in that quality of sleep can be adversely affected. Having an alcoholic drink in the hour before bed may disrupt the second part of the sleep cycle. Surprisingly, even having a drink much earlier in the evening at 'happy hour' (about six hours before retiring) can still interrupt an evening's sleep. This suggests that alcohol, even after it has been recently metabolised, can exert lasting influences over sleep regulation (Vitiello, 1997). After a few hours of sleep, those who have been drinking even modest amounts can suffer rebound wakefulness which leads to difficulty getting back to sleep. The depth of sleep is also adversely affected, leading to fatigue the next day. Elderly people who rely on a little alcohol to sleep also have an increased risk of injuries and falls during the night (Aldrich, 1998).

Certainly the extent of sleep disturbance is often related to how much alcohol is consumed, but if sleep problems are a concern, even small amounts of alcohol consumption need to be considered. A small amount of alcohol can also uncover accumulated sleep debt, which may make it dangerously easy to lapse into sleep or microsleeps (Dement, 1999). When combined with sleep debt, alcohol becomes a potent sedative that can have dangerous repercussions, for example, in traffic and work injuries (Taylor and Dorn, 2006). A large sleep debt and even a small amount of alcohol can cause fatal fatigue.

Alcohol-dependent sleep disorder is diagnosed when a patient needs alcohol to get to sleep on at least thirty consecutive days. The problem can lead to early wakening, poor sleep quality and greater alcohol tolerance, leading to more and more alcohol being required to get to sleep. Specialist care is required (Dement, 1999).

Sleep, exercise and inactivity

Initial research on exercise and sleep showed the complexity of this relationship. Sleep following exercise was found to be disturbed. However, the results were influenced by the fact that the subjects used in the research did not exercise regularly. When regular exercisers (joggers) were tested, sleep quality generally improved. Exercise just before bedtime, however, may decrease alertness and decrease sleep capacity; however, once again this may be less so in highly fit individuals (Youngstedt et al., 1999), who, incidentally, are less likely to present to a clinician with a sleep problem.

Data from the US National Health and Nutrition Survey (NHANES III) showed that people with insufficient physical activity were two to four times more likely to report feeling tired or exhausted compared to the group that reported feeling fresh (Resnick, 2006). Exercise in fit individuals has also been found to increase the deepest stages of sleep (Youngstedt, 2005). Excessive exercise, on the other, hand can lead to disturbed and shortened sleep. Patients should be advised that regular exercise will improve sleep as fitness increases but that this should not be carried out in excess and usually not just before retiring.

Sleep and diabetes

Type 2 diabetes can be a cause of disturbed sleep. More importantly, however, it could result from sleep loss. This association has been shown epidemiologically (Al-Delaimy et al., 2002), but there are also physiological explanations related to the modulatory effect of sleep on glucose metabolism and the molecular mechanisms for the interaction between sleeping and feeding (Spiegel et al., 2005). Restless legs syndrome (RLS), a relatively common sleep disorder, is also increased in diabetic patients and those with impaired glucose control, possibly through the activation of small neural fibres associated with peripheral neuropathy (Gemignani et al., 2007). Decreased glucose tolerance and insulin sensitivity have been found with increased sleep deprivation and hunger-related hormones such as leptin and ghrelin change in a way conducive to greater food intake.

Obesity and sleep loss are related and sleep-disordered breathing is linked to obesity; this suggests a feedforward cascade of negative events generated by sleep problems which are likely to exacerbate the severity of metabolic problems.

Sleep, bedding and airconditioning

As discussed in Chapter 17, bedding can have a significant impact on skin, as well as sleep patterns. Overheating under a continental quilt or with an electric blanket, for example, can cause disturbed sleep, sleep debt, consequent daytime sleepiness and mood changes.

Sleep disorders

Sleep disorders represent the extreme of sleep-related problems. Over eighty different types of such disorders have now been identified and described in the *International classification of sleep disorders and coding manual* published by the American Sleep Disorders Association. The major classifications are shown in Table 16.1.

Those disorders associated with lifestyle are mainly dyssomnias. The two most common problems considered here are insomnia and obstructive sleep apnoea.

TABLE 16.1 Classification of sleep disorders

Major category	Subcategories	Examples
dyssomnias (disorders that cause difficulty initiating or maintaining sleep or excessive sleepiness)	intrinsic sleep disorders (originating in the body)	obstructive sleep apnoea insomnias narcolepsy restless legs syndrome
	extrinsic sleep disorders (originating outside the body)	alcohol-dependent sleep disorder altitude insomnia inadequate sleep hygiene
	circadian rhythm sleep disorders	'jet lag' syndrome shiftwork sleep disorder delayed sleep phase syndrome.
parasomnias (disorders of partial arousal or those that interfere with sleep stage transitions)	arousal disorders	sleepwalking night terrors confusional arousal
	sleep-wake transition disorders	sleep talking nocturnal leg cramps rhythmic movement disorders
	parasomnias usually associated with REM sleep	nightmares sleep paralysis REM sleep behaviour disorder
	other parasomnias	sleep bruxism enuresis abnormal swallowing syndrome SIDS
medical and psychiatric sleep disorders	sleep disorders associated with medical disorders	alcoholism nocturnal cardiac ischaemia COPD
	sleep problems associated with neurological disorders	degenerative brain disorders sleep-related epilepsy sleep-related headache
	sleep disorders associated with psychiatric disorders	psychoses mood disorders anxiety disorders panic disorders
proposed sleep disorders (not yet formally categorised as discrete sleep disorders)		short sleeper long sleeper menstrual-associated disorder sleep choking syndrome

What is insomnia?

Insomnia is not so much a condition as a symptom. It is defined as difficulty getting to sleep or staying asleep, waking through the night, waking up earlier in the morning, or not getting the amount or quality of sleep needed (Neubauer, 2005). Short-term or transient insomnia lasting days or a couple of weeks may be triggered by stress, temporary illness, excitement at an upcoming event, travel or environmental factors, such as light, heat or noise. Chronic insomnia lasts 2–3 weeks or more. It can be related to lifestyle issues, beliefs or attitudes about sleep, or an underlying medical problem. The list shown in Table 16.2 contains just some of the factors to consider when someone presents with chronic insomnia.

TABLE 16.2 Triggers and medical conditions that can cause insomnia

Triggers	Medical conditions
attitudes and beliefs about sleep	sleep-related epilepsy
poor sleep habits	cerebral degenerative disorders
feelings of loss of control about sleep	thyroid disease
inadequate exercise	anxiety/depression
trying to control sleep	alcohol abuse
stress/worrying	Parkinson's disease
lying in bed tense and frustrated	obstructive sleep apnoea
too much light or noise in the bedroom	pain disorders
excess caffeine or stimulant intake	gastrointestinal diseases
drugs and alcohol	hormone imbalances
	medication side effects
	urological conditions
	itching/allergies
	fibromyalgia

In order to establish the source of insomnia, it is vital that a full medical history is taken paying attention to any potential underlying medical conditions, recreational drugs, stimulants, prescription medications, beliefs about sleep, and lifestyle factors. Getting to the root of the problem is vital, as this will govern the management of the problem. It is important to determine the pattern of and beliefs about sleep and to work out the impact of sleep deprivation on the individual. For example, exercise before sleep at the time of arrival at a destination (if this is during the daylight) is a way of dealing with insomnia from jet lag.

For chronic insomnia relating to lifestyle issues, sleeping medications are usually inappropriate because they fail to deal with the underlying triggers for poor sleep. However, for transient insomnia relating to travel or a change in life circumstances, short-term sleeping medication use may be an appropriate option along with lifestyle/sleep habit modification. Careful review, dispelling myths about sleep and providing practical healthy sleep tips, can be vital in improving sleep. Lifestyle change prescriptions such as increasing daytime physical activity, winding down in the evening, eating less, watching caffeine and alcohol intake, trying to avoid accumulating a sleep debt, and using sleep hygiene practices (see *Practice tips*) can all help to dramatically improve sleep for many patients.

The value of sleep diaries in determining sleep patterns

Just as patients are regularly asked about their diet and exercise habits as part of lifestyle medicine, it is also appropriate to review sleep patterns. One of the most effective ways of doing this is to get patients to keep a sleep diary (mental recall alone is notoriously inaccurate when trying to assess a prior week's sleep patterns). Ideally this should include:

- daytime lifestyle factors (exercise, caffeine intake, alcohol and drugs, wind down routine in the hour before bed);
- getting into bed time;

- sleep time;
- any night-time wakening;
- time awake in the morning;
- time out of bed in the morning; and
- mood on waking (e.g. refreshed, tired, exhausted).

Patterns quickly emerge that can then be targeted with healthy lifestyle changes, counselling and CBT. Maintaining the sleep diary can then help chart progress and improvements (see *Professional resources* for an example of a sleep diary).

Snoring and obstructive sleep apnoea (OSA)

Apnoea is a classical Greek word for absence of breath. With sleep apnoea, a person stops breathing repeatedly during sleep for at least ten seconds and sometimes for a minute or more. The most common type of sleep apnoea, which has a strong lifestyle link, is obstructive sleep apnoea (OSA). With this condition, the soft tissue at the back of the throat collapses and obstructs the airway, which stops or impedes air flow. The sufferer usually snores, then stops breathing. This is followed by arousal, a gasp for breath, and breathing resuming. This exhausting cycle can happen hundreds of times a night, leading to fractured, poor quality sleep along with fatigue and sleepiness the next day.

The exact number of people affected by OSA remains controversial, although some sleep researchers like Dement (1999) estimate that up to 20% of people could have clinically significant apnoea. What is agreed, however, is that the incidence is on the rise, coincident with the increase of one of its most prominent causes: obesity. Because of its link with disease, sleep apnoea has even been defined as a manifestation of the metabolic syndrome (Vgontzas et al., 2005).

Sleep apnoea is known to increase blood pressure (Wolf et al., 2007) and is therefore a risk factor for heart disease. However, a more immediate danger is the large sleep debt accumulated by sufferers from their brief (usually unrecognised) wakening. This increases risks from driving or using machinery and is the reason apnoea sufferers are excluded from becoming professional drivers in some countries. Other problems common to people with apnoea are reflux, nocturnal urination, sweating at night, morning headaches, raspy voice, personality changes, loss of hearing, and even male impotence and reduction of sex drive in men and women (Ting and Malhotra, 2005). Risk factors for apnoea identified from the prospective Bussleton study in Western Australia are being male, obesity and weight gain (Knuiman et al., 2006). Development of asthma over time (also associated with obesity and taking up smoking) may also play a role.

Snoring is highly associated with sleep apnoea, although not all snorers have OSA (Knuiman et al., 2006). In general, the louder the snoring, the more likely it is that the sleeper has apnoea. Treatment for OSA and snoring can require surgery, but opening of the airways through continuous positive airway pressure (CPAP) machines has become standard treatment since their invention by Dr Colin Sullivan at the Royal Prince Alfred hospital in Sydney in the 1980s (Kaparianos et al., 2006). Another technique, which is cheaper and useful in some cases, involves dental devices to move the lower jaw forward. While highly successful, these techniques should be seen as treating the symptoms, not the cause. Weight loss, a moderate amount of physical activity, and reduction of alcohol before retiring are the primary lifestyle prescriptions in conjunction with these devices where they assist in reducing sleep debt and hence daytime sleepiness (which otherwise reduces the desire to be active during the day). If this does not occur, a vicious circle can be created, leading to greater weight gain and more severe apnoea and disease risk.

Sleep hygiene

The following are the key points in an effective patient sleep hygiene program. All should undertaken together for best effect.

- *Establish a routine.* Babies and children love sleeping routines, but adults also benefit from regular bedtime and wake up times, including weekends. Sleeping in on the weekend can reset the body clock and lead to a type of weekend jet lag. Sleeping in on a Sunday can mean going to bed later on Sunday night, making Monday morning particularly tough.
- *Wind down before bed.* Particularly in the hour before bed, it is useful to engage in soothing, calming activities. Avoid activities that stimulate, for example, watching TV, searching the internet, reading emails or newspapers, paying bills or exercising. Instead, focus on enjoying a warm shower or bath, listening to calming music or relaxing.
- *Keep the bedroom for sleep and sex only.* Avoid working, eating or other activities in bed and try to keep computers and TV out of the bedroom. Reading, however, may be helpful to help wind down.
- *Get comfortable.* Sleep on a comfortable mattress and pillow. Make sure the bedroom is dark, quiet and cool. Eyeshades and earplugs may be useful additions.
- *Control caffeine (coffee, tea, cola and energy drinks) and limit alcohol before bed.* Keep in mind that caffeine can still create a buzz in some people up to twelve hours after consumption. Avoiding caffeine at least in the eight hours prior to bed can help improve sleep quality. Alcohol should be limited to 1–2 drinks for women and 3–4 drinks for men, in line with other recommendations for alcohol consumption.
- *Get regular physical activity.* Regular daily exercise promotes sleep. Avoid exercise in the few hours prior to bed, however, because the adrenaline released increases alertness.
- *Finish dinner at least a couple of hours before bed.* Eating too late or eating spicy foods (that trigger heartburn) or heavy meals can interfere with sleep.
- *Avoid nicotine.* Nicotine is a stimulant, so smoking close to bedtime can make it more difficult to fall asleep.
- *Avoid long daytime naps if insomnia is a problem.* Napping for more than 20–30 minutes may disrupt evening sleep. Shorter naps, however, may be advantageous.
- *Develop healthy thinking about sleep.* Controlling worry and 'racing thoughts' through relaxation practices can facilitate sleep.

Summary

While the reasons for our physiological need for sleep are unknown, the need for a consistent amount is unquestioned. And while there are big individual differences in sleep requirements, less than around seven hours or more than around 8.5 hours appear to have negative health outcomes for the majority of the population. Sleep problems can begin as mild forms of insomnia or hypersomnia, often associated with lifestyle habits, but can also include serious disorders or signs of other problems, such as snoring and sleep apnoea, which are linked to heart disease. At the even more serious end of the spectrum are major disturbances such as narcolepsy or night terrors. Sleep (or, more usually, lack of it) is thus a significant cause of modern lifestyle-related ill health and should be included in any considered lifestyle analysis.

practice tips

PRACTICE TIPS: IMPROVING SLEEP QUALITY

	Medical practitioner	Practice nurse
Assess	Sleep as part of a routine check-up. Underlying lifestyle factors including exercise, eating patterns and stress levels. Underlying medical conditions such as depression or thyroid disease. Use of sleeping medications including over the counter preparations. Intake of drugs, alcohol, stimulants and caffeine.	Sleep as part of a routine check-up. Underlying lifestyle factors including exercise, eating patterns and stress levels.
Assist	By recommending a sleep diary. By providing tips for healthy sleep habits (see below). By reviewing sleeping medication and reducing/eliminating it where appropriate.	By explaining and assisting in completion of a seven-day sleep diary.
Arrange	Referral for treatment of co-morbidities where appropriate. List of other health professionals for a care plan. Sleep specialist review if further assessment required. Sleep laboratory or home monitoring investigations if a disorder such as sleep apnoea is suspected. Follow-up to monitor sleep improvements (first follow-up session with the seven-day sleep diary completed) and a timetable for ongoing review. Psychologist referral for CBT if appropriate.	A discussion of tactics with other involved health professionals. A sleep therapist, psychologist or life coach if appropriate. Contact with self-help groups.

KEY POINTS FOR CLINICAL MANAGEMENT

- Consider sleep as an issue in other lifestyle-related illnesses, for example, obesity, diabetes and fatigue,
- Discuss sleep-related problems such as snoring, early wakening, late onset to sleep and regular wakening.
- Relate excessive regular daytime sleepiness with sleep problems/patterns.
- Consider bedding, airconditioning and other environmental factors as potential contributors to poor sleep.

REFERENCES

Al-Delaimy WK, Manson JE, Willett WC et al. (2002) Snoring as a risk factor for type II diabetes mellitus: a prospective study. *Am J Epidem* 5: 387–93.

Aldrich MS. (1998) *Effects of alcohol on sleep. Alcohol problems and aging. NIAAA research monograph no 33. National Institutes of Health publication no. 98-4163.* Bethesda, Maryland: National Institutes of Health.

Alvarez GG, Ayas NT. (2004) The impact of daily sleep duration on health: a review of the literature. *Prog Cardiovasc Nurs* 19(2): 56–59.

American Sleep Disorders Association. (2006) *International classification of sleep disorders and coding manual.* Westchester, IL: American Sleep Disorders Association.

Bixler EO, Vgontzaz AN, Lin HM et al. (2005) Excessive daytime sleepiness in a general population sample: the role of sleep apnoea, age, obesity, diabetes and depression. *J Clin Endocrin Metab* 90: 4510–15.

Cappuccio F, Taggart F, Kandala N-B et al. (2007) short sleep duration and obesity: meta-analysis of studies world-wide. Paper presented to 5th Congress of World Federation of Sleep Research, cairns, Australia, 2007.

Carmelli D, Swan GE, Bliwise DL. (2000) Relationship of 30-year changes in obesity to sleep-disordered breathing in the Western Collaborative Group Study. *Obes Res* 8(9): 632–37.

Dawson D, Reid K. (1997) Fatigue, alcohol and performance impairment. *Nature* 388(6639): 235.

Dement WC. (1999) *The promise of sleep*. NY: Delacort Press.

Dhand R, Sohal H. (2006) Good sleep, bad sleep! The role of daytime naps in healthy adults. *Curr Opin Pulm Med* 12(6): 379–82.

Dujardin K, Guerrien A, Leconte P. (1990) Sleep, brain activation and cognition. *Phys & Behav* 47: 1271–78.

Gangwisch JE, Malaspina D, Boden-Albala B et al. (2005) Inadequate sleep as a risk factor for obesity: analyses of the NHANES I. *Sleep* 28(10):1289–96.

Gangwisch P, Heymsfield (2005). Columbia University's Mailman School of Public Health and the Obesity Research Centre, Analysis of National Health and Nutrition Examination Survey 1 (NHANES 1), 28(10): 1289–96.

Gemignani F, Brindani F, Vitetta F et al. (2007) Restless legs syndrome in diabetic neuropathy: a frequent manifestation of small fiber neuropathy. *J Periph Nerv Syst* 12(1): 50–53.

Haack M, Mullington JM. (2005) Sustained sleep restriction reduces emotional and physical well-being. *Pain* 119(1–3): 56–64.

Kaparianos A, Sampsonas F, Karkoulias K et al. (2006) The metabolic aspects and hormonal derangements in obstructive sleep apnoea syndrome and the role of CPAP therapy. *Eur Rev Med Pharmacol Sci* 10(6): 319–26.

Knuiman M, James A, Divitini M et al. (2006) Longitudinal study of risk factors for habitual snoring in a general adult population: the Busselton health study. *Chest* 130(6): 1779–83.

McEwan BS. (2006) Sleep deprivation as a neurobiological and physiologic stressor: Allostasis and allostatic load. *Metab* 55(10 Suppl 2): S20–23.

Naska A, Oikonomou E, Trichopoulou A et al. (2007) Siesta in healthy adults and coronary mortality in the general population. *Arch Intern Med* 167: 296–301.

National Sleep Foundation. (2002) *'Sleep in America' poll*. National Sleep Foundation: Washington DC.

Neubauer DN. (2005) Insomnia. *Prim Care* 32(2): 375–88.

Patel SR, Malhotra A, Gottlieb DJ et al. (2006) Correlates of long sleep duration. *Sleep* 29(7): 881–89.

Reilly J, Armstrong J, Dorosty A et al. (2005) Early life risk factors for obesity in childhood. *Brit Med J* 330(7504): 1357.

Resnick HE. (2006) Cross-sectional relationship of reported fatigue to obesity, diet and physical activity: results from the Third National Health and Nutrition Examination Survey. *J Clin Sleep Med* 2: 163–69.

Roth T. (2005) Prevalence, associated risks, and treatment patterns of insomnia. *J Clin Psychiatry* 66 (Suppl 9): 10–13.

See CQ, Mensah E, Olopade CO. (2006) Obesity, ethnicity, and sleep-disordered breathing: medical and health policy implications. *Clin Chest Med* 27(3): 521–33.

Spiegel K, Knutson K, Leproult R et al. (2005) Sleep loss: a novel risk factor for insulin resistance and type 2 diabetes. *J Appl Physiol* 99(5): 2008–19.

Taylor AH, Dorn L. (2006) Stress, fatigue, health, and the risk of road traffic accidents among professional drivers: the contribution of physical inactivity. *Ann Rev Public Hlth* 27: 371–79.

Ting L, Malhotra A. (2005) Disorders of sleep: an overview. *Prim Care* 32(2) 305–18.

Vitiello MV. (1997) Sleep, alcohol and alcohol abuse. *Addict Biol* 2(2): 151–58.

Vgontzas AN, Bixler EO, Chrousos GP. (2005) Sleep apnoea is a manifestation of the metabolic syndrome. *Sleep Med Rev* 9(3): 211–24.

Vgontzas AN, Bixler EO, Chrousos GP. (2006) Obesity-related sleepiness and fatigue: the role of the stress system and cytokines. *Ann NY Acad Sc* 1083: 329–44.

Wolf J, Lewicka J, Narkiewicz K. (2007) Obstructive sleep apnoea: an update on mechanisms and cardiovascular consequences. *Nutr Metab Cardiovasc Dis* 17(3): 233–40.

Youngstedt SD. (2005) Effects of exercise on sleep. *Clin Sports Med* 24(2): 355–65.

Youngsted SD, Kripke DF (2004) Long sleep and mortality: rational for sleep restriction. *Sleep Med Rev, 8(3): 159–74.*

Youngstedt SD, Kripke DF, Elliott JA. (1999) Is sleep disturbed by vigorous late-night exercise? *Med Sci Sports Exerc* 31(6): 864–69.

professional resources

PROFESSIONAL RESOURCES: MEASURING SLEEP

Assessing sleep problems

To work out how successful a patient is at meeting his or her sleep requirements, try asking these simple questions:

- How many hours a night do you sleep through the week?
- Do you fall asleep the instant your head hits the pillow?

- Do you struggle to get out of the bed in the morning?
- Do your eyelids droop (or do you even drop off) during a boring presentation or meeting at work?
- Do you sleep extra on weekends to catch up?
- Do you rely on coffee to stay alert?
- Do you need an alarm to wake up in the mornings?
- Do you regularly use the snooze function?
- Do you often feel drowsy while driving?
- Do you have trouble concentrating or remembering?

If the answer to some of these questions is yes, the patient may be getting insufficient sleep or have a sleep debt. While nodding off during a meeting may not be life threatening, falling asleep at the wheel definitely is—heeding warning signs of sleepiness and fatigue is vital.

Briefly assessing for sleep apnoea

Two useful questions to determine whether someone should be tested for sleep apnoea are:

- Are you excessively tired during the daytime?
- Have you been told that you snore?

A sample sleep diary

A sleep dairy is an excellent way of monitoring sleep patterns and charting progress. To begin, the diary should be kept for a minimum of two weeks to establish initial sleep patterns. Maintaining the diary helps keep track of progress.

	MONDAY	TUESDAY	WEDNESDAY	THURSDAY	FRIDAY	SATURDAY	SUNDAY
What time did you go to bed?							
How long did it take to fall asleep?							
How many times through the night did you wake?							
What time did you get up?							
How many hours did you sleep in total?							
Caffeine/alcohol (number drinks and time consumed)							

other resources

OTHER USEFUL RESOURCES

www.sleepfoundation.org

National Sleep Foundation, USA; a non-profit independent organisation dedicated to research and providing information to the general public; sleep diaries can be downloaded; online questionnaires regarding sleepiness and general information are available.

www.newcastle.edu.au

University of Newcastle Sleep Disorders Centre.

www.aasmnet.org

American Academy of Sleep Medicine.

CHAPTER 17

Saving your patient's skin: environmental influences on skin care

HUGH MOLLOY, GARRY EGGER

It's skin that keeps us in.

Introduction

Little more than a decade ago, it would have been appropriate to start this chapter by stating that the skin is the body's biggest organ. Laid out on the ground it would cover an area of roughly 4 × 3 m in the average sized human. As a structural unit responsible for different functions in the body (the definition of an organ), it would seem there are none bigger. It was only when adipose tissue (fat), endothial tissue and even muscle were classified as endocrine organs in recent times that skin was seen as one of a number of active 'new' organs in the body (Scherer, 2006). Still, this does not detract from the often overlooked fact that skin is an organ and it covers a large area of the human body. Its roles include keeping us contained, exerting an even pressure on all the tissues enclosed within the deep fascia (body stocking), protecting us against the rigors of the outside world, and assisting awareness of what is happening around us (Balin and Balin, 1997).

Why skin in lifestyle medicine?

This chapter is not concerned with infectious skin diseases or skin conditions with internal origins. Instead, it aims at providing a new way of looking at the many common skin problems related to the modern environment and highlighting what lifestyle medicine can do about these. It is our contention that three factors—overheating, excessive dryness and an over-obsession with cleanliness, alone or in combination—are responsible for a large proportion of modern skin problems, ranging from persistent acne to certain forms of eczema and psoriasis (this is spelled out in more detail in Molloy and Egger, 2008).

Unfortunately, these factors have been all but ignored in skin care education. It should be stressed that not all the approaches discussed here have a strong evidence base (as yet) and much of what is discussed is based on logic and clinical experience.

Nevertheless, our premise is that much, although obviously not all, of what happens to the skin in modern times results from our way of life rather than any mysterious or unknown microbes. Lifestyle medicine is a way of helping to manage and deal with skin problems such as those shown in Table 17.1

TABLE 17.1 A 'skindex' of modern skin problems with possible lifestyle causes

dry, rough or scaly skin, which may or may not be itchy
redness, greasiness, rashes or persistent acne with no obvious cause
unexplained morning sneezing, runny nose and/or dry throat
limp, lifeless, stringy or greasy hair
dark, baggy rings around the eyes ('doona eyes')
comedones ('whiteheads') on the forehead, cheeks and chin
redness and itchiness between the breasts
recurrent tinea
disturbed sleep
feeling tired/washed out on waking up

Source: Molloy and Egger, 2008

Dermatitis: the biggest lifestyle-based skin problem

Dermatitis—literally meaning an inflammatory condition ('itis') of the skin ('derma')—is a general term given to a range of non-infectious skin disorders. These are subdivided in many ways, for example, based on appearance, location or underlying cause. The approach we use here (not necessarily accepted by all dermatologists) is to consider most types of dermatitis to be reactions to skin 'insult(s)' of some form, either external or internal, psychological or physical. The skin then reacts in a variety of ways (e.g. eczema, acne, psoriasis, urticaria, rashes, pimples) but typically there are patterns of reaction. No one pattern is necessarily discrete or as clear cut as its name may suggest.

Causes of dermatitis and other modern skin problems

Although the causes of skin problems can be many and varied, we are concerned here only with those associated with lifestyle factors that can be easily recognised and modified with clinical advice and assistance, without recourse to expensive treatment options. We do not review the role of medication.

Environmental factors

It is now thought that the effects of heat and drying on skin, which is often inherently dry anyway, are among the most unrecognised causes of skin damage seen today (Morris-Jones et al., 2002). There are a number of contributing environmental factors, both natural and unnatural.

THE OUTDOOR ENVIRONMENT

- **Sunlight** While sunlight is necessary for an optimal level of vitamin D, excessive sunlight can cause skin problems (Janda et al., 2007). Skin cancers, which result from excessive years of 'baking' in the sun, are more common in fair-skinned than dark-skinned people but are still possible in those with totally black skin (Gloster and Neal, 2006). Good quality sunglasses with 100% UV protection (price is no indication) and a broad-brimmed hat are recommended as the best lines of defence. Sun damage to skin can range from relatively benign solar keratoses (sunspots) to highly malignant melanomas.

- **Cold** Winter reduces the potential for skin cancers through sun exposure but cold, dry winter air can dry the skin, leading to xerosis, which in turn can cause 'winter itch'. This is most common in older people with good or even excessive hygiene but who, through ageing, have increasingly dry skin. However, it can also exist in younger and more active people (Adams, 2002). Dryness from cold can also be the cause of a range of other skin insults (Wolf et al., 2004). Regular use of an inexpensive moisturiser can help overcome this.

THE INDOOR ENVIRONMENT

- **Bedding** Modern bedding and the overheating resulting from this are often unrecognised causes of skin problems in the indoor environment (Okamoto-Mizuno et al., 1999). The standard continental quilt (duvet, doona), which was developed for the European climate but has been taken up widely in Australia, is equivalent in insulation to 5–6 blankets, but unlike blankets it cannot be discarded in sections during the night. Because heat cannot escape from under a doona, body heat during sleep rises to where it can be released (i.e. from the nipple line to the head) as sweat into the open air. This occurs during periods of light sleep and often causes rubbing of the face and head scratching.

  Problems that can result from this are poor sleep, 'doona eyes' (the term given to the darkening of skin around the eyes), facial and peri-oral dermatitis, Grover's disease (itchy red lumps on the upper chest), facial excrescences, atopic eczema, lank hair and scalp problems, acne and dry itch (Molloy et al., 1993). The severity of many of these problems is reduced by using blankets instead of doonas, not using electric blankets or hot water bottles, wearing light bed clothing, and not wearing bed socks. Some early discomfort from an initially cool bed is better than the later skin problems that can result.
- **Workplaces** The modern work environment can be another source of skin troubles. Office airconditioning systems extract water vapour from the air before it is circulated, thereby creating a 'hostile' environment for the skin (Morris-Jones et al., 2002). 'Screen dermatitis' is the name given to an increasingly common skin problem associated with electric equipment, particularly video display terminals (Johansson et al., 2001). General symptoms can include dizziness, tiredness, headache, and erythema or skin flushing. The effects may simply be the result of the dryness of the office environment, giving rise to irritation of the skin and consequent facial rubbing.

  Unlike in the home, it is often difficult to change the work environment. Some changes that may be helpful include having large bowls of water around the office, opening windows where possible instead of using airconditioning, taking regular breaks outside the office, avoiding cigarette smokers and regularly waterproofing the skin with a moisturiser.

- **Travelling** Long haul flights mean sitting for hours in planes where the relative humidity can get below 5% (the ideal for skin is 40–65%). This, together with dehydration (or at least lack of hydration), can dry out the skin and mucous membranes and helps explain the washed-out, tired look when arriving at a destination.

  The local traveller is also not exempt. Cars, which used to have side windows to allow air for cooling while the main window was closed, now have airconditioning for summer and heaters for winter, both of which dry out the interior of the car and cocoon it from the natural atmosphere. One way of rectifying this is a fine spray of water into the air every now and then from a spray bottle left in the car over long journeys, particularly in winter when the air is drier (Lu et al., 2007).

  In many large hotels, the windows cannot be opened and the room becomes a veritable drying pit, even though it might be cool. The dryness requires turning off the airconditioning (if you can find it), which then often means getting cold while sleeping. In many hotels the only sleeping cover is a doona or continental quilt, which increases overheating and cannot be peeled off in stages. Once uncovered, the body gets too cold and the cycle is then repeated, making the modern hotel room not only a blight on the environment (see Chapter 22) but a potential insult to skin. Propping open the bathroom door and putting a 2 cm base of water in the bathtub may go some way towards relieving this, and regular use of a skin moisturiser both while on the plane and on the ground can help. Otherwise, it is prudent to advise travelling patients to look for hotels with windows that can open and blankets that can be peeled off.

MODERN TECHNOLOGY

Changes in living environments for humans over the past century have been caused and accompanied by big advances in technology. And while there is no doubt that this has improved the living conditions of the human race, there are downsides, including insults to the skin. Problem technologies include heaters, airconditioning, modern fabrics and chemicals.

- **Heating and airconditioning** As discussed above, dryness caused by artificial heating or cooling can cause dermatitis with roughness, flaking, scaling, fissuring and apparent lack of moisture (Sunwoo et al., 2006). Avoiding excessively dry places and minimising airconditioning and heating can help reduce these problems. The most common cause of physical irritant dermatitis in one major English study was low humidity due to airconditioning, which caused dermatitis of the face and neck in office workers due to the drying out of skin (Morris-Jones et al., 2002)
- **Clothing** Synthetic fibres are now incorporated into much modern clothing and bedding. They are cheaper than natural fibres, wear better, are lighter and less bulky, and are often better insulators. Over 5–10% of these fibres, even when mixed with natural fibres, tend to cause a build-up of heat.

Synthetic exercise clothing, for example, can reduce the natural functional effects of sweat (i.e. cooling the body). A build-up of heat on the skin that is not dissipated can cause itchiness and irritation which is worsened by washing and scrubbing to get rid of the itch. Exercise clothing is best derived from natural fibres with the extremities (i.e. arms and legs) kept bare and a bare midriff. It should also be as loose as possible to avoid frictional damage (Ricci et al., 2006).

The same applies to childrenswear. Parents often fail to understand that heat loss from the hands and feet is important for the control of body temperature in children and that covering these with gloves, bootees and bonnets in may parts of the country where this is not necessary may damage the child's skin. In a normally placid climate such as Australia's, it is possible that this can upset the normal thermoregulatory mechanisms. The head, and more specifically the face, become the main sites for heat loss from the over-clothed child, and this is made worse if the head is also covered. Atopic eczema in infants aged 6–12 months frequently presents on the cheeks and chin. Although not proven, it is feasible to suggest that over-clothing/heating may play a part in this.

Modern footwear can also present problems for the skin (Springett, 2002). Contemporary shoes are often 'hot boxes' from which heat has difficulty escaping. The uppers are often made of synthetic material or, if made from leather, are sprayed with anti-scuff applications to reduce the need for polishing. As a result, air is unable to circulate and the inside of the shoe is turned into a kind of steam bath, providing an ideal environment for all forms of skin problems, including tinea pedis and pitted keratolysis. In obese patients, the problem is exacerbated by the extra weight transferred to the feet, reducing the natural arch which may otherwise allow an air pocket, causing an irritating itch under the feet. This is often why big men prefer sandals or thongs. The problem can be overcome by ventilating the shoes through a few small holes in the instep, approximately 1 cm above the welt. This allows air to circulate in the shoe and can reduce the internal temperature by up to three degrees Celsius.

- **Chemicals** Modern household chemicals also have great potential for skin damage. Detergent for washing dishes, for example, is usually over-used, and any ill effects are compounded by the use of occlusive gloves made of synthetic materials as these allow the hands to be inserted into much hotter water than usual. The resultant overheating and excessive sweating of the hands within the gloves can cause dermatitis that will not respond to the usual therapies. A more preferable option is to use minimum detergent in comfortably warm water, without gloves but with the hands protected by a layer of moisturiser.

THE OBSESSION WITH CLEANLINESS

If the modern environment and modern technology are problems for the skin, what we do to counter these often makes the problem worse. The immediate reaction for someone with dry skin, greasy hair or an itchy scalp is to have regular showers, scrub down with soap, and shampoo the hair repeatedly, often not realising that this is only drying the skin and scalp out more and leaving it open for the vicious circle of 'dermatitis'. There are a number of things we do that causes this to happen (Wolf et al., 2001).

- **Showers and cleaning** Regular showering is obviously necessary and good for the skin, provided showers are brief and not too hot. Strong soaps, however, tend to take away the surface layer of natural grease which serves a barrier function on the skin. This is a common cause of perianal dermatitis. Washing with water only, on the other hand, dries out the epidermis and causes chapping. A simple and inexpensive moisturising lotion can provide a solution to this (Draelos, 2005), used in the shower or bath and applied to the skin after as an all-over moisturiser (Simion et al., 2005). A relatively cheap mix of sorbolene and glycerol is usually as good as the more expensive versions, although different moisturisers may be required for different reasons, for example, such as forming a barrier or reducing dryness (Loden, 2003).
- **Shampoos** While the advertisements tell us that shampoos are a must for lovely hair, the famous French dermatologist Dr Aron-Brunetiere has likened shampoo to industrial strength detergents, not unlike those used to 'scrape' the grease off plates in dishwashing (Aron-Brunetiere and Kilmartin, 1978). It 'scrapes' the natural grease out of hair and can cause damage to the hair, scalp, face, shoulders, upper trunk and hands.

  Hair can be easily managed by using conditioner alone. Conditioners contain surfactants (spreading agents), some of which have mild detergent capacities, enough to remove the normal grease in the hair but not enough to remove the thick tacky emulsion that can result from overheating at night (and which can be prevented by reducing night-time heating). Conditioners can be used as often as desired because the level of detergent activity is much less than in shampoo. During the transition period from shampoo to conditioner, some increase in greasiness may be noted, perhaps along with a little itching and flaking, but this usually settles in a matter of weeks. The condition of the hair becomes noticeably better by the end of 6–8 weeks, provided overheating at night is avoided.
- **Soap** Soap is made from oil and alkalines. It works by washing the grease (sebum) off the skin, in the process changing it from its usual slightly acid state to one of alkalinity. Unfortunately, no soap made has been able to differentiate between the skin's natural oils and exogenous dirt. Thus, washing with soap always involves the removal of the uppermost layer of oil from the skin, as well as changing the pH. Yeasts, fungi and some forms of bacteria, especially gastrointestinal bacteria, grow better in alkaline situations and hence this is a recipe for bacterial 'insult' to the skin. The use of moisturising soaps is of intermediate value only. They should also be used minimally and are less effective than the use of moisturising cream and water (Wolf et al., 2001).
- **Scrubbing and drying** It is better to treat skin with tender loving care than to scrub it and to waterproof it than to dry it out. If skin is adequately waterproofed, it can look after itself. Drying talcum powder tends to collect in skin creases and become abrasive (although some special powders such as diphemanil methylsulfate can be useful for sweat rashes); scrubbing the skin with a towel

and the aggressive use of scourers such loofahs are masochistic and have no real role in skin care.

- **Hair dryers** Although hair dryers are not as damaging as may be thought, their excessive use can contribute to hair damage. One useful way of reducing this is to dry the hair first with a synthetic chamois, such as a sports towel or car washer. This will remove the bulk of the moisture quickly, particularly if the hair is long and thick. If a dryer is still necessary, it can be used relatively briefly at a mild temperature so it is less likely to set up later damage in the hair follicle.
- **Deodorants and antiperspirants** When our skin care recommendations are adopted, there is less need to use deodorant in temperate climates (although admittedly it may be necessary in warmer parts of the country). Those who sell deodorant are usually those who sell soap. It is possible that the regular use of soap brings about minor alterations in the composition of the bacteria that are normally resident on the skin, in turn giving rise to changes in body odour: a deodorant may be the obvious solution to counteract this effect. It may be wiser to not produce the effect in the first place, if this is the case.

  Antiperspirants work by blocking the outer portion of the sweat duct. This forms a physical barrier preventing sweat from escaping to the outer surface of the skin where it would normally be evaporated and hence aid in heat loss. Although there are some idiosyncratic smells associated with individual sweat, the main offensive smells that come from it result from all the conventional approaches to soaping, drying and cleansing outlined earlier, which make the body respond in an 'unnatural' way.
- **Cosmetics** In general, cosmetics have little overall effect on the skin. But the damage inflicted on the skin by some cosmetics or medicaments can be a problem for some women (Orton and Wilkinson, 2004). Various combinations of showering, shampooing, cleansing and drying mentioned above are capable of aggravating, augmenting and prolonging any instability already present in the skin. Adding a cosmetic, which may consist of dozens of ingredients, can raise the chances of sensitivity to one or a combination of ingredients, resulting in dermatitis in some form. Quite often this leads to medicines being prescribed, but unless the causes are considered in their own right, these are unlikely to have any long-term effect. Indeed, they may just add to the problem because of the addition of yet another potential skin irritant. And while few would support the total elimination of cosmetics, there is a definite case to be made for careful and perceptive use.
- **'Natural' cosmetics** Most so-called natural products are mixtures of many ingredients. Lanolin from sheep's wool is claimed to have particular benefits for the skin because it is a natural product. Yet lanolin contains more than sixty different components and thus has a high potential for skin reactions. Most plant extracts also consist of many ingredients. They may be natural but they are also little different to products consisting of exactly the same chemicals made up in a laboratory. A good example of this is the commonly used tea tree oil, with which a significant incidence of skin sensitivities is associated.

What can be done in a standard consultation

Observe skin disturbances that may be related to lifestyle.

Observe skin type and possible environmental effects (e.g. sun).

Use the skin behaviour check list (see *Professional resources*), if appropriate.

Ask about use of shampoo, soap, astringent and deodorants/antiperspirants.

Check obese/overweight patients for diabetic dermopathy and acanthosis.

Discuss effects of constant dryness/overheating on skin.

Investigate lifestyle habits (scratching, medicating) as a cause of specific skin insult.

LIFESTYLE

The modern environment, technological advances and lifestyle behaviours can affect the skin. The most obvious contributor is obesity, which is responsible for changes in skin barrier function, sebaceous glands and sebum production, sweat glands, lymphatics, collagen structure and function, wound healing, microcirculation and macro-circulation, and subcutaneous fat (Yosipovitch et al., 2007). It is also a cause of a wide spectrum of dermatological diseases including acanthosis nigricans, intertrigo, acrochordons, keratosis pilaris, hyperandrogenism and hirsutism, striae distensae, adiposis dolorosa and fat redistribution, lymphoedema, chronic venous insufficiency, plantar hyperkeratosis, cellulitis, skin infections, hidradenitis suppurativa, psoriasis, insulin resistance syndrome and tophaceous gout.

Diabetic dermopathy is the most common cutaneous marker of diabetes and presents as single or multiple well-demarcated brown atrophic macules, predominantly on the shins. This has also been shown to be associated with *diabetic retinopathy* (Abdollahi et al., 2007), supporting the need for optical care in diabetic patients. Smoking can also affect skin and enhance wrinkling, giving the appearance of ageing.

A skin care package for patients

For best effect, the skin care techniques discussed here should be seen as a package. If some suggestions only are taken up, and the rest ignored, the results are likely to be less than totally satisfactory. It should also be realised that this is unlikely to provide an overnight remedy. Patience and perseverance are necessary. An effective outcome can take at least 3–4 months (Molloy and Egger, 2007). Under the principle of 'do no harm', the following are not likely to have any adverse effects, even if they do not have a substantial evidence base in some cases.

Showering/bathing

If the skin is irritable, no soap should be used and oatmeal baths should be substituted.

Moisturising cream mixed with water may be used as soap. It will adequately clean *all* areas of the skin.

Keeping soap to a minimum will reduce the need for deodorants, which themselves can have a damaging effect on the skin.

Showers may be taken as often as desired, but they should be brief and tepid. Very hot water should be avoided. Any soap used should be rinsed off well before drying.

Avoid spa baths and other heat treatments such as saunas.

Avoid bubble baths or bath salts and do not use antiseptics such as Dettol™ in the bath water.

If desired, use an oatmeal bath (not oatmeal soap), by doing the following:

1. Put 1 cup of rolled oats in an old nylon stocking or muslin bag.
2. Fill a bath with tepid water so the whole body can be immersed.
3. Swish the bag around in the water until it goes white.
4. Soak in the bath and squeeze bag against infected skin (10–15 minutes).
5. After the bath, pat the skin dry gently.

Drying

After each shower, half dry the skin by patting, rather than rubbing.

Soak up most of the moisture from the hair with a chamois or absorbent towel. It is not necessary to have the skin completely dry.

Moisturising

Use a simple, inexpensive moisturiser (such as sorbolene cream with glycerine) regularly after showering or washing.

Half dry the skin by patting before applying moisturiser.

Take approximately one teaspoon of moisturising cream and four teaspoons of water.

Mix these well in the hands until a nice simple lotion is formed and then rub this all over the body.

Since the cream neither smells nor stains (except silk) and washes out of clothing by normal means, it is unnecessary to wait for the skin to dry before dressing.

Occasionally, when very dry skin is being moisturised, small red spots (some with minute pustules in the centre) may develop, especially on the thighs and forearms. These are caused by blockage of hair follicles. Such spots should be ignored. They are not infectious. Squeezing or rubbing will make them worse.

Clothing

Aim to keep comfortably cool both during the day and at night. When the body is warmed up enough, consider taking some clothing off. (After some weeks of doing this the body adjusts, and it becomes easier to cope with temperature changes.)

Punch holes in the insteps of leather shoes to enable them to breathe.

Sports clothing

Avoid synthetic, full-body clothing, such as lycra. Wear light cotton clothing that breathes to allow sweat to be evaporated off the body.

Do not over-dress. There is no such thing as 'sweating weight off' by overdressing during exercise.

Where possible, keep the extremities (such as arms and legs) and the midriff bare to allow for maximum sweat evaporation.

Wear chunky acrylic socks during exercise to wick away moisture created by overheating the feet.

Hair care

Avoid shampoos. Use 1–2 tablespoons of hair conditioner for washing hair.

Avoid the frequent use of hair dryers, especially if these are on hot.

Skin care

Avoid the use of aftershave, toners, tonics, astringents and cleansers.

Do not try to exfoliate the skin, particularly if exposure to sunlight is imminent.

Avoid chemicals and over-use of antiseptics and medicated skin care items.

Use moisturising cream as a 'soap', hand cream, shaving cream, facial cleanser, moisturiser and shampoo if desired (mix with a little water and run into the scalp at night, then rinse out the next day).

Reduce body fat (not necessarily weight).

Reduce the amount of chemicals (in cosmetic products) applied to the skin.

Do not be fooled by cosmetics that claim to be natural.

Use basic lipsticks and lip creams for moisturising and protecting of the lips.

Learn techniques of stress management.

Indoors

Where possible, avoid situations of constant overheating such as airconditioned rooms and cars.

Avoid rubber gloves while washing up.

Do not use excessive detergent when washing up.

Use a bowl of water to increase humidity in an airconditioned office.

Take frequent breaks outdoors.

Outdoors

Use a maximum protection sunscreen at all times if exposed to the sun.

Move around if it is necessary to stay in the sun. Do not sunbake.

Use sun protective clothing if exposed to the sun over long periods.

Regularly wear a sun-protective hat.

Use moisturiser after sun and salt water or chlorine exposure.

Wear sunglasses when in the outdoors, but choose a brand based on UV protection level (preferably 100%) rather than price.

Night-time

Use blankets and sheets instead of a doona or quilt.

Avoid electric blankets, hot water bottles and heated water beds.

Use light, natural fibre blankets such as wool (but not Angora or mohair).

Avoid over-using blankets or continental quilts that cause night-time overheating. Become used to 'sleeping light'.

Do not use bed socks.

If cold feet are a problem, heat a damp towel in a microwave and place under the feet.

Wear light night attire all year round.

Travelling

If possible in a hotel/motel room, turn off the airconditioning and open the window. If this is not possible, fill the bath full of water and leave overnight.

If spending long periods in an airconditioned or heated car, use a light spray mist to increase the humidity.

Carry a moisturiser in hand luggage for use on long distance airplane flights.

Ask the hotel if it is possible to have blankets instead of a doona or continental quilt.

Summary

Skin is one of the body's largest organs. As such it reacts to insults, both physical and psychological, and this is reflected in the general term 'dermatitis'. While much of this may come from physiological sources, a good deal of modern skin damage is currently caused by the modern environment, particularly through excessive heating, drying, modern technology and our obsession with cleanliness. A skin care package incorporating a range of simple lifestyle changes can help overcome many modern environmentally induced skin care problems.

practice tips

PRACTICE TIPS: SKIN CARE

	Medical practitioner	Practice nurse
Assess	Signs of skin cancer and other non-lifestyle related skin damage. ABCD* of moles and nevae. Lifestyle/environmental causes. Underlying disease (e.g. diabetes with acanthosis; obesity with heat rash).	Environmental causes of skin insult in detail. ABCDE* of moles and nevae. Lifestyle (conduct a lifestyle check list; see *Professional resources*). Possible underlying diseases.
Assist	By providing medication for skin treatment only where required. By advising on possible influences of lifestyle factors.	Modification of lifestyle factors that could be related to skin insult; this requires a 'package' approach (see *Professional resources*). By providing ongoing support.
Arrange	Referral to dermatologist where indicated. List of other health professionals for a care plan (e.g. dietitian).	Care plan. Contact with and coordination of other health professionals (e.g. dermatologist, dietitian).

*ABCD = assymetry, border irregular, colour, diameter

key points

KEY POINTS FOR CLINICAL MANAGEMENT

- Consider lifestyle factors as potential cause of skin problems (e.g. smoking, sleep, office/home/sleep environment).
- Investigate possible modern causes of skin insult, physical or psychological.
- Explain the relationship between the modern environment and possible skin problems.
- Consider treatment for modern environmental skin problems as a package, requiring attention to all factors.

references

REFERENCES

Abdollahi A, Daneshpazhooh M, Amirchagmaghi E et al. (2007) Dermopathy and retinopathy in diabetes: is there an association? *Dermatology* 214(2) :133–36.

Adams BB. (2002) Dermatologic disorders of the athlete. *Sports Med* 32(5): 309–21.

Aron-Brunetiere R, Kilmartin J. (1978) *Beauty and medicine.* London: Oxford Press.

Balin AK, Balin LP. (1997) *The life of the skin: what it hides, what it reveals, and how it communicates.* NY: Bantam Books.

Draelos ZD. (2005) Concepts in skin care maintenance. *Cutis* 76(6 Suppl): 19–25.

Gloster HM, Neal K. (2006) Skin cancer in skin of colour. *J Am Acad Dermatol* 55(5): 741–60

Janda M, Kimlin MG, Whiteman DC et al. (2007) Sun protection messages, vitamin D and skin cancer: out of the frying pan and into the fire? *MJA* 186 (2): 52–53.

Johansson O, Gangi S, Liang Y et al. (2001) Cutaneous mast cells are altered in normal healthy volunteers sitting in front of ordinary TVs/PCs–results from open-field provocation experiments. *J Cutan Pathol* 28(10): 513–19.

Loden M. (2003) Do moisturizers work? *J Cosmet Dermatol* 2(3–4): 141–49

Lu CY, Ma YC, Lin JM et al. (2007) Oxidative stress associated with indoor air pollution and sick building syndrome-related symptoms among office workers in Taiwan. *Inhal Toxicol* 19(1): 57–65.

Molloy HF, Egger G. (2008) *Good skin*, 2nd edn. Sydney: Allen and Unwin.

Molloy HF, LaMont-Gregory E, Idzikowski C et al. (1993) Overheating in bed as an important factor in many common dermatoses. *Int J Dermatol* 32(9): 668–72.

Morris-Jones R, Robertson SJ, Ross JS et al. (2002) Dermatitis caused by physical irritants. *Br J Dermatol* 147(2): 270–75.

Okamoto-Mizuno K, Mizuno K, Michie S et al. (1999) Effects of humid heat exposure on human sleep stages and body temperature. *Sleep* 22(6): 767–73.

Orton DI, Wilkinson JD. (2004) Cosmetic allergy: incidence, diagnosis, and management. *Am J Clin Dermatol* 5(5): 327–37

Ricci G, Patrizi A, Bellini F et al. (2006) Use of textiles in atopic dermatitis: care of atopic dermatitis. *Curr Probl Dermatol* 33: 127–43.

Scherer PE. (2006) Adipose tissue: from lipid storage compartment to endocrine organ. *Diabetes* 55(6): 1537–45.

Simion FA, Abrutyn ES, Draelos ZD. (2005) Ability of moisturizers to reduce dry skin and irritation and to prevent their return. *J Cosmet Sci* 56(6): 427–44.

Springett K. (2002) Introduction to some common cutaneous foot conditions and their management. *J Tissue Viability* 12(3): 100–01, 104–07.

Sunwoo Y, Chou C, Takeshita J et al. (2006) Physiological and subjective responses to low relative humidity in young and elderly men. *J Physiol Anthrop* 25(3): 229–38.

Wolf R, Orion E, Parish LC. (2004) A scientific soap opera and winter itch. *Skinmed* 3(1): 9–10.

Wolf R, Wolf D, Tuzan B et al Y. (2001) Soaps, shampoos and detergents. *Clin Dermatol* 19(4): 393–97.

Yosipovitch G, DeVore A, Dawn A. (2007) Obesity and the skin: skin physiology and skin manifestations of obesity *J Am Coll Dermatol* 56(6): 901–16.

PROFESSIONAL RESOURCES: A SKIN BEHAVIOUR CHECK LIST

Do you

- Try to stay as warm as possible at all times?
- Work in an airconditioned office?
- Drive an airconditioned car?
- Sleep with a doona, electric blanket or heated waterbed at night?
- Shampoo your hair daily or every two days?
- Frequently use soap, antiperspirant/deodorant, astringents, aftershave, tonics or toners?
- Regularly stay in hotels/motels without external ventilation?
- Travel regularly in aeroplanes?
- Work, play or lie in the sun?

Affirmative answers to all or most of these questions could suggest the need for an environmental approach to skin care problems.

CHAPTER 18

Sex and lifestyle

MICHAEL GILLMAN, GARRY EGGER

The phrase 'use it or lose it' is particularly appropriate for the genitalia.

MEULEMAN, 2002

Introduction

According to Australian sex therapist Dr Rosie King, the prevalence of sexual dysfunction in men roughly corresponds to the decade of age in which this occurs. Hence, 40% of forty-year-olds will experience some problem, 50% of fifty-year-olds and 60% of sixty-year-olds. It is this knowledge, she claims, that makes no man want to live to a hundred!

While this may reflect some medical licence, it does indicate the importance of age in sexual functioning. Age is perhaps the most predictable determinant of sexual dysfunction (where dysfunction is defined as 'an issue of concern for a particular individual'), with problems typically increasing proportionately with age. Other factors are biology, illness, psychological health, past experience and education. However, the next most common cause is lifestyle, and this can exacerbate or ameliorate the effects of ageing.

Sex and lifestyle are linked in a number of ways, from sexually transmitted infections to sexual performance malfunction. Because the former is more of a conventional health problem, which has an extensive literature of its own, it is only the latter with which we concern ourselves here. This is still an extensive field covering a wide variety of conditions, including erectile dysfunction, hypoactive sexual desire, and ejaculatory, orgasmic, sexual aversion, and hormonal disorders, to name but a few. As can be seen from the list, the biggest problems—at least in terms of performance—are likely to occur amongst males, hence the greater concentration on male sexual performance and lifestyle in this chapter. We do not ignore issues of performance or desire for females, and where there is clear evidence for these being associated with lifestyle, they are considered. However, the bulk of the discussion will concern lifestyle and sexual performance in men.

Prevalence of sexual problems

Because of the sensitivity of the topic, the prevalence of sexual problems in the community is difficult to detect accurately. Generally accepted figures suggest that around one in three men aged 18–59 report dissatisfaction with some aspect of their sexual function (Foresta et al., 2003). This continues to rise over age sixty, despite the fact that sexual desire may remain high. Erectile dysfunction (ED) appears to be the most common problem, with surveys suggesting a prevalence of close to 20% of men over twenty years of age (Selvin et al., 2007). The rate of ED in men with type 2 diabetes is estimated to be two to three times higher than those without diabetes (Selvin et al., 2007) but, more critically, the changes in lifestyle and lifestyle-based aetiology of many of these problems has led to predictions of a doubling in prevalence by the year 2025 (Fabbri et al., 2003).

ED, sometimes called impotence, is the repeated inability to obtain or maintain an erection firm enough for sexual intercourse. Erectile dysfunction can be *global*, in which case all erections are decreased, or *situational*, where strong erections may be obtained during rapid eye movement sleep but not with sexual stimulation. In older men, ED usually has a physical cause, such as disease, injury or side effects of drugs. The most common cause is vascular disease and it has the same risk factors as for cardiovascular disease. Diseases such as diabetes, kidney disease, chronic alcoholism, multiple sclerosis, atherosclerosis, other vascular diseases and neurologic disease account for about 70% of all cases.

Sexual drive, ejaculatory function, sexual problem assessment and sexual satisfaction are the other main areas where lifestyle can affect male sexuality. Medical awareness of a patient's sexual health, however, is probably not high, and often health professionals do not pay sufficient attention, probably because of their conservative attitudes, lack of skill in addressing sexuality problems and, of course, time constraints within the consultation setting.

Causes—general

There is now clear evidence that lifestyle factors have a direct impact on the development of many sexual problems. Clearly, stress, anxiety and depression will impact on many of the conditions listed above and addressing these will improve patient outcomes. Cardiovascular risk factors, such as type 2 diabetes mellitus (T2DM), hypertension, smoking, alcohol or drug abuse, a sedentary lifestyle and obesity, as well as chronic diseases such as arthritis, renal and hepatic failure, and pulmonary disease, have all been linked to the development of sexual problems in general and ED in particular. Many medications used to treat these problems have paradoxically been implicated in reducing sexual function (Chapter 21). Finally, sleep deprivation (Chapter 16) has also been suggested to inhibit nocturnal erections, thus decreasing the normal oxygenation of the corpora cavernosa necessary to maintain endothelial function (Kamp et al., 2005).

While less commonly reported, lifestyle factors can also have an impact on female sexuality. As with men, ageing is an inhibitory factor on sexual desire and ability, but according to Professor Beverly Whipple, an author of *The Science of Orgasm*, the adage of 'use it or lose it' is as relevant for women as it is for men, in this case for maintaining high oestrogen levels and reducing vaginal dryness. Obesity, smoking and inactivity are also lifestyle factors likely to have a dampening effect on female arousal. A small study of thirty women with ischaemic heart disease suggested that sexual dysfunction was common (30%) and, in fact, 23% of these women experienced sexual problems before developing cardiac symptoms (Salonia et al., 2002). Larger studies are required, however, before any definite links between cardiovascular disease and female sexual dysfunction can be made. Medications can also affect female sexuality, with a significant proportion of females having problems with arousal or orgasm due to certain medications (see below).

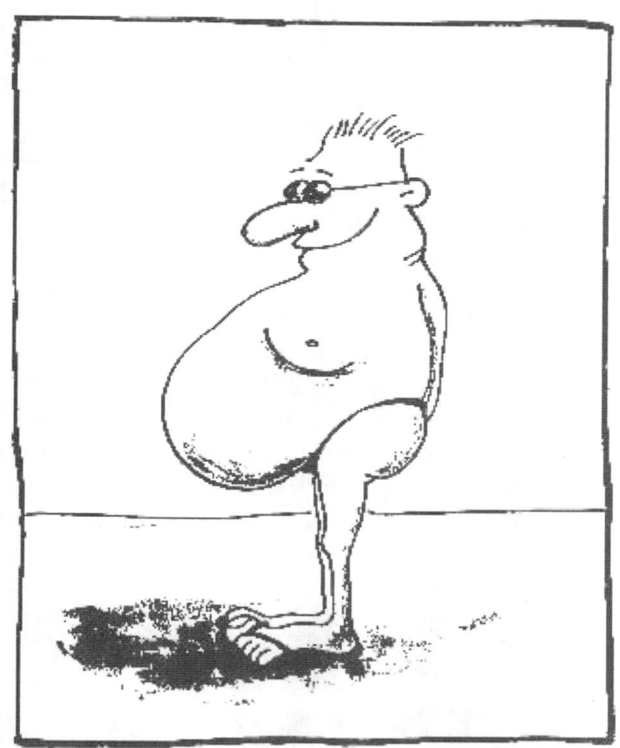

SEXUAL ORGAN HARASSMENT

Causes—specific

Individual lifestyle factors that can cause sexual problems include inactivity, obesity, T2DM, depression, smoking, alcohol and medications.

Inactivity

Several studies have shown a higher risk of sexual problems, including ED, among those who are sedentary or inactive, with a dose–response relationship. One Australian study has shown that a history of vigorous exercise is protective against ED across all ages (Pinnock et al., 1999). The reasons for this are not clear but it may be an evolutionary development, with a consistent level of physical activity resulting in a feedforward mechanism for maintaining sex hormone levels, and this is disrupted with inactivity.

Obesity

The scientific literature is unequivocal about ED and obesity. In the Massachusetts Male Ageing Study, having a BMI >28 doubled the incidence of ED at follow-up (Feldman et al., 2000). An increase in BMI has been shown to reduce the quality of erections as demonstrated using the IIEF-5 (International Index of Erectile Dysfunction), a validated questionnaire-based method of assessing erectile dysfunction. Just by increasing the BMI by 1 kilogram per metre squared, the IIEF-5 score can decrease by 0.141 independent of age (Derby et al., 2000). However, obesity per se may not be the issue and, as with metabolic health in general, remaining fit and active, even in the presence of obesity, may help reduce the problem.

Obesity is associated with polycystic ovaries in women, probably through insulin resistance (Orio et al., 2007), and consequent fertility problems. Obesity in couples has also been shown to result in subfecundity, with the time to pregnancy increasing with the level of obesity of both male and female partners (Ramlau-Hansen et al., 2007). There is also an inverse relationship between bioavailable testosterone levels in men, sexual performance and waist circumference (Kapoor et al., 2007).

Type 2 diabetes

As T2DM results from several of the risk factors discussed above, it is not surprising that it is a major risk factor for sexual dysfunction in itself. As with obesity, there is a clear and unequivocal relationship between T2DM and sexual function, ED and ejaculatory problems in men, but also problems with arousal, genital sensation, lubrication and dyspareunia in up to 50% of women (Muniyappa et al., 2005). This can occur through the narrowing of peripheral arteries, as well as the development of insulin resistance and its effects on sex-based hormones. Hypogonadism affecting all aspects of sexual performance in men has been shown to be higher in diabetic than non-diabetic men (Kapoor et al., 2007). Screening for ED and other sexual problems in T2DM patients may therefore be warranted.

What can be done in a standard consultation

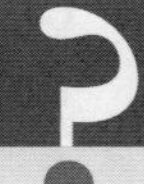

Ask about sexual performance in patients with other metabolic risk factors.

Determine whether this is a problem for the patient.

Discuss specific aspects of the problem (e.g. ED, ejaculation).

Explain the lifestyle basis of many sexual performance problems.

Consider changes in female desire as well as changes in male performance.

Explain possible adjunctive treatments.

Order pathology tests (e.g. EUCs, LFTs, serum testosterone, TSH).

Refer or make another appointment for further consideration of the issues.

Depression

Depression can be both a cause and a consequence of sexual problems, and both can be co-morbid with other diseases (Shabsigh et al., 2001). Although little has been published on the non-drug-induced effects of depression on sexual performance, some studies suggest that 25–75% of both men and women with unipolar depression suffer either loss of libido, disorders of arousal or erection, or lubrication problems (Williams and Reynolds, 2006). One study has shown that the link in men, at least, may be through the mediation of decreased sexual activity occurring in single, widowed or divorced men, as well as smoking, age and physical inactivity (Nicolosi et al., 2004).

Smoking

Smoking is a risk factor for ED in particular because of the narrowing of the pudendal artery through atherogenesis. This reduces blood flow and velocity in smokers as well as the penile nitric oxide synthase activity required for an adequate erection. Data from the Massachusetts Male Aging Study shows that cigarette smoking doubled the risk of ED (Feldman et al., 2000).

Alcohol

While alcohol in moderation may have a stimulatory effect on sexual arousal, its excessive use, as Shakespeare put it, 'provokes the desire but takes away the performance'. Alcohol can cause orgasmic delay in women and can depress testosterone concentrations in men (Mueleman, 2002). While short-term effects from social drinking may not be of concern, chronic drinking can lead to systemic disturbances such as liver and pancreatic problems, which can interfere with performance. Chronic alcoholism can also result in permanent impotence even after the cessation of drinking for many years.

Medications

One of the most common side effects of medication is sexual dysfunction, either in desire or performance ability. Ironically, many of the medications used to treat diseases—or risk factors that can also be risk factors for sexual problems such as heart disease, hypertension, hypercholesterolemia, diabetes or depression—can cause or exacerbate sexual problems. Perhaps the most commonly used of these are the antidepressants, which can set up a vicious cycle where sexual inadequacy can lead to depression, leading to further sexual inadequacy (Clayton and Montejo, 2006). While some antidepressants (e.g. bupropion) appear to have less adverse effects on sexual performance, they are also generally less effective for depression treatment. Trying a different antidepressant, using cognitive therapy for mild depression, and using sildenafil as antidote therapy (Rudkin et al., 2004) can help overcome these problems.

Medications, such as some antidepressants, also affect female sexuality, with a significant proportion of females having problems with arousal or orgasm. Antihistamines can also cause vaginal dryness.

Management

In a study of around 600 men aged 30–70 years, midlife appeared to be too late for lifestyle modification to reverse the adverse effects of nicotine, obesity and alcohol consumption on sexual function, but physical activity appeared to be effective in reducing the risk of ED (Esposito et al., 2004). A controlled study of obese men (BMI > 30) revealed that an increase in physical activity from 48 to 195 mins per week and a decrease in BMI from 37 to 31 over two years resulted in an increase of the IIEF-5 score from 13.9 to 17 (Salonia et al., 2004). It does appear, however, that identification and correction of vascular ED and regular physical activity and normalising BMI will help both in the prevention and the treatment of this disorder.

Healthcare professionals are seeing an increasing number of male patients wanting to know whether they have low testosterone levels and whether medication can correct this. True male hypogonadism—with unequivocal symptoms and signs of androgen deficiency and at least two separate early morning serum testosterone levels of less than 8 nmol/L—is quite rare. This condition needs to be treated with testosterone replacement therapy to avoid longer-term consequences such as osteoporosis. However, it is unlikely to be the panacea for men's health problems.

It is known that testosterone levels decrease with increasing age in men, with levels going down by around 0.8% per year over the age of forty (Morales and Lunenfeld, 2002). Many terms have been coined for this condition such as 'andropause', 'male climacteric', ADAM (androgen deficiency in the ageing male) and most recently 'late onset hypogonadism'. It is unclear whether these men should be managed with hormone therapy.

Ageing is also often associated with an increase in abdominal fat mass, a decrease in muscle mass and a decrease in activity levels, and these can independently affect testosterone levels. It is also known that testosterone disorders are implicated in metabolic derangements such as obesity, insulin resistance and the metabolic syndrome. It has become apparent that visceral obesity leads to a decrease in insulin receptor numbers which result in hyperinsulinaemia; hyperinsulinaemia leads to decreased levels of sex hormone binding globulin and thus a decrease in available serum testosterone. Furthermore, it has been demonstrated that insulin receptor numbers can be restored to normal if insulin levels are decreased by weight loss (Bar et al., 1976).

Testosterone undergoes aromatisation to oestradiol, particularly in adipose tissue. Therefore, men with increased visceral fat will have higher levels of oestradiol. This can lead to effects on the male breast tissue resulting in gynaecomastia. Interestingly, physical activity appears to decrease this process of aromatisation. Hence, a slightly reduced serum testosterone level may merely reflect increased visceral fat mass and the initial treatment should involve lifestyle behavioural modification aimed at decreasing the percentage of visceral fat before resorting to testosterone replacement therapy. PDE5 inhibitors (e.g. sildenafil) are less effective in men with hypogonadal levels of testosterone (such as men with diabetes) and testosterone replacement in these cases can convert sildenafil non-responders into responders (Kapoor et al., 2007)

Other treatments may involve medication substitution or reduction; medications to enhance the sexual response such as the PDE5 inhibitors; cognitive behaviour therapy; counselling; vacuum therapy treatments; injections; and, as a last resort, surgery. There are no approved medications for women for sexual problems, and lifestyle changes might be expected to have less effect here than with males.

The final word goes to Meuleman (2002), who suggested that, 'given the fact that current symptomatic treatments are invasive, are costly, or have unproved long-term benefits, in daily practice, too little attention is paid to the modification of risk factors and secondary prevention. A more physically active lifestyle, quitting smoking, reduction of overweight and a moderate alcohol intake may be viewed as integral components of a comprehensive risk reduction program'.

Summary

Lifestyle factors play a significant role in sexual performance. Key pervasive factors—such as obesity, poor nutrition, inactivity and smoking—once again stand out as the predominant influences, but other factors such as poor sleep, depression and some forms of medication may also play a part. Sexual activity, desire and performance, where these are seen as problems, should be considered in any overall lifestyle analysis.

PRACTICE TIPS: MANAGING LIFESTYLE-RELATED SEXUAL PROBLEMS

	General practitioner	Practice nurse
Assess	Sexual function in those with cardiovascular and metabolic risk (sensitively). Possible co-morbidities. Medication effects and possible alternatives. Pharmacotherapy options.	Smoking, drinking, activity levels and obesity for any impact on sexual function. BP, height, weight, waist circumference and dipstick urinalysis.
Assist	With first-line treatments such as lifestyle change, counselling, patient education and medication changes. With advice on the 'use it or lose it' principle. With PDE5 inhibitors, vacuum constriction devices or intracavernosal injections if appropriate.	With written materials for patient education. With counselling, if experienced in this area.
Arrange	List of other health professionals for a care plan. Referral to a mental health professional, endocrinologist, urologist or sex therapist where appropriate	Care plan. Contact with and coordination of other health professionals. Discussion of options with other professionals

KEY POINTS FOR CLINICAL MANAGEMENT

- Check sexual function as part of other major chronic disease symptoms.
- Consider problems such as ED as multifactorial conditions that may require a multidisciplinary approach to treatment (especially when depression is present).

- Consider adjuvant or drug substitution treatment approaches to depression where this is associated with sexual dysfunction.
- Discuss the range of treatment approaches available (e.g. PDE5 inhibitors, intracavernosal injections, vacuum constriction devises).

REFERENCES

Bar RS, Gorden P, Roth J. (1976) Fluctuations in the affinity and concentrations of insulin receptors on circulating monocytes of obese patients: effects of starvation, refeeding and dieting. *J Clin Invest* 58: 1123–35.

Clayton AH, Montejo AL. (2006) Major depressive disorder, antidepressants and sexual function. *J Clin Psychiatry* 67(Suppl 6): 33–37.

Derby CA, Mohr BA, Goldstein I et al. (2000) Modifiable risk factors and erectile dysfunction: can lifestyle changes modify risk? *Urology* 56(2): 302–06.

Esposito K, Giugliana F, Di Palo C et al. (2004) Effect of lifestyle changes on erectile dysfunction in obese men. *JAMA* 291: 2978–84.

Fabbri A, Caprio M, Aversa A. (2003) Pathology or erection. *J Endocrinol Invest* 26(3Suppl): 87–90.

Feldman HA, Johannes CB, Derby CA et al. (2000) Erectile dysfunction and coronary risk factors: prospective results from the Massachusetts Male Aging Study. *Prev Med* 30: 328–38.

Foresta C, Argiolas A, Bassi P et al. (2003) Clinical and diagnostic approach to erectile dysfunction. *Ann Ital Med Int* 18(4): 204–18.

Kamp S, Ott R, Knoll T et al. (2005) EM-sleep deprivation leads to a decrease of nocturnal penile tumescence (NPT) in young health males: The significance of NPT-measurements (611.13). *XVII World Congress of Sexology*, July 10–15, 2005, Montreal, Canada.

Kapoor D, Aldred H, Clark S et al. (2007) Clinical and biochemical assessment of hypogonadism in men with type 2 diabetes. *Diab Care* 30(4): 911–17.

Komisaruk BR, Beyer-Flores C, Whipple B. (2006) *The science of orgasm.* Baltimore: Johns Hopkins University Press.

Morales A, Lunenfeld B. (2002) Investigation, treatment and monitoring of late onset hypogonadism in males. *Official recommendations of the International Society for the Study of the Aging Male* 5: 74–86.

Meuleman EJH. (2002) Prevalence of erectile dysfunction: need for treatment? *Int J Impot Res* 14(Suppl 1): S22–S28.

Muniyappa R, Norton M, Dunn ME et al. (2005) Diabetes and female sexual dysfunction: moving beyond 'benign neglect'. *Curr Diab Rep* 8(2): 515–22.

Nicolosi A, Moreira ED Jr, Villa M et al. (2004) A population study of the association between sexual function, sexual satisfaction and depressive symptoms in men. *J Affect Disord* 82(2): 235-2-3.

Orio F, Falbo A, Grieco A et al. (2007) Polycystic ovary syndrome and obesity: non pharmacological options. *Minerva Ginecol* 59(1): 63–73.

Pinnock CB, Stapleton AM, Marshall VR. (1999) Erectile dysfunction in the community: a prevalence study. *MJA* 171: 353–57.

Ramlau-Hansen CH, Thulstrup AM, Nohr EA. (2007) Subfecundity in overweight and obese couples. *Hum Reprod* 2(6): 1634–37.

Rosen RC. (1999) Development and evaluation of an abridged, 5-item version of the International Index of Erectile Function (IIEF-5) as a diagnostic tool for erectile dysfunction. *International J Impot Res* 11: 319–26.

Rudkin L, Taylor MJ, Hawton K. (2004) Strategies for managing sexual dysfunction induced by antidepressant medication. *Cochrane Database Syst Rev* 18(4):CD003382.

Salonia A, Briganti A, Montorsi P. (2002) Sexual dysfunction in women with coronary heart disease. *Int J Impot Res* 14(suppl 4): S80.

Seftel AD. (2006) Diagnosis of sexual dysfunction. Porst H, Buvat J (eds). *Standard practice in sexual medicine.* Blackwell Publishing Ltd: Massachusetts.

Selvin E, Burnett AL, Platz EA. (2007) Prevalence and risk factors for erectile dysfunction in the US. *Am J Med* 120(2): 151–57.

Shabsigh R, Zakaria L, Anastasiadis AG et al. (2001) Sexual dysfunction and depression: etiology, prevalence, and treatment. *Curr Urol Rep* 2(6): 463–67.

Williams K, Reynolds MF. (2006) Sexual dysfunction in major depression. *CNS Spectr* 11(8 Suppl 9): 19–23.

professional resources

PROFESSIONAL RESOURCES: MEASURING SEXUAL FUNCTION

Sexual Health Inventory for Men (Rosen, 1999)

Patient instructions: Please answer the following questions, ticking the number that most applies from 1 = least functional to 5 = most functional.

	1 least functional	2	3	4	5 most functional
How do you rate your confidence that you could get and keep an erection?					
When you had erections with sexual stimulation, how often were your erections hard enough for penetration?					
During sexual intercourse, how often are you able to maintain your erection after you had penetrated (entered) your partner?					
During sexual intercourse, how difficult was it to maintain your erection to the completion of intercourse?					
When you attempted sexual intercourse, how often was it satisfactory for you?					

Professional instructions: Each question is rated on a Likert scale of 1 = least functional to 5 = most functional. Total scores range from 5 to 25:

- 22–25 normal erectile function
- 17–21 mild erectile dysfunction
- 12–16 mild to moderate erectile dysfunction
- 8–11 moderate erectile dysfunction

Brief points to cover in the physical examination of a male patient with erectile dysfunction (Seftel, 2006)

Check the following:

- gynaecomastia
- body hair distribution
- penis size

- femoral pulses
- inguinal hernia
- the foreskin and glans and urethra for STIs, other infections or pathology
- the tunica for plaques
- the testes for size and consistency and lie and the presence of two testes
- varicocoeles
- the rectum for anal tone, anal pathology and prostate (after informed consent)

CHAPTER 19

Lifestyle and oral health: wild animals don't floss

BERNADETTE DRUMOND, GARRY EGGER

Unlike most human organs, teeth need a rest.

Introduction

Imagine a serene afternoon on a Serengeti plain. All that is left of a big cat's meal is a steaming carcass and some blood dripping from its powerful jaws. As always, the remnants remain in the teeth for some time. Lions don't floss. Yet they usually maintain strong, healthy, teeth throughout the duration of their lives and die with their choppers intact. Most humans, on the other hand, are lucky to get to three-score-and-ten with a full mouthful of teeth; those who do have often had significant 'work' done.

So what does this tell us about human oral health? That many of the dental problems suffered by humans result from the lifestyle we lead and the way we care for our teeth. Obviously, dental problems are not all to do with the modern way of life, and images of toothless serfs from earlier days testify to the great strides made in dentistry with modernity. However, as with many aspects of health canvassed in this book, there comes a time when positive advances are often overwhelmed by environmental changes that, while providing greater material prosperity, can have a hidden cost in human wellbeing.

Oral health is a large vista, with several professions dedicated to its management. We do not intend here to tramp the whole field, but merely to sample some oral health problems specifically associated with our way of life. The two main forms of oral disease considered are dental decay/erosion and periodontal (gum) disease. The main culprits are all too familiar—inadequate diet, sweetened beverages, inactivity, obesity, smoking and diabetes. Their links with health become even more obvious when we open our mouths.

Lifestyle, dental caries and tooth erosion

Dental caries is a contagious bacterial disease, with children generally gaining the infection from their mothers (or possibly it is passed between teenagers). Having said this, the bacteria which cause the problem (mutans streptococci and lactobacilli, in particular) exist in all humans and do not necessarily cause problems unless a number of conditions coexist. The bacteria require fermentable carbohydrate as a nutrient (not just simple sugar, as is the general public perception) and produce acids that demineralise (dissolve) teeth on a particular area of a tooth covered by dental plaque. Coupled with acidic foods and beverages with a pH below 5.5, these acids can cause dental caries and erosion of tooth enamel (Bartlett, 2005). When erosion occurs, the whole surface of the tooth dissolves, leaving the enamel very thin and the tooth extremely sensitive to cold and hot foods.

Decay cannot occur without food and bacteria, but protection is afforded by saliva, which acts as a buffer (with calcium, fluoride and other minerals) to protect against acidosis, saliva contains protective antibodies and antibacterial action, and helps remineralise teeth (Hara et al., 2006). However, several factors in the modern lifestyle mitigate the protective effects of saliva; these include medications that decrease the salivary flow and eating habits that do not allow saliva time to bathe the teeth and remineralise the enamel. Consequently, protective actions need to be consciously taken or decay will occur.

Erosive factors in the diet

While fermentable carbohydrate is the key nutritive factor for dental bacteria, this is only relevant if there is enough for bacterial metabolism: total food intake as well as the quality of that intake can be relevant. Eating a whole chocolate bar can have the same effect on mouth bacteria as eating just one piece, as long as it is eaten all at one time. If it is eaten in several bursts, bacteria make acid for longer and this has a worse effect on the tooth. Carbohydrates that 'stick' to the teeth, such as toffee, will have a greater effect on decay production. This is not necessarily because of their sugar content but because they are likely to be around and between the teeth for longer, and because they require flossing as well as brushing to remove.

A growing issue is the carbohydrate—acid mix provided by some beverages, such as soft drinks, sports drinks, flavoured sparkling water drinks, packet mixes and fruit juices. Contrary to popular opinion, cola and other soft drinks are sometimes less acidic than fruit juices, so it is important to understand that all drinks containing acids can potentially erode teeth if they are used inappropriately. It has been shown that the sugared version of both cola and non-cola drinks are more corrosive than their 'diet' counterparts (Jain et al., 2007) but these are still not risk free. Removing the sugar will remove the risk of decay but it will not remove the risk of erosion.

The childhood trick of placing a tooth in a glass of cola to see the enamel erodes overnight works equally well for most fruit juices: the food or drink product itself is important for erosion and decay, but these are most corrosive when the teeth are left to bathe in such solutions. Sipping drinks over an extended period—for example, when long distance cyclists use 'sports' drinks or babies are left to sip juice in the cot—can have the most damaging effects (Zero and Lussi, 2006). Wine tasters and judges are particularly at risk because of the regular contact of wine with teeth (Lussi and Jaeggi, 2006).

Tips for good teeth

Take at least two hours between eating or drinking, if at all possible.

Eat (or drink) sweet foods with meals, not between.

Avoid sticky sweet foods and carbohydrates before bedtime.

Chew (unsugared) gum (for at least twenty minutes) after a main meal.

Do not sip soft drinks, fruit juices, flavoured water or sports drinks over time.

Floss as well as brush to make sure plaque is removed between the teeth.

Eat a variety of foods, including the recommended intake of dairy protein.

Do not smoke; get regular exercise; and reduce obesity.

Drink fluoridated water or ask your dentist for advice about the best way to use fluoride to improve your teeth.

Wear a mouthguard if playing a contact sport.

Protective factors

Teeth take time to recover from a carbohydrate onslaught. Hence, breaks in eating and drinking of at least two hours are recommended, something uncommon in young children in the modern environment. The belief that a constant intake of liquid is needed to avoid dehydration is discussed in Chapter 9. It is certainly not a good practice when trying to protect the teeth from damage.

The timing of eating is also important. Carbohydrate-rich foods (particularly those that are sweet and/or sticky) should be avoided before bedtime when the salivary flow is at its lowest and will therefore not provide the best tooth protection. Sweet drinks, such as soft drinks, sports drinks, wine and fruit juices, if drunk at all, should be taken with meals or other foods. A variety of foods, as encouraged in a healthy diet, is also best for teeth, preferably avoiding frequent use of sticky carbohydrate-rich foods.

As well as brushing (and preferably flossing) teeth, chewing unsugared gum after a meal or snack can help stimulate saliva with anti-acidic and antibacterial protective benefits. However, this appears to require at least twenty minutes of chewing. Some foods in the diet, such as dairy products, also have a protective effect, possibly through the qualities of proteins such as casein phosphopeptide that can coat the teeth, providing a rich source of calcium and phosphate to decrease demineralisation and enhance remineralisation (see below). Even sweetened, flavoured milk does not cause the same increase in acidity as other sweetened drinks. Again, this supports the benefits of a higher protein diet in weight control, as discussed in Chapter 4. Fluoride, added to many water supplies, also acts to slow down the demineralisation process and enhance the remineralisation process.

Periodontal disease and diabetes

A key feature of insulin resistance and type 2 diabetes (T2DM) is endothelial dysfunction and systemic inflammation, particularly in the small vessels of the body. This can lead to infection and reduced blood flow to the peripheral vessels leading to peripheral neuropathy, nephropathy, retinopathy and other problems associated with diabetes. Less well known is that the inflammation and endothelial dysfunction of small vessels of the gums and tissues surrounding the teeth—and the effects of this on the periodontal structure—often result in loss of teeth and in tooth, gum and mouth disease (Amar et al., 2003). Periodontal problems are thus linked with systemic health problems including heart disease, chronic infections, respiratory disease and diabetes (Joshipura et al., 2000), although the link is possibly bidirectional (Mealey and Rethman, 2003).

In particular, the link between periodontal disease and diabetes is becoming increasingly clear (Mealey and Oates, 2006), and hence it is not unexpected that these problems are also associated with diabetes risk factors such as obesity (Pischon et al., 2007). Inactivity, which itself is a cause of T2DM, has been linked to tooth loss in older people (Tada et al., 2003), presumably from periodontal problems. Unhealthy diet is also an issue both for diabetes risk and dental problems (Lussi et al., 2006).

Last, but definitely not least, cigarette smoking is thought to be the main risk factor associated with chronic destructive periodontal disease, and the risk is five to twenty times higher in smokers (Bergstrom, 2004).

What can be done in a standard consultation

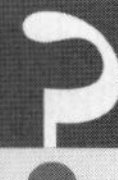

Check for potential periodontal problems in obese, inactive or patients who smoke.

Ask about pattern of use of drinks and food (i.e. sipping, snacking).

With parents, check on the pattern of fluid intake of their children as well as teeth care, including flossing.

Check that fluoride is used either in the drinking water or in other vehicles such as toothpaste or mouth rinse.

Explain the 5–20-fold risk of periodontal disease and tooth loss in smokers.

Sports and dental health

While an active sporting involvement is to be recommended for a healthy lifestyle, engagement in sports comes with injury risks. Mouthguards to protect against orofacial injury were first introduced in boxing in the U.S. in the 1920s. Since then, they have been made compulsory by sporting bodies in a number of sports. Modern materials and design have made a range of products effective in reducing the number of fractured teeth and providing some protection against jaw fracture as well. Studies comparing mouthguard users with non-users in a range of sports have shown a relative risk of injury 1.6–1.9 times greater when a mouthguard is not used. Hence, these are recommended for all sports with a potential for impact or fall injuries (Knapik et al., 2007).

Summary

The lifestyle factors that cause poor oral health are generally the same culprits responsible for other metabolic diseases discussed in this book—poor nutrition, excessive sugary foods and drinks, smoking, obesity and inactivity. The links between poor oral health and T2DM are also becoming clearer with new research, but whether this is a cause or an outcome is yet to be determined. Good oral health requires attention to diet, body weight and activity level. However, brushing, flossing, chewing sugarless gum, giving the teeth a rest between meals and avoiding sticky carbohydrate foods before retiring all add up to good oral health.

PRACTICE TIPS: IMPROVING ORAL HEALTH

	Medical practitioner	**Practice nurse**
Assess	Teeth in association with lifestyle information. Periodontal damage in patients with diabetes risk. Oral health in obese/overweight patients. Oral health practices.	Use of food and drinks in relation to teeth. Oral health practices in the obese/overweight. Need for mouthguards in sports participants, particularly children.
Assist	By explaining about lifestyle factors and their association with dental health. By explaining how poor dental health can affect general health. By explaining how parents' poor dental health can put children at risk.	By providing written materials for oral health. By informing where dental care can be obtained. By explaining the links between oral health and lifestyle practices leading to metabolic problems.
Arrange	Referral to dentist or dental specialist.	Referral.

KEY POINTS FOR CLINICAL MANAGEMENT

- Consider oral health as a significant aspect of lifestyle medicine.
- Consider the dental as well as calorific implications of food and fluid intake.
- Associate dental decay and periodontal disease with other forms of metabolic problems (i.e. hypoglycaemia).
- Become proactive on dental health with overweight children and their parents.
- Bring dental health into nutritional advice and obesity and weight control management.

REFERENCES

Amar S, Gokce N, Morgan S et al. (2003) Periodontal disease is associated with brachial artery endothelial dysfunction and systemic inflammation. *Arterioscler Thromb Vasc Biol* 23(7):1245–49.

Bartlett DW. (2005) The erosion in tooth wear: aetiology, prevention and management. *Int Dent J* 55(Suppl 1): 277–84.

Bergstrom J. (2004) Tobacco smoking and chronic destructive periodontal disease. *Odontology* 92(1): 1–8.

Hara AT, Lussi A, Zero DT. (2006) Biological factors. *Mongr Oral Sci* 20: 88–99.

Jain P, Nihill P, Sobkowski J et al. (2007) Commercial soft drinks: pH and in vitro dissolution of enamel. *Gen Dent* 55(2): 150–54.

Joshipura K, Ritchie C, Douglass C. (2000) Strength of evidence linking oral conditions and systemic disease. *Comp Contin Educ Dent Suppl* (30): 12–23.

Knapik JJ, Marshall SW, Lee RB et al. (2007) Mouthguards in sport activities: history, physical properties and injury prevention effectiveness. *Sports Med* 37(2): 117–44.

Lussi A, Hellwig E, Zero D et al. (2006) Erosive tooth wear: diagnosis, risk factors and prevention. *Am J Dent* 19(6): 319–25.

Mealey BL, Oates TW. (2006) Diabetes mellitus and periodontal disease. *J Periodontol* 77(8): 1289–303.

Mealey BL, Rethman MP. (2003) Periodontal disease and diabetes mellitus. Bidirectional relationship. *Dent Today* 22(4): 107–13.

Pischon N, Heng N, Bernimoulin JP et al. (2007) Obesity, inflammation, and periodontal disease. *J Dent Res* 86(5): 400–09.

Tada A, Watanabe T, Yokoe H, Hanada N, Tanzawa H. (2003) Relationship between the number of remaining teeth and physical activity in community-dwelling elderly. *Arch Gerontol Geriatr* 37(2): 109–17.

Zero DT, Lussi A. (2006) Behavioral factors. *Mongr Oral Sci* 20: 100–05.

CHAPTER 20

Preventing and managing injury at the clinical level

KEVIN WOLFENDEN, GARRY EGGER

Accidents aren't 'accidents'.

Introduction

In 1974 William Haddon, an engineer from the New York Health Department, redefined an area of health when he proposed that there was no such a thing as an 'accident', that injuries were in epidemic proportions, and that injuries could be treated just like any other epidemic, by dealing with a host, a vector and an environmental cause, all of which need to be considered in a global approach to the problem (Haddon, 1974). Using this method, motor vehicle injuries are dissected not just in terms of treating the victim but modifying vectors (e.g. speed) and changing environments (e.g. dangerous roads). This brought injury into the realm of preventable health-related problems.

The epidemic of injury

Injury is the fourth leading cause of death in Australia and the fifth leading cause of hospitalisation (Berry and Harrison, 2006; Kreisfeld et al., 2004). Injury is also the most common cause of death from early childhood through to middle age, being responsible for approximately 50% of all deaths in people aged 1–44 years (Kreisfeld et al, 2004), and hence the leading cause of lost years of potential life. The World Health Organization predicts that road accidents alone will be the third most burdensome health problem worldwide in 2020 (Murray and Lopez, 1996).

The most common causes of injury deaths in Australia are suicide (30%), transport related (24%), falls (19%), poisoning (6%), homicide (4%) and drowning (3%) (Kreisfeld et al., 2004). The leading causes of hospitalisation are unintentional falls (34%), transportation (15%), self harm (7%), assault (6%) and poisoning (3.1%) (Berry and Harrison, 2006). Injuries can be categorised into unintentional (e.g. falls) or intentional (arising from self harm or harm to others).

This chapter focuses on injuries that commonly present to GPs and that can be managed within a lifestyle medicine model. We focus here particularly on:

- injuries occurring from falls (in the young and the elderly), transportation, drowning and poisoning;
- the intentional injury of suicide;
- developing a framework within which to understand the causes of these injuries, one that can leading to understanding of, and intervention for, injury at the clinical level; and
- a framework to guide practitioners in addressing injury issues within the context of lifestyle medicine.

Understanding injury

Injury differs from the common term accident in that the latter implies something that can neither be understood nor altered. 'Accident' fails to distinguish between the outcome (damage) and how it arose. Injury, on the other hand, is both understandable in cause and preventable.

The most common framework for understanding the causes and causal sequence leading to injury is the matrix developed by Haddon (1980). This model includes the factors associated with an injury event (e.g. those related to the person injured—the 'host'; the means by which the physical damage was inflicted—the 'vector'; and the physical and social environment leading to the injury) and the time sequence of these factors (before the injury, during the injury, after the injury event). This is shown as it may apply to falls in the elderly in Table 20.1.

TABLE 20.1 An example of a Haddon matrix for falls in the elderly

	Pre-event	Event	Post-event
Host (human)	musculoskeletal integrity intoxication medication personal fitness judgment fatigue	vision flexibility bone integrity imbalance eyesight	age physical condition pre-existing illness
Vector	surface condition (e.g. slipperiness, slope, moisture)	speed of action hardness of surface	contaminants on the surface (e.g. infections resulting)
Physical environment	home/institutional environment step distance support (e.g. rails) safety design	guard rails fall surface	recovery opportunities (rails) communications emergency services rehabilitation services
Sociocultural environment	alcohol attitudes family arrangements attitudes to safety	warning system family/institutional support	trauma support personnel training

The matrix provides a means of understanding the causal factors leading to injury, as well as factors that might be modified to prevent or mitigate against injury.

The matrix also provides a framework for practitioners to:

- *assess* a patient who may be injured and the injury process over time (by identifying factors that may have played a role in a patient's injury);
- *assist* in treating, preventing or minimising injury (by changing causal factors at the pre-event, event or post-event phases);
- *arrange* for patients to access those activities that counteract causal factors or mitigate damage.

The role of the clinician in anything other than the treatment of injury may seem limited. However, in this chapter we consider aspects of a number of injuries—including falls, transportation, drowning, avoidable sports injuries, poisoning and suicide—where lifestyle interventions may help reduce the injury rate.

Falls and injuries

Falls causing injuries are a particular problem for the elderly and the young. Deaths and hospitalisation rates due to falls are high in the elderly (rising rapidly over seventy years of age), with elderly males having a higher rate of deaths than females but the reverse being the case for hospitalisations (Berry and Harrison, 2006; Kreisfeld et al., 2004). Falls are also the most common cause of injuries leading to childhood admission to hospital, where male children have almost twice the level of fall injuries (Berry and Harrison, 2006).

Not surprisingly, the pattern of injuries differs between the young and elderly. For the elderly admitted to hospital, falls commonly involve slipping, tripping and stumbling, with a considerable number suffering falls from stairs, steps, ladders and beds (Berry and Harrison, 2006). A frequent type of injury for the elderly is the fracture of the femur, particularly for females (Cripps and Carman, 2001).

For children admitted to hospital, falls involving playground equipment (particularly climbing apparatus and trampolines) are the most common, particularly in the 5–9 year age bracket. Common equipment involved in falls also includes ice or roller skates and skateboards. Fractures to the forearm are common in this age group. Where the injury happens varies with age. Overall, the home is the most common location for all age injuries. Young children (0–10 years) most commonly sustain fall injuries at home or school; for young men (15–24 years), injuries most commonly occur in sport areas (Berry and Harrison, 2006).

There are a variety of activities that have been shown to reduce falls in the elderly and the young, with the best results being obtained when a range of initiatives are undertaken in combination (Norton, 1999).

For the elderly, there are both intrinsic and external factors that can be modified. Intrinsic factors often relate to the person's general health status, including deteriorated mobility and gait, poor muscle tone and strength, decreased sensation in lower limbs, reduced bone density, decreased vision, and poor balance or dizziness (often from the effects of medication).

There is literature to indicate that the clinician may modify these factors (NSW Health, 2001) through:

- regular monitoring and treatment of pre-existing conditions (such as cardiovascular disease, depression, arthritis, cataracts/vision problems);
- encouraging resistance and other appropriate exercise training;
- reducing osteoporosis/enhancing bone density;
- hormone replacement therapy for post-menopausal women;
- vitamin D and calcium supplementation; and
- medication review, particularly antidepressants, antipsychotics, antihypertensives and diuretics, and especially polypharmacy, which seems to increase the risk of falls.

External factors that pose an injury risk to the elderly include slippery floors, loose carpets, rugs, slippery shoe soles and poor lighting (NSW Health, 2001). As a result, check lists for identifying hazards in households inhabited by older people have been developed, such as the *Stay on Your Feet* check list, which provides a comprehensive list of potential hazards in the home and suggested actions (NSW Health, 2004a). Clinicians can assist in modifying these factors through encouraging the use of these check lists, reminding patients of the importance of appropriate footwear, considering the use of hip protectors in high-risk patients, and encouraging the use of personal alarms and alerts to avoid the 'long lie' experience of the fallen.

Falls in children usually result from heights. Prevention usually requires parental supervision, protective equipment (e.g. pads), and awareness of hazards in the home and play environment. Clinicians can assist by encouraging parents to obtain and apply a check list of fall hazards in the home and play areas available through Kidsafe or Farmsafe (see *Other resources*).

Transportation injuries

Transportation injuries occur in a range of transportation modes, the most common of which for deaths and hospitalisations are motor vehicles (66% transport deaths; 40% transport hospitalisations), pedestrians (12% deaths; 9% hospitalisations); cyclists (10% deaths; 16% hospitalisation) and motor cyclists (2% deaths; 22% hospitalisation). Injury rates for males are twice that of females, with adults having the highest injury rates (Berry and Harrison, 2006; Kreisfeld et al., 2004).

Over the last twenty years, there has been a significant reduction in overall transport injury rates (Kreisfeld et al, 2004). This can be attributed to a range of initiatives developed to address factors identified in the matrix on p. 254, most notably the introduction of seatbelt legislation and enforcement, drink driver legislation and enforcement, improved car safety design, improved road design, speed reduction initiatives, cycle helmet legislation and enforcement, and driver education, restriction and reinforcement (e.g. driver's licence point systems).

Medical practitioners have been at the forefront in advocating for these broad social policy changes, but individual practitioners can also play a leading role at an individual and at a local community level by testing drivers' eyesight, coordination and general health (e.g. epilepsy, coronary risk) during medical examinations for licences and by encouraging healthy attitudes to drink driving, children's use of bicycle helmets and protective gear for skating/skateboards, and the use of authorised baby capsules.

What can be done in a standard consultation

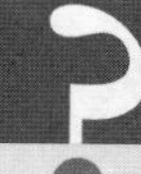

Consider individual patient risks for injury in older adults and children.

Discuss the potential for falls and falls prevention tactics in older patients.

Discuss with parents the importance of preventing poisoning and drowning in children.

Offer advice on sports injury prevention (e.g. using mouthguards).

Empathetically weigh up risks and consider risk factors for suicide.

Drowning

Drowning and near drowning account for a small percentage of all injury deaths and hospitalisations but are the major injury causes of death for children under five years of age, representing 33% of injury deaths in this age group. The highest rates of drowning are in the very young and very old (Kreisfeld et al., 2004).

The place of drowning differs with age. Private swimming pools (and bathtubs for the very young) are the most common site for children; for adults the most common setting is natural water. For all-age unintentional drowning, men have more than three times the drowning rate of women (Kreisfeld et al., 2004).

Attention can be given to this at the clinical level by checking with parents on toddlers' access to water and their swimming skills, referring to swim schools, increasing parental awareness of risk, encouraging parents to learn resuscitation skills, asking about appropriate pool fencing and advising about bathing practices in infants.

Poisoning

Unintentional poisoning death rates are somewhat difficult to identify because of coding complexities and the difficulty of differentiating intentional from unintentional (occurring in the setting of drug dependence) poisoning. For unintentional poisoning deaths by drugs, the overall rates vary with age, with young to middle aged adults (20–50 years) having the highest rates. Males account for two-thirds of the deaths (Kreisfeld et al, 2004).

The pattern of hospitalisation for unintentional poisoning by drugs differs from the death patterns. For hospital admissions, a quarter occur in children 0–4 years. Rates are low in older children (5–14 years) but rise for young people (15–24 years) before gradually declining with age. Interestingly, more females than males are hospitalised for poisoning. The drugs most commonly involved are benzodiazepines and 4-aminophenol derivatives such as paracetamol. The home is by far the most common location of poisoning (Berry and Harrison, 2006). Many medicinal poisonings for very young children arise from incorrect administration from parents, increasing the importance of correct advice from clinicians to parents.

The incident pattern for hospital admissions for unintentional poisoning with substances other than medicines, although this is much less frequent, shows similar patterns to medicinal poisonings, with highest rates in the 0–4 years age group (particularly toddlers), rising for young adults, and tapering with age. However, more males are hospitalised than females. The most frequent agents of injury are toxic food, alcohol and pesticides, and the most frequent location is the home (Berry and Harrison, 2004).

Reducing the accessibility of the poisoning agents has been shown to be a key strategy for reducing poisoning, particularly childhood poisoning. Clinicians can also help by advising parents of the accessibility risks (e.g. the potential dangers of household cleaning agents, correct labelling of containers), providing clear information on child medication use and providing literature on the immediate management of poisoning.

Sports injuries

While encouraging sporting involvement for good physical health is wise, and most sport injuries are not severe, they can be prevented or the damage limited by early treatment.

Most hospitalisations occur in the young, with overall sport injury rates doubling after age 12 and increasing 6–7-fold after age 16 (Egger, 1990). Most sporting injuries come from contact sports (e.g. football codes, netball, basketball) and occur in the lower limb joints, namely, the knees and ankles (Australian Bureau of Statistics, 2003; Flood and Harrison, 2006).

These injuries can only partly be avoided by appropriate strengthening and, where there is an evidence base, the use of protective clothing such as ankle strapping (Australian Rules), knee protection (netball) and shin pads (soccer). Compulsory use (e.g. shin pads in soccer) reduces the clinician's need to be involved here. However, questioning about the use of mouthguards, headgear (cricket, rugby) and padding can help prevent some of the major causes of injury.

Suicide

More Australians die from suicide each year than from motor vehicle accidents, with around 2000 suicides annually (Kreisfeld et al., 2004). Suicide is highest among 15–34-year-olds and accounts for about 25% of deaths in 20–24-year-olds (Kreisfeld et al., 2004). For every completed suicide there are estimated to be many times that number of attempts made.

Most people seek help prior to a suicide attempt, and the majority of those who die have consulted a primary healthcare professional in the weeks prior to their death (Pirkis and Burgess, 1998). It is here where the astute clinician may be able to have an effect.

Suicide attempts are influenced by a range of risk factors including the person's history (e.g. abuse victim, previous attempts, mental illness) and current mental state (e.g. depression), current external stresses (e.g. recent divorce, financial problems), access to the means of self harm (e.g. firearms, medications), and access to protective factors such as family or peer support. Risk factors and warning signs are shown in Table 20.2.

TABLE 20.2 Risk factors and warning signs for suicide

Risk factors	Warning signs
change in illness status	depression, despair, feeling of uselessness
history of mental illness	impulsivity, agitation
history of abuse (sexual, physical, neglect)	anger, feelings of rejection
family disruption	psychosis, psychotic thought
violence in family	putting self down
change in dwelling location	feeling unsupported
change in finances	being distant/remote
loss of employment	talk about suicide
change in relationships	giving away possessions
abuse at home/school	being on edge
access to suicide implements	excessive drug/alcohol use

The overall suicide rate in Australia has trended downwards in recent years, (Kreisfeld et al., 2004). However, suicide prevention at the individual level is complex. NSW Health has provided some useful guidelines for the assessment of suicide risk and its management (NSW Health, 2004b) which highlight the importance of the clinician in:

- engaging the client;
- assessing the risk factors;
- conducting a preliminary risk assessment (history, presentation, psychiatric assessment);
- implementing immediate action to ensure patient's safety, if at significant risk; and
- referral, if appropriate.

There is no current rating scale that has proven predictive value, but Table 20.3 is provided as a guide to assessing the level of current risk.

TABLE 20.3 Suicide risk assessment guide

Issue	High risk	Medium risk	Low risk
At-risk mental state: depressed psychotic hopelessness guilt, shame anger, agitation impulsivity	severe level exists (particularly hopelessness)	moderate level exists (particularly hopelessness)	low level or absent
History of suicide attempt	any previous attempt or gesture	possible attempt or family/friend attempt	no history of attempt

CONTINUED OVERLEAF

Suicide risk assessment guide (Continued)

Suicidal thoughts: extent intention lethality	thoughts of suicide persistent clear plan and lethal means	frequent thoughts of suicide threats with low lethality	nil or vague thought of suicide no plans
Substance disorder: current alcohol or drug misuse	current intoxication or dependence	risk of intoxication or abuse	nil or infrequent use
Means: knowledge of and access to means	access to lethal means (e.g. firearms)	sought knowledge of lethal means	no evidence of seeking access to lethal means
Strengths and supports: help seeking support of others	patient refusing help lack of supportive relationships	patient ambivalent; limited supportive relationships	patient accepting help insightful
Assessment confidence: information quality changeability of the assessment	clinician not confident/unable to verify information from patient patient's condition dynamic	some areas of limited confidence in the information from patient patient's condition stable	good patient engagement information verified from other sources low changeability

Note: This is a guide only and does not replace clinical decision making.

Source: adapted from NSW Health *Suicide risk assessment guideline,* 2004b (www.health.nsw.gov.au/pubs/2005/suicide_risk.html)

The level of risk will assist the clinician in determining the patient's management. Those patients at high risk may need to be provided with actions to ensure their safety and be reassessed within twenty-four hours. Understanding and utilising listening skills is valuable, along with recognition of warning signs and careful control of medications. Referral to specialist services where necessary is, obviously, also vital.

Summary

Injury is the fourth leading cause of death in Australia. Risks that can be reduced in the clinical setting involve older adults and children. Morbidity from injury becomes more important with ageing, with falls being one of the major causes of hospitalisation and health costs in older people. Transportation injuries, drownings, poisoning and sports injuries are all preventable causes of injury in children. Suicide and violence (not covered here) are the two main forms of injury involving older adolescents and the middle aged. Contrary to popular opinion, injuries are not accidents: they are largely preventable using an epidemiological approach to their management. Clinicians can aid in this by adopting a few basic lifestyle-oriented principles and adopting a modern approach to injury prevention.

practice tips

PRACTICE TIPS: REDUCING INJURY

	Medical practitioner	Practice nurse
Assess	Risk factors in the elderly (as in RACGP *Red book*). Eyesight, bone density, functional coordination and musculoskeletal integrity of older people (assess opportunistically). Prescribed medications with regard to a potential role in injury. Use of correct baby capsules. Use of swimming pool fencing. Swimming skills of toddlers and resuscitation skills of parents. Suicide risk.	In-home falls risk (provide check list). Medication use (perform home medication review in the elderly where feasible). Use of appropriate footwear. Home hazards (encourage parents to conduct a hazard check in the home and play areas). Signs of suicide risk.
Assist	By encouraging parents to take preventive action with young children (e.g. scalds, poisoning, drowning prevention). By encouraging a view of 'accidents' as non-preventable. By encouraging use of protective gear in play and sport (e.g. helmets, strapping, mouthguards).	By encouraging parents to take specific preventive action (e.g. turning hot water down to <50 degrees Celsius, safe storage of poisoning agents). By reinforcing use of protective gear (e.g. helmets, strapping, mouthguards) in sport. By providing literature on the prevention and immediate management of injuries (e.g. falls injuries, water safety). By providing information (e.g. from the Consumers Association) on safety products such as baby capsules.
Arrange	Appropriate exercise programs for the elderly for falls protection. Vitamin D/sunlight treatment for bone density if necessary. Occupational therapist for home environment check of the aged. Referral to mental health specialist for those at risk of suicide.	Exercise specialist/physiotherapist for exercise program for the elderly. Referral to accredited swim schools for toddlers. Referral to safety information sources (e.g. Kidsafe, Farmsafe, bike safety organisations) where appropriate.

key points

KEY POINTS FOR CLINICAL MANAGEMENT

- Work towards changing patients' perception of injury so they are seen as preventable and not synonymous with accidents.
- Regard injury management as within the ambit of lifestyle medicine.
- Undertake regular medication and mobility review in elderly patients and consider injury risk.
- Be alert to the risk factors for suicide in patients experiencing stress or mental illness.
- Use opportunistic counselling to assist in injury awareness and prevention.
- Encourage parents to identify hazards in the home, travel and play environments.
- Have available a range of information pamphlets and resource directories on injury in the surgery.

references

REFERENCES

Australian Bureau of Statistics. (2003) *National health survey. Injuries*. Canberra: ABS.

Berry J, Harrison J. (2006) *Hospital separations due to injury and poisoning, Australia 2001–02. Injury research and statistics series number 26.* Canberra: Australian Institute of Health and Welfare.

Cripps R, Carman J. (2001) *Falls in the elderly in Australia. Trends and data for 1998. Injury research and statistics series.* Canberra: Australian Institute of Health and Welfare.

Egger, G. (1990) Sports injuries in Australia: causes costs and prevention. *Health Promotion Journal of Australia* 1(2): 28–33.

Flood I, Harrison J. (2006) *Hospitalised sport injury, Australia 2002–2003. Injury research and statistics series number 27.* Canberra: Australian Institute of Health and Welfare.

Haddon W. (1974) Strategies in preventive medicine: passive v active approaches to reduce human wastage. *Journal Trauma* 4: 353–54.

Haddon W. (1980) Advances in the epidemiology of injuries as a basis for public policy. *Pub Health Rep* (5): 411–20.

Kreisfeld R, Newson R, Harrison J. (2004) *Injury deaths, Australia 2002.* Injury research and statistics series number 23. Canberra: Australian Institute of Health and Welfare.

Murray C, Lopez A. (1996) *Global burden of disease—a comprehensive assessment of mortality and disability from diseases, injuries and risk factors in 1990 and projected to 2020.* World Health Organization. Boston: Harvard University Press.

Norton R. (1999) Preventing falls and fall related injuries among older Australians. *Australasian J Ageing* 18: 4–10.

NSW Health. (2001) *Preventing injuries from falls in older people.* Sydney: NSW Department of Health. Available from ww.health.nsw.gov.au/pubs/p/pdf/prevent_falls_old.pdf.

—— (2004a) *Stay on your feet—your home safety checklist.* Sydney: NSW Department of Health. Available from www.health.nsw.gov.au/pubs/s/pdf/stay_on_feet.pdf.

—— (2004b) *A framework for suicide risk assessment and management for NSW Health staff.* Sydney: NSW Department of Health. Available from www.health.nsw.gov.au/pubs/2005/suicide_risk.html.

Pirkis J, Burgess P. (1998) Suicide and recency of health care contacts—a systematic review. *British Journal of Psychiatry* 173(12): 462–74.

other resources

OTHER RESOURCES

Water safety and skills	Royal Life Saving Society, Australia (www.royallifesaving.com.au); state department of sport and recreation; local council.
Prevention and immediate management of childhood injury	Kidsafe (www.kidsafe.com.au)—provides fact sheets, home safety check lists and first aid advice for various forms of poisoning.
Farm safety	Farmsafe (www.farmsafe.org.au)—provides information on farm safety including chemicals such as pesticides.

Poisons information	Poisons Information Centre 13 11 26—provides expert advice in the event of a poisoning, 24 hours, 7 days a week.
Suicide information	Beyond Blue (www.beyondblue.org.au).
Suicide assessment	www.health.nsw.gov.au/pub/2005/suicide risk.html
Injuries	National Injury Surveillance Unit (www.nisu.flinders. edu.au)—provides a large number of publications on Australian injury, including the consequences of injury (death, hospitalisation), causes and settings (animal, assault, falls, health complications, sport/recreation, self harm, transport, occupation), types (brain, burns, drowning, fractures, spinal cord), populations (children, youth, adults, elderly, Aboriginal, males, females and rural) and risk factors (alcohol, firearms).

CHAPTER 21

Medicines: the good, the not so good and the over-used

JULIAN HENWOOD, STEPHAN ROSSNER, ANDREW BINNS, GARRY EGGER

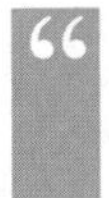

The tragedy of science is the slaying of a beautiful hypothesis by an ugly fact.

T.H. HUXLEY

Introduction

In the mid 1990s, *TIME Magazine* featured a cover story on the new wonder drug combination for weight loss, dexfenfluramine (Redux) with phentermine, or 'phen-fen' as it was affectionately known. According to *TIME* (and some significantly influenced academic proponents), the combination was a 'miracle' cure set to significantly impact the obesity epidemic. The rest, as they say, is history. Less than two years after the feature, dexfenfluramine was taken off the market to short-circuit a number of potential lawsuits for the rise in primary pulmonary hypertension (PPH) and mitral valve problems in users (Connolly et al., 1997).

Without doubt, medications—whether they are based on plant compounds (e.g. digitalis, atropine) or derived from laboratory synthesis (e.g. penicillin, statins)—are among the greatest success stories of modern medicine. We only have to look to the development of antibiotics and their huge impact on disease in the early part of the twentieth century to see this. There is also no doubt that, while the human body is well equipped to self-correct much disease through a highly sophisticated immune system, the addition of medicines both natural and synthetic has significantly aided this process throughout human history. However, to reverse an old proverb, for every silver lining, there is a cloud. It is easy to forget that, although drugs can be selective, they can be non-specific with respect to effects on other organs, causing side effects or adverse drugs reactions, which may also impact on lifestyle.

Medications and side effects

Just about every drug that has a therapeutic effect also has a side effect. While there is immense value in the use of appropriate medication, the benefits of each medication need to be weighed against the risks of their side effects. In some situations, very serious side effects can be accepted because they may cure potentially lethal diseases. For drugs treating cancer, for example, even life-threatening side effects may be acceptable if they significantly increase the chances of survival. The more benign the condition, the fewer the acceptable side effects.

It is also obvious that compliance to a medication schedule is dependent on the ability of a patient to put up with the side effects. This is more likely where these are outweighed by the benefits. Hypertension illustrates this point. Fifty years ago, hypertension was treated with mutilating surgery, when nerves were cut on both sides along the spine to produce modest effects on blood pressure. Barbiturates were then prescribed, which calmed patients to the extent that they could not perform their work. Gradually, drugs were developed that controlled blood pressure with fewer and fewer side effects. However, as late as the 1970s methyldopa was the most common drug used. It reduced mental alertness, caused drowsiness, impaired autoimmune function and affected liver function. Despite these relatively common serious side effects, physicians found methyldopa to be the most effective and least objectionable drug for the majority of patients with moderate degrees of hypertension.

It is obvious that with conditions related to lifestyle-based causes, medication—if necessary—should have a profile with minimal side effects. In many cases, this will result in a decision to continue with that medication (albeit cautiously). An alternative may simply be a change in lifestyle. Early-stage type 2 diabetes, for example, may be treated with an insulin-sensitising drug or a graded exercise program with dietary changes.

In this chapter, we look at potential problems that can arise from *only* going down the drug path with medications that impact on lifestyle and health (excluding over-the-counter and alternative/complementary therapies). We believe that side effects of treatment need to be considered in lifestyle medicine as part of the outcome and that drug use cannot always be justified by treatment outcomes.

Common side effects

Almost all drugs may cause side effects; however, a number of side effects are characteristic of many different drugs. These include headaches, nausea, reductions in libido, impotence, dryness of the mouth, weight gain (or loss), fatigue, muscular pain and dizziness.

We concentrate here only on those medications that either are widely used in the population but carry a small and significant risk of side effects, or those that have a small number of users but produce significant adverse effects that may interfere with a lifestyle medicine approach. As with the doctor who is taught to suspect pregnancy in every fertile woman, the underlying principle is to treat *every* medication as having potential side effects and *every* decision to treat as a balance between benefits and risk. We have not looked extensively at herbal and non-prescription medications because, unlike medications that have to go through extensive clinical trials, there is often no reliable evidence base for these.

Iatrogenesis and medicines

The term iatrogenesis literally means 'doctor-induced disease'. It was popularised by Ivan Illich in the 1970s when discussing the influences of modern health services. In the current context, iatrogenesis is used to describe the less than positive outcomes of medication use under certain circumstances (Illich, 1976). This includes medications that may:

- cause weight gain;
- cause other side effects which may be counterproductive to a lifestyle-based solution; or
- interact adversely with other medications/foods or substances.

Medications that can cause weight gain

Weight gain is a common side effect of many medications (Ness-Abramof and Apovian, 2005). However, the precise mechanism of action that leads to this remains surprisingly unclear in most instances. According to Kopelman (2006), it is likely to involve a number of interlinked mechanisms that include altered mood, enhanced hunger and altered metabolic processes (including thermogenesis). Such weight gain is likely to occur on a background of genetic predisposition, as shown in Figure 21.1.

FIGURE 21.1 A schematic illustration of the linkages between mood, hunger regulation and metabolic pathways in relation to drug-induced weight gain

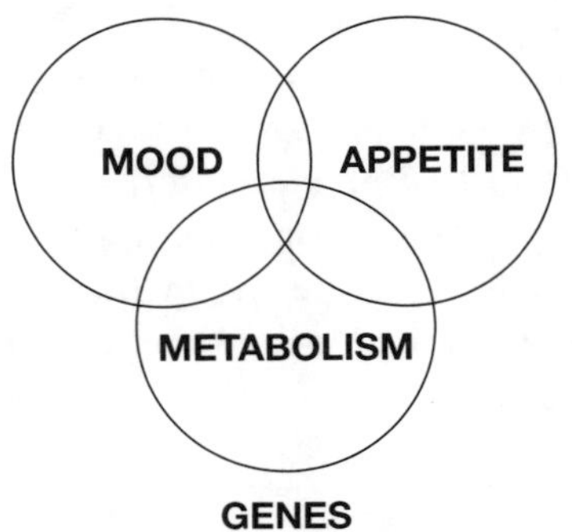

Source: Kopelman, 2006

A list of medication categories and examples of common generic and brand names known to cause weight gain is shown in Table 21.1.

Prescription medications causing the most weight gain are the antipsychotics (almost all), anti-diabetics (almost all except metformin), oral corticosteroids (all, if taken long enough) and certain antidepressants (varies with medication andreaction to depression). Lesser effects come from the anxiolytics, some antihypertensives such as beta-blockers, and some anticonvulsants. Indeed, one anticonvulsant (topiramate) is currently being tested as a weight loss medication.

TABLE 21.1 Common medications that can have weight gain as a side effect

Category	Use	Some common generic names	Some common brand names
anxiolytics	reducing anxiety	alprazolam diazepam oxazepam nitrazepam	Xanax Valium Serepax Mogadon
corticosteroids	anti-allergy anti-inflammatory	dexamethasone prednisone	Dexmethasone Predsone
anti-diabetics	reducing blood sugars/insulin resistance	sulfonylureas insulin glitazones Insulin	Diamicron Many brand names
phenothiazines	antipsychotic	chlorpromazine olanzapine risperidone quetiapine	Largactil Zyprexa Risperdal Seroquel
tricyclic antidepressants	reduce depression	amitriptyline clomipramine imipramine	Tryptanol Anafranil Tofranil
SSRIs/SNRIs	reduce depression	fluoxetine sertraline	Prozac Zoloft
oral contraceptives	contraception	oestrogens progesterones	Many brand names
beta-blockers	antihypertensive	atenolol metoprolol	Tenormin Betaloc
anticonvulsants	control seizures	carbamazepine sodium valproate phenytoin	Tegretol Epilim Dilantin

While hormone replacement therapy (HRT) has been widely touted as causing weight gain, there is clear evidence that this is not the case (Kongnyuy et al., 1999). Weight gain is common during menopause. Women on HRT actually have less weight gain compared to women of the same age not using HRT, although there may still be some absolute weight gain. Restriction of HRT may be based on other concerns (e.g. breast cancer risk), but weight gain should not be a consideration.

When the prescription of drugs that can cause weight gain will provide clear clinical benefit, clinician and patient should anticipate the possibility of weight gain. Methods to avoid weight gain should be pre-planned and implemented to minimise any detrimental effect of additional body weight at the time.

Medications that cause side effects counterproductive to lifestyle change

There are a number of categories of medication that need to be considered under this heading, including weight loss medications, medications for managing cholesterol and antidepressants.

WEIGHT LOSS MEDICATIONS

There are only a limited number of medications prescribed specifically for weight loss, and all were discovered by serendipity—none of the current batch of weight loss medications was developed specifically for this purpose. All have potential side effects.

- Sibutramine (Reductil), which was initially marketed as an antidepressant, is now used as an appetite suppressant and may be contraindicated in uncontrolled hypertension (it increases blood pressure and heart rate in some patients). Some early deaths were reported, but the association has yet to be proved.
- Orlistat (Xenical) is a gastric lipase inhibitor, the side effects of which are actually part of the treatment (steatorrhoea). The long-term effects of this on the other aspects of health are not yet clear.
- Rimonabant (Accomplia), a cannabinoid receptor blocker which reduces hunger, can cause depression in some individuals, which may be counterproductive to weight loss.
- A caffeine/ephedrine mix (which is not available in many countries) has resulted in some cardiac deaths from the ephedrine or ephedra (ma huong) additive.
- Phentermine (Duromine) is one of the oldest weight loss medications and may have less side effects than most, perhaps because it is usually only prescribed over short periods (three months maximum). However, insomnia and tachycardia make it unsuitable for use in a small proportion of overweight patients.

All weight loss medications still require a lifestyle change for a successful outcome and hence should be seen as adjuncts to treatment, rather than the main approach.

CHOLESTEROL LOWERING/MODIFYING MEDICATIONS

The discovery of statins for modifying heart disease risk levels of blood lipids has been equated in importance with the development of antibiotics in the early twentieth century. Study after study has shown their value in reducing mortality and morbidity from heart disease and stroke and even in reducing risk of related problems such as type 2 diabetes (Jones, 2007), although it should be noted that the 'beatification' of the statins has been questioned (Mascitelli and Pezetta, 2007) because of a failure to compare their effects with those of lifestyle change.

One significant side effect of the statins, however, and another group of lipid lowering medications, the fibrates, is myalgia or muscle-related pain or soreness, including cramping and increased muscle tears (Baer and Wortmann, 2007; Gaist et al., 2001). At the extremes, this may manifest as rhabdomyolysis, although the risk of this is very rare, less than 3 in 100 000 patient years (Law and Rudnicka, 2006; Muhktar and Reckless, 2005). Of particular concern is the higher rate of myalgia and myositis in exercising individuals (Urso et al., 2005), such as athletes (Sinzinger and O'Grady, 2004), although this may have a genetic component (Vladutiu et al., 2006). Given that physical activity is a lifestyle recommendation for lipid lowering, this class of drug, particularly in heavily exercising individuals, may counteract this.

One alternative in susceptible individuals may be a reversion to an older form of cholesterol lowering medication, nicotinic acid, which is often not tolerated because of flushing side effects (Capuzzi et al., 1998). There is now available a slow release form (inositol hexanicotinate), which may have a lower incidence of flushing. Lowering the dosage or trying alternative statins may also help. If this does not work, an assessment of benefit-to-side effect ratio will need to be made for each individual.

ANTIDEPRESSANTS

Although the new generations of SSRI and SNRI antidepressants appears to be effective and have a milder side effect profile than previous medications of this type (TCAs, MAOs), they can still have side effects that may be counterproductive in some cases. Reduced libido and erectile dysfunction in many men, for example, may add to depression (Shabsigh et al., 1998) and sexual functioning is often decreased in those with depression (Seidman and Roose, 2001). Weight gain from some of this class of medications is also common. Alternatives include choosing anti-depressants that do not cause weight gain (e.g. sertraline), psychological approaches (at least in mild depression), or alternative OTC medications with an evidence base, such as St John's wort (Williams and Holsinger, 2005) or SAMe (Papakostas et al. 2003). Exercise is a non-drug alternative with proven benefits for mild to moderate depression.

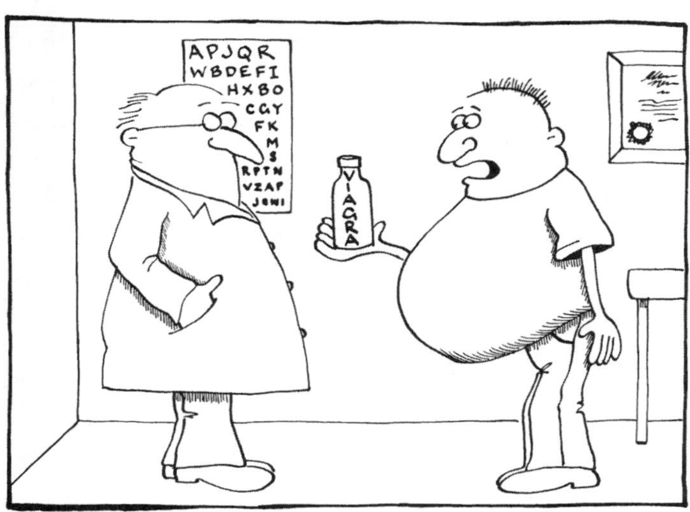

"WHEN I SAID I'D LIKE TO SEE IT AGAIN I WAS THINKING MORE IN TERMS OF A DIET."

Without elaborating on the wide range of medications available and their minor side effects (and remember all drugs may have side effects), it is worth pointing out some potential problematic interactions between lifestyle change and medication.

Modern exercisers, sports participants and patients with arthritis, for example, are often heavy users of painkillers such as NSAIDs (e.g. ibuprofen, naproxen) to reduce pain and, in the case of athletes, maintain performance in increasingly long and heavy contact playing seasons. Some studies have shown an increase in erectile dysfunction as a result of NSAID use in men (Shiri et al., 2006), elevated hypertension in men who use several forms of NSAIDs, and gut problems such as abdominal pain and nausea. NSAIDs may also adversely affect renal function. Reduced NSAID use following increased awareness of the problems is probably the best approach, as these are usually taken on a discretionary basis anyway. However, paracetamol 1 g every 4–6 hours is a sufficient analgesic without these side effects in many cases.

Similarly, glucocorticoids can increase the risk of osteoporosis and bone fractures from activity if used for longer periods (Compston, 2003) and should be used cautiously. Mania (and paradoxically depression), psychosis and diabetes risk can also be increased with steroid use. Short-term use is usually not a problem, but alternatives may need to be sought over the longer term.

While antihypertensive medications have improved significantly in their side effect profiles since the 1960s and '70s, there are still potential problems, with some diuretics carrying a risk of diabetes and some beta-blockers carrying the risk of fatigue or weight gain and muscle pain that could limit physical activity involvement.

Medications that interact adversely with other drugs/food

As expected, many medications can interact with other medications or indeed with chemicals in food and may cause side effects or adverse reactions. Of these, the most relevant for our discussion here is the potential synergistic effect of prescribed and OTC antidepressant medications. The combination of St John's wort and certain SSRIs or SNRIs may lead to serotonin syndrome (Hu et al., 2005); other potential risk in this area are shown in Table 21.2.

TABLE 21.2 Common medications that may lead to serotonin syndrome

Drug class	Examples
antidepressants	mirtazapine
	monoamine oxidase inhibitors (MAOIs)
	selective serotonin reuptake inhibitors (SSRIs)
	tricyclics
	venlafaxine
antiparkinson's drugs	amantadine
	bromocriptine
	cabergoline
	levodopa
	pergolide
	selegiline

CONTINUED OVERLEAF

Common medications that may lead to serotonin syndrome (Continued)

Drug class	Examples
migraine therapy	dihydroergotamine
	naratriptan
	sumatriptan
	zolmitriptan
illicit drugs	cocaine
	hallucinogenics (MDMA, LSD)
other agents	bupropion
	carbamazepine
	lithium
	morphine
	pethidine
	reserpine
	sibutramine
	St John's wort
	tramadol

Grapefruit juice, which is normally considered a healthy addition to a nutritional diet, is contraindicated with certain statins (e.g. simvastatin) because it causes an approximate doubling of the plasma levels of the drug (the result of increased absorption from a decreased metabolism in the gut wall), increasing the chance of myalgia and other side effects. Alcohol, which is recommended in moderation for a healthy heart, is known to have adverse effects with a list of medications too numerous to mention here.

In addition, to improve compliance, there is a trend towards combining medications in the one 'polypill'. While the drugs making up these combinations have usually been tested in separate prescriptions, the effects of combination will not be known until they are tested in large numbers.

What can be done in a standard consultation

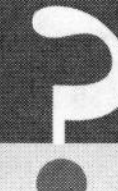

Attempt lifestyle change before initiating drug treatment, where possible.

Check possible side effects of any medication and limitations for the patient.

Discuss any side effects that may limit lifestyle change.

Consider drug interaction possibilities, which may not be covered in the product information.

Consider/discuss effects of weight gain with medication.

Other potential problems

Because a low incidence of side effects is not picked up until a medication is used much more widely than in the clinical trials that allowed it to be marketed, long-term problems are often not immediately obvious. This was the case with the fen-phen combination discussed earlier. Although highly successful in weight loss, the severe side effects were ultimately seen as too risky for continued use.

Pharmaceutical business interests also play no small role in drug-related iatrogenesis. The industry (and its shareholders) has a vested interest in increased prescribing, because of the profits at stake. Minor reductions in risk, for example, in terms of mmol/L of cholesterol, should be viewed in their proper context. For instance, an absolute reduction of risk from 4% to 3% might be advertised as a 25% improvement (in relative risk), although the clinical significance of this may be relatively insignificant.

Small changes in the chemical formula of a medication for competitive gain may also lead to complications that come to light only after the medication has been used in the population at large. This was seen with cervistatin (Lipobay), which increased the risk of rhabdomyolysis beyond an acceptable level for a statin. The COX-2 inhibitors rofecoxib (Vioxx) and lumiracoxib (Prexige) was withdrawn because of an increased risk of heart attack and stroke. One of the glitazones—a new class of antidiabetic insulin sensitisers used in diabetes—was withdrawn because of the potential risks of liver damage (troglitazone); and cautions have been issued against another glitazone (rosiglitazone, Avandia) because of a rise in apparent heart disease rates (Nissen and Wolski, 2007). As seen in Chapter 5, most antidiabetic medications cause weight gain, which may ultimately reduce glycaemic control. The glitazones raised hopes of a pharmaceutical solution for prevention of progression from pre-diabetes to diabetes. The DREAM (Diabetes Reduction Assessment with Ramipril and Rosiglitazone Medication) study tended to support this suggestion (DREAM, 2006); however, the drug has been widely criticised on the basis of outcomes important to patients (Montori et al., 2007). Others drugs in this class are still widely used, such as pioglitazone (Actos). Although this class of drugs does cause weight gain, it is subcutaneous rather than visceral fat and therefore not such a metabolic risk. Another glitazone side effect is fluid retention and resulting cardiac failure.

Finnish researchers have shown that a more effective solution to diabetes prevention is a greater emphasis on lifestyle change, which has now been shown to be effective over five years from a single dose, compared to medication which is required on an ongoing basis (Tuomilehto, 2007). Any side effects from changes such as increased exercise or improved nutrition are likely to be positive, and the economic costs are less. Modelling outcomes, Dutch workers have shown that both community and individual approaches to prevention and early stage treatment are more cost effective than intensive treatment options (Jacobs-van de Bruggen et al., 2007).

The problem of non-adherence

On a different level to iatrogenesis is the problem of non-adherence to appropriately prescribed medication (Heidenreich, 2004). Indications are that less than half of all patients prescribed a lipid lowering medication, for example, are still taking it six months later. This is of special concern considering that it may take from six months to a year for the beneficial effects of certain medications such as statins to become apparent (Blackburn et al., 2005). Barriers to medication adherence include complex regimens, treatment of asymptomatic conditions (e.g. hypertension) and convenience and cost factors. These barriers are particularly prevalent in the elderly, making them especially at risk for medication non-adherence. Where genuine efficacy is established, and the risks and benefits of treatment are evaluated, adherence through targeting motivation, as discussed in Chapter 3, is particularly relevant.

What can the clinician do?

Lifestyle medicine involves the wise (and creative) use of medications as an adjunct to lifestyle interventions. Where medications present a potential problem, however, there are a number of options available to the clinician:

- reducing or even eliminating some medications, if possible, assuming the patient can change his or her lifestyle;
- eliminating the need for medication in the first place by early intervention through a lifestyle change in pre-diabetes and early diabetes (i.e. exercise as an alternative to some early stage antidiabetics);
- substitution with a medication with fewer side effects that impact on lifestyle change, if available (e.g. SSRIs instead of MAOIs or TCAs for depression; ACE inhibitors or angiotensin receptor blockers instead of beta-blockers for hypertension);
- lowering dosage to a level that better balances side effects and benefits (e.g. reduced statin dosage for myalgia);
- using drugs in combination where they have a combined lower risk (e.g. a statin and ezetimibe); and
- if no option is available, informing the patient about the risk of side effects and the side effects–benefit ratio. If a drug that causes weight gain must be used, early preventative lifestyle measures should be recommended.

Summary

Pharmaceutical advances have been a boon to modern health. However, the rise in lifestyle-related diseases has meant a re-evaluation of the benefits of some medications where these are used as a substitute for lifestyle change and cause side effects which may outweigh the benefits of the drug. Where possible, lifestyle change should be attempted before medication use, and drugs that have least impact on potential lifestyle change should be favoured over those that make lifestyle change difficult.

practice tips

PRACTICE TIPS: PREVENTING MISUSE OF MEDICATIONS

	Medical practitioner	**Practice nurse**
Assess	Side effects of current medication usage. Possible interactions of different drugs (including non-prescription therapies) and potential effects on lifestyle change. Current literature and respected information sources for an update on side effects.	Medication and complementary therapy use in conjunction with prescribing doctor. Role of recommended lifestyle changes (e.g. exercise) on side effects of medication.

Assist	Changing lifestyle instead of using medication where possible. Monitoring potential risk factors resulting from a change/decrease in medication use.	By providing advice about changing lifestyle instead of using medication where possible. Monitoring of dosages used.
Arrange	Use of lowest effective doses to minimise any side effects where possible. Changing medication where this is likely to help in lifestyle change. Pharmacist involvement/advice where feasible.	Follow-up visits. Referrals to other allied health professionals.

key points

KEY POINTS FOR CLINICAL MANAGEMENT

- In cases of lifestyle-related disease, consider medication as an adjunct to lifestyle change rather than vice versa.
- Where possible, look for a lifestyle alternative to medications that may have side effects that interfere with lifestyle change.
- Concentrate on patient's motivation and readiness to change (see Chapter 3) to improve compliance with lifestyle change.
- Consider and discuss potential side effects of a medication and alternatives.
- Monitor lifestyle-related side effects and their impact on lifestyle change (e.g. potential muscle soreness effects on exercise with statins).
- If medication is necessary, change the medication or dose to enable better compliance with lifestyle change.

references

REFERENCES

Baer AN, Wortmann RL. (2007) Myotoxicity associated with lipid-lowering drugs. *Curr Opin Rheumatol* 19(1): 67–73.

Blackburn DF, Dobson RT, Blackburn JL et al. (2005) Cardiovascular morbidity associated with nonadherence to statin therapy. *Pharmacotherapy* 25: 1035–43.

Capuzzi DM, Guyton JR, Morgan JM et al. (1998) Effect and safety of an extended-release niacin (Niaspan): a long-term study. *Am J Cardiol* 82: 74U–81U.

Compston J. (2003) Glucocorticoid-induced osteoporosis. *Horm Res* 60(Suppl 3): 77–79.

Connolly HM, Crary JL, McGoon MD et al. (1997) Valvular heart disease associated with fenfluramine-phentermine. *N Engl J Med* 337: 581–88.

DREAM (diabetes reduction assessment with ramipril and rosiglitazone medication) Trial Investigation. (2006) Effect of rosiglitazone on the frequency of diabetes in patients with impaired glucose tolerance or impaired fasting glucose: a randomised control trial. *Lancet* 368: 1096–105.

Gaist D, Rodriguez LG, Huerta C et al. (2001) Lipid-lowering drugs and risk of myopathy: a population-based follow-up study. *Epidemiol* 12: 565–69.

Heidenreich PA. (2004) Patient adherence: the next frontier in quality improvement. *Am J Med* 117: 130–32.

Hu Z, Yang X, Ho PC et al. (2005) Herb–drug interactions: a literature review. *Drugs* 65: 1239–82.

Illich I. (1976) *Medical nemesis. The expropriation of health.* NY: Pantheon Books.

Jacobs-van der Bruggen MAM, Vijgen SM, Hoogenveen RT et al. (2007) Lifestyle interventions are cost effective in people with different levels of diabetes risk: results from a modeling study. *Diab Care* 30: 128–34.

Jones PH. (2007) Clinical significance of recent lipid trials on reducing risk in patients with type 2 diabetes mellitus. *Am J Cardiol* 99: 133B–140B.

Kongnyuy EJ, Norman RJ, Flight IHK, Rees MCP. (1999) Oestrogen and progestogen hormone replacement therapy for peri-menopausal and post-menopausal women: weight and body fat distribution. *Cochrane Database of Systematic Reviews* 1999, Issue 3. Art. No. CD001018. DOI: 10.1002/14651858.CD001018.

Kopelman P. (2006) Iatrogenesis and weight gain. *Paper presented to the Tenth International Congress on Obesity*, Sydney, September, 2006.

Law M, Rudnicka AR. (2006) Statin safety: a systematic review. *Am J Cardiol* 97(Suppl): 52C–60C.

Mascitelli L, Pezetta F. (2007) Questioning the 'beatification' of statins. *Int J Cardiol* Published online Feb 26, 2007.

Montori V, Isley W, Guyatt G. (2007) Waking up from the DREAM of preventing diabetes with drugs. *BMJ* 334: 882–84.

Mukhtar RY, Reckless JP. (2005) Statin induced myositis; a commonly encountered or rare side effect? *Curr Opin in Lipid* 16: 640–47.

Ness-Abramof R, Apovian CM. (2005) Drug-induced weight gain. *Drugs Today* (Barc). 41: 547–55.

Nissen SE, Wolski K. (2007) Effect of rosiglitazone on the risk of myocardial infarction and death from cardiovascular causes. *NEJM* 356: 1–15

Papakostas GI, Alpert JE, Fava M. (2003) S-adenosyl-methionine in depression: a comprehensive review of the literature. *Curr Psychiatry Rep* 5: 460–66.

Seidman SN, Roose SP. (2001) Sexual dysfunction and depression. *Curr Psychiatry Rep* 3: 202–08.

Shabsigh R, Klein LT, Seidman S et al. (1998) Increased incidence of depressive symptoms in men with erectile dysfunction. *Urology* 52: 848–52.

Shiri R, Koskimaki J, Hakkinen J et al. (2006) Effect of nonsteroidal anti-inflammatory drug use on the incidence of erectile dysfunction. *J Urology* 175: 1812–15.

Sinzinger H, O'Grady J. (2004) Professional athletes suffering from familial hypercholesterolaemia rarely tolerate statin treatment because of muscular problems. *Br J Clin Pharmacol* 57: 525–28.

Tuomilehto J. (2007) Counterpoint: evidence-based prevention of type 2 diabetes: the power of lifestyle management. *Diab Care* 30: 435–38.

Urso ML, Clarkson PM, Hittel D et al. (2005) Changes in ubiquitin proteasome pathway gene expression in skeletal muscle with exercise and statins. *Arterioscler Thromb Vasc Biol* 25: 2560–68.

Vladutiu GD, Simmons Z, Isackson PJ et al. (2006) Genetic risk factors associated with lipid-lowering drug intensive myopathies. *Muscle & Nerve* 34: 153–62.

Williams JW Jr, Holsinger T. (2005) St John's for depression, worts and all. *BMJ* 330: E350–1.

CHAPTER 22

The big issue for society: tackling distal causes

GARRY EGGER, ANDREW BINNS, STEPHAN ROSSNER, MAXIMILIAN DE COURTEN

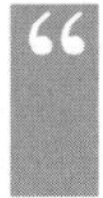

If civilisation is to survive, it must live on the interest of nature, not the capital.

RONALD WRIGHT, 2004

Causality revisited

In Chapter 2, levels of causality for the modern epidemic of lifestyle-related diseases were dissected, step by step. This pointed to distal factors that initially seemed far removed from culpability, such as industrialisation, population pressures and economic growth. The paradox, which becomes apparent from this, is that the underlying system of growth and development that has allowed great advances in human living conditions has become a Damoclean sword, from which we need to find a safe and expedient escape. In the words of one writer, 'we behave like someone spending wildly on their credit card, in the belief that the bill will never come. But it's already in the mail' (Mass, 2006).

In the intervening chapters we discussed the management of lifestyle-related risk factors and the proximal and medial causes of these, with an emphasis on interventions more immediate to the realm of a clinician. In this chapter we pull back again to look at the broader distal factors that need to be considered for a more global perspective on the problem. This may not appear immediately relevant to the clinician, but it is necessary for a deeper understanding of the future of lifestyle medicine and a better understanding of solutions to the problem at the public health, as well as the clinical level.

Dealing with epidemics

Lifestyle-related diseases, as we have seen, are in epidemic proportions in developed as well as many developing countries. Typically, epidemics are dealt with by considering all three points of an epidemiological triad—host, vector and environment (Figure 22.1); the host being the sufferer of the disease, the vector the deliverer of an infective agent, and the environment the situation in which the vector is allowed to flourish (Leowell and Clark, 1966).

FIGURE 22.1 The epidemiological triad

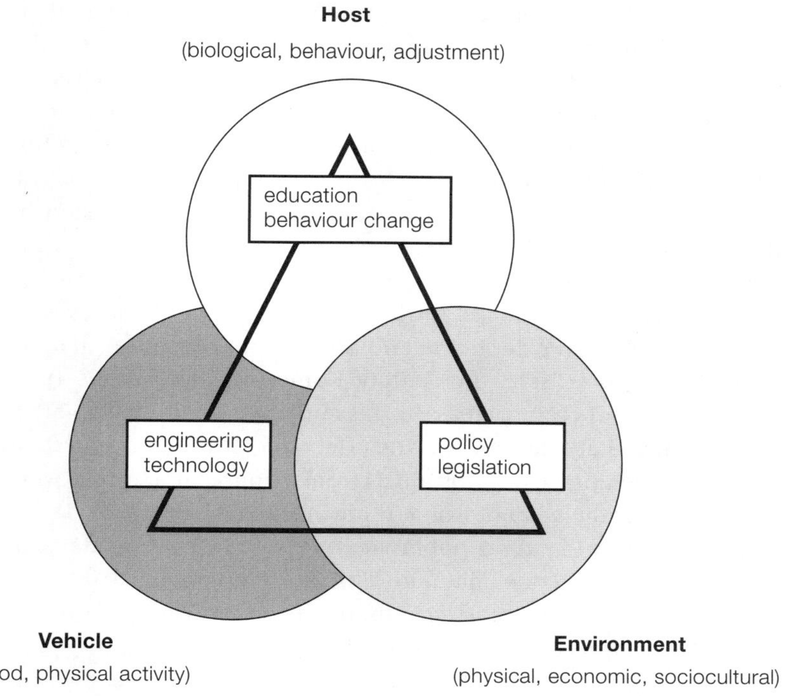

In the case of infectious diseases, these are clearly defined. With bird flu, for example, the host is the person suffering the disease, the vector is the bird carrying the infective agent/virus and the environment is the crowded living conditions in which the virus is able to mutate. With non-communicable or lifestyle diseases, on the other hand, an epidemic is often considered as something different, and the host is usually the only component treated. Recognition of the importance of vectors and environments has led to big improvements in epidemic outcomes (Egger et al., 2003). Using this triad, Haddon's (1980) re-assessment of motor vehicle accidents, for example, led to a paradigm shift in dealing with injury (see Chapter 20) with consequent big improvements in motor vehicle injury rates. Similarly, big inroads into the smoking epidemic did not happen until changes occurred in the cultural environment making smoking less socially acceptable in the workplace and public places (Chapman, 1995).

In previous chapters we have concentrated mainly on the host, some vectors (e.g. high energy-dense foods, effort-saving technology, stress) and some micro-environments (peer pressure, social pressure), while implying a major role for distal factors such as industrialisation and economic development in overall epidemiology. Here we look more at one of the biggest threats to both health and humanity in the coming years: macro-environmental change resulting from unbridled technological and economic development.

Development as a cause of lifestyle-related diseases

While economic growth has had enormous advantages for humanity, the implication is that this can, and should, continue indefinitely. Yet in all exponential growth there comes a point of diminishing marginal rate of returns. Even the definition of 'growth'—*expansion to maturity*—suggests a finite limit that has to be reached at some point. Depending on the measures used, it is debatable as to whether advances in the biological aspects of medical science have already reached this point. Our analysis of the growth of lifestyle-related diseases to the level of approximately 70% of all clinical visits indicates this now may be the case, and this has been suggested by James Le Fanu (2002) in *The rise and fall of modern medicine.* Certainly, forecasters of the modern environmental crisis 3-4 decades ago, such as Rachel Carson (*Silent spring*), the Club of Rome (*Limits to growth*) and Paul Ehrlich (*The population bomb*) forewarned of significant problems if resource depletion and throughput continued at an exponential rate. One possibility, forecast by the Club of Rome (Meadows et al., 1974), was that 'sources' of energy resources, such as oil, gas and coal, would dry up at an exponential rate. Not predicted at that time was the effect uncontrolled resource usage would have on 'sinks', or the uptake of by-products from resource usage, as now suggested in a thirty-year update of the Club of Rome report (Meadows et al., 2004).

Overpopulation as an issue in public health no longer seems debatable. A total world population of around one billion in 1800 took more than 500 000 years to reach. It doubled in the next 125 years and again in the next fifty years (four billion by 1975). The six-billion level was passed by the end of the second millennium. A predicted peak of more than nine billion people by 2040 is certain to put added stresses on a finite environment, many of which will be manifest in human disease (McMichael et al., 2003). This rapid population growth plus the declining per capita availability of land, water and energy resources also brings into question the sustainability of our diet and its environmental impact (Pimentel et al., 2003). As with energy use, for example, it could be argued that a less meat-based (ie. energy dense) diet would be beneficial to both the global environment and personal health (Goodland, 1997).

Population growth is stimulated by a number of factors including poverty, lack of education and religious belief. However it is also driven, at least in the early transition stages of development of a country, by economic growth that requires constantly increased consumption, irrespective of type, for ongoing expansion. Growth has been the raison d'être of the macro-economic system throughout the twentieth century. However, even JM Keynes, the architect of the modern economic system, stated that growth cannot continue indefinitely. Keynes claimed in the first part of the twentieth century that the current growth system may serve for around a hundred years but then an alternative would need to be sought, as nothing can continue to grow exponentially.

Economic growth has been and is predicated on three main factors: population growth, technological advancement and the discovery of new resources. While the last option is still feasible, this has been largely reduced by the expansion of populations into new territories. The first option, population growth, is reaching (or may have already exceeded) its limits for a sustainable planet. This leaves technological development to not only drive the economy but solve the problems of over-consumption and concomitant waste and pollution. To date, however, as we have seen, technology has been a two-edged sword for human health. While adding enhancement through medical discovery, it has contributed to lifestyle diseases through easy access to high energy-dense foods and energy-saving devices. Unlike all other animal species, we have successfully managed to defeat all predators: we have become our own worse enemies. A race against time occurs to see if technology can solve more problems than it creates.

An overall elimination of the distal causes of lifestyle-related disease is going to be difficult. Some reprieve, however, may be gained through current recommendations coming from Europe for dealing with the energy crisis and climate change.

Energy is the underlying factor in three current world issues: obesity (and consequent metabolic diseases), resource depletion and climate change. In the case of obesity, too little human energy is expended and too much food energy is being consumed. In the case of resource depletion and climate change, too much non-renewable fossil fuel is being used and too much carbon dioxide emitted. This is having a major impact on climate change, which itself is expected to change the worldwide spread of disease (McMichael et al., 2003). However energy use is also a cause of many of the lifestyle-related 'chronic' diseases discussed in this book. Any proposal that results in an increase in personal human energy expenditure and a decrease in carbon emitting energy use would therefore not only have benefits for health but also environmental benefits. A proposal to introduce a personal carbon-trading scheme may provide a 'stealth intervention' opportunity for doing this (Egger, 2007).

Carbon trading and health

A scheme for Personal Carbon Allowances (PCAs)—also known as Tradable Energy Quotas (TEQs)—was initially proposed by Aubrey Meyer of the Global Commons Institute in 1996 and has been expanded on by others (Flemming, 2005; Roberts and Thumin, 2007; Starkey and Anderson, 2007). It is based on the notion that a sustainable level of carbon emissions is dependent on limiting emissions to a level of around two tonnes of carbon per person per year with the current world population. Current emissions are as high as ten tonnes in countries such as the UK, sixteen tonnes in Australia and up to twenty-four tonnes in the USA. A plan for 'contraction' and 'convergence' has been developed to provide gradual reduction to a sustainable level in an equitable fashion across individuals and countries. TEQs involve the setting of carbon quotas each year by a centrally appointed carbon council. Individuals within a country (and then hopefully worldwide) would be given a set number of carbon units (based on 1 unit being the equivalent energy use resulting in 1 kg of carbon emissions). Individuals would hold their emissions credits in electronic accounts and would surrender them when they make carbon-related purchases, such as electricity, heating fuel and petroleum. TEQs would also be used by individuals as credit for public transport and air flights.

Those who are frugal in their energy use (i.e. by decreasing use of energy or using totally renewable energy sources such as solar) would then be able to trade their unused carbon units to those who may be less frugal but who would then pay an increasingly higher premium for such use as the number of units is contracted to the sustainable goal. The scheme could use the established credit card system and operate through a central marketplace, probably administered through the banks. Fraud could not be totally ruled out but would be about the level of current credit card fraud.

Several reports on TEQs have shown that the scheme is not only feasible and accessible but also equitable, both within and between countries (Stott, 2006). High energy using countries such as the U.S.A., for example, would purchase carbon units from poorer and lower energy using countries such as Africa, thus mitigating the need for untied economic aid.

A particular advantage of personal carbon trading is that it operates not on consumer sentiment and goodwill, or even legislative restriction, but on personal economics, which is known to be a great modern driver of human behaviour (as any politician vying for election knows). It also applies an effective dictum for health promotion, which has been successful in lifestyle change such as smoking, seat belt legislation, drink-driving and childhood injury: 'Legislate and regulate where this is possible; educate and motivate where it is not' (Egger, 2007).

A reduction in energy usage generated by such a trading scheme have not only have the obvious physical advantages of reducing fossil fuels and hence carbon emissions but of attitudinal change within the population. There would be greater incentives and rewards to become more physically active rather than rely on non-renewable energy resources. Because carbon allowances would also be provided to commercial operators, the price of processed high energy-dense foods relative to those (generally more low energy-dense) naturally produced foods would increase. As only a minor change in energy balance (e.g. up to 100 kcals or 440 kJ per day) can lead to significant long-term reductions in obesity, the implications of this for population health are obvious. Hopefully, attitudes towards exhaustible fuel use would also change: 'keeping up with the Joneses' would no longer mean driving a bigger car and using more unnecessary consumables but managing more within a frugal energy budget.

Public and political acceptance is obviously the main barrier to such a scheme. However, it is vital that a 'tipping point' in political attitudes be achieved before the tipping point of carbon emissions into the atmosphere (thought to be around 450 ppm in contrast to the current level of 380 ppm with an annual increase of around 2 ppm/year; Stott, 2006) and health costs from lifestyle-related diseases are reached.

A system of personal carbon trading allowances is, of course, just one proposal for dealing with major environmental issues. But, unlike many others, it could simultaneously address major issues of human health by managing distal or 'upstream' causes of disease. The introduction of such a scheme would require time, effort, goodwill and considerable change among human populations, probably heralding a third major human shift, an 'ecological' revolution to rival the agricultural and industrial revolutions of the last millennium. The alternative, however—the continuation of our current growth—is unthinkable, both from an environmental and a health perspective.

In the meantime, clinicians must play an important, albeit limited, role in dealing with risk factors and proximal and medial causes of disease. The role of the health professions as advocates of stealth interventions such as this is vital if we are to make a dent in the rising tide of lifestyle-related diseases. It adds to the rapidly expanding requirements of medicine to include the broader issues of lifestyle and environmental and even economic factors in health management under the broad umbrella of 'lifestyle medicine' discussed here. If nothing else, it should stimulate a healthy debate in an increasingly unhealthy environment.

REFERENCES

Chapman S. (1995) Unwrapping gossamer with boxing gloves. *BMJ* 311: 989.

Egger G, Swinburn B, Rossner S. (2003) Dusting off the epidemiological triad: could it apply to obesity. *Obes Rev* 4(2): 115–20.

Egger G. (2007) Personal carbon trading: A potential 'stealth intervention' for obesity reduction? *Med J Aus* 187(3): 185–7.

Flemming D. (2005) *Energy and the common purpose*. London: Lean Economy Connection.

Goodland R. (1997) Environmental sustainability in agriculture: diet matters. *Ecolog Econ* 23: 189–200.

Global Commons Institute: www.gci.org.uk.

Haddon W. (1980) Advances in the epidemiology of injuries as a basis for public policy. *Pub Health Rep* 95(5): 411–20.

Le Fanu J. (2002) *The rise and fall of modern medicine*. London: Carroll Graf.

Leowell HR, Clark EG. (1966) *Preventive medicine for the doctor in his community,* 3rd edn. NY: McGraw-Hill.

Mass B. (2006) Quoted in *Planet earth: the future,* p 172. London: BBC Books.

McMichael A, Campbell-Lendrum DH, Corvalan CF et al. (eds). (2003) *Climate change and human health: risks and responses*. Geneva: WHO.

Meadows D, Randers J, Meadows D. (1974) *Limits to growth.* White River Junction, Vt: Chelsea Green Publishing Co.

Meadows D, Randers J, Meadows D. (2004) *Limits to growth: the 30-year update*. White River Junction, Vt: Chelsea Green Publishing Co.

Pimentel D, Pimentel M. (2003) Sustainability of meat-based and plant-based diets and the environment. *Am J Clin Nutr* 78: 660S–663.

Roberts S, Thumin J. (2007) *A rough guide to individual carbon trading: The issues, ideas and the next steps. Centre for Sustainable Energy Report to DEFRA.* Available from www.defra.gov.uk/environment/climatechange/uk/individual/pca/pdf/pca-scopingstudy.pdf.

Starkey R, Anderson K. (2007) *Domestic tradable quotas. A policy instrument for reducing greenhouse gas emissions from energy use. Tyndall Centre Technical Report No 39.* Available from www.tyndall.ac.uk/publications/tech_reports/tech_reports.shtml.

Stott R. (2006) Contraction and convergence: healthy response to climate change. *Brit Med J* 332: 1385–87.

Wright R. (2004) *A short history of progress.* NY: Carroll Graf.

APPENDIX

Making lifestyle medicine work and pay in general practice

BARBARA O'TOOLE

In Chapter 1 the question was asked, 'Who is best qualified to practice lifestyle medicine?' After considering the various disciplines, it seems that, for the foreseeable future at least, the GP will be the coordinator of a team of health professionals providing multidisciplinary care to those who have a chronic condition. This is facilitated by the Enhanced Primary Care system (EPC) in Australia, which includes the Chronic Disease Management Plan (CDMP), Case Conferencing (CC) and Practice Incentive Programs (PIP). This chapter looks at these item numbers in some detail and outlines how they can best be utilised in general practice to improve client outcomes and self-management.

What are EPC, CDMP and PIP?

The EPC system was introduced in 1999 and consisted of health assessments, case conferencing and care plans. The health assessments were a useable item number but the care plans were very time consuming, labour intensive, poorly understood and unwieldy. The uptake of these and case conferencing was slow and low and had to be done by the GP without input or assistance from a practice nurse except in an administrative capacity.

The PIP came into being in 2001 and provided incentives in areas such as after-hours care, information technology, cervical screening and quality prescribing (although these areas will not be discussed here) and for appropriate treatment of asthma, diabetes, and mental health. According to Medicare Australia, the PIP was an attempt to compensate GPs for the limitations of the fee-for-service arrangement by offering an incentive to provide comprehensive, quality care for clients with asthma, diabetes and mental health problems. Once a cycle of care was completed for these chronic conditions, a Service Incentive Payment (SIP) was made to the practice and, in the case of diabetes, an outcomes payment would sometimes be applicable.

In response to collaboration with major GP organisations, the 2003 Red Tape Taskforce recommended changes to the EPC and PIP to simplify the care planning system to improve useability. This was done by overhauling the PIP system and by the introduction of CDMP item numbers in July 2005. The other item number worthy of mention here is the Medication Management Review (MMR), Item 900, which will be discussed later.

Health assessments

A health assessment is defined by Medicare Australia as 'the assessment of a patient's health and physical, psychological and social function, and whether preventative health care should be offered to the patient to improve that patient's health and physical, psychological and social function'.

The various health assessments available for use are summarised in the table below.

MBS health assessments (as at 1 July 2007)

Group	Item no	Location	Medicare fee (100%)	Recommended frequency
Over 75 year olds	Item 700	In surgery	$164.00	Yearly
	Item 702	In home	$232.00	Yearly
ATSI and over 55 years	Item 704	In surgery	$164.00	Yearly
	Item 706	In home	$232.00	Yearly
ATSI and under 15 years	Item 708	In surgery or in home	$164.00	Yearly—as early as 9 months old
ATSI and between 15 and 54 years	Item 710	In surgery or in home	$195.50	2 yearly—as early as 18 months old
Comprehensive medical assessment (for clients in RACFs)	Item 712	In surgery or residential aged care facility	$187.65	Yearly
Refugees and other humanitarian entrants	Item 714	In surgery	$195.50	Once only assessment
	Item 716	Not in surgery	$195.50 + $22.50/number of clients, for each client	
45–49 year olds (who are at risk of developing a chronic disease)	Item 717	In surgery	$100.00	Once only assessment
Clients with an intellectual disability	Item 718	In surgery	$199.60	Yearly
	Item 719	In home	$222.05	Yearly

The health assessment includes a mandatory assessment of a client's blood pressure, pulse rate and rhythm, medications, continence status, and immunisation status for influenza, pneumococcus and tetanus. It is also mandatory to assess the client's physical function, activities of daily living, falls in the past three months, psychological function, cognition and mood, social function, the availability and adequacy of paid and unpaid help, and whether or not the client is or has a carer.

There are other areas that may be assessed, if appropriate, including diet and nutritional status, smoking and alcohol use, home safety, foot care, sleep, vision, hearing and oral health. A client's fitness to drive, cardiovascular risk factors and need for community services may also be assessed. There are also some additional specific areas to cover Aboriginal and Torres Strait Islander (ATSI) clients and those with an intellectual disability.

Comprehensive medical assessment

This assessment is available only to residents of an aged care facility and is available initially on admission to a facility and then yearly after that if the client's condition warrants it.

Refugee and other humanitarian entrants

This health assessment differs from the others in that it includes a physical examination of the client that is in addition to taking the client's medical history, undertaking or arranging any required investigations, assessing the client using information gained from the history, ordering appropriate investigations, developing a management plan (not a GPMP) to deal with any issues or problems, and organising any referrals to other health providers or any interventions. A copy of this management plan must be given to the client.

This once-only assessment is a means of introducing the client to the Australian preventative healthcare areas of immunisation, breast and cervical screening, and maternal and child health.

45–49 year old health check

This item number, introduced in November 2006, is designed to help prevent chronic disease. With this assessment, it is mandatory to take a history and to perform relevant examinations and investigations based on the client's medical, social and family history. Relevant interventions in the form of referrals and follow-ups are done, and advice and information is given to the client regarding strategies for lifestyle and behavioural changes. Particular attention should be paid to lifestyle risk factors of smoking, physical inactivity, poor nutrition and alcohol misuse. This is a once-only assessment.

Chronic Disease Management Plan

The various CDMP items available for use are summarised in the table below.

MBS Chronic Disease Management Plan items (as at 1 November 2006)

Name	Item no	Medicare fee (100%)	Recommended frequency	Minimum claiming period (exceptional circumstances)
Preparation of General Practice Management Plan (GPMP)	721	$124.95	2 yearly	12 months
Preparation of Team Care Arrangement (TCA)	723	$98.95	2 yearly	12 months

CONTINUED OVERLEAF

MBS Chronic Disease Management Plan items (as at 1 November 2006) (Continued)

Name	Item no	Medicare fee (100%)	Recommended frequency	Minimum claiming period (exceptional circumstances)
Review of GPMP	725	$62.50	6 monthly	3 months
Coordination of review of TCA	727	$62.50	6 monthly	3 months
Contribution to a multi-disciplinary care plan	729.	$43.40	6 monthly	3 months
Contribution to a multi-disciplinary care plan by an aged care facility	731	$43.40	6 monthly	3 months

General Practice Management Plan

A General Practice Management Plan (GPMP) is available to any client with a chronic condition that has been in place for at least six months, or is likely to be in place for at least six months, or who has a terminal condition. The client must be living in the community or privately funded and living in an aged care facility.

The GP develops the GPMP without input from other service providers. The practice nurse may assist by developing the plan on behalf of the GP but the GP must see the client to review the plan and sign off on it.

Steps involved in preparing a GPMP include:

- assessing the client to identify healthcare needs, problems and relevant conditions;
- setting management goals with the client for the changes to be achieved by the treatment and the services identified in the plan;
- identifying any actions to be taken by the client;
- identifying tests, treatment and services that the client is likely to need;
- arranging for provision of these services and ongoing management;
- documenting the client's needs, goals, client actions and treatment/services; and
- setting a review date.

The client's progress against the plan should be reviewed six monthly using the GPMP Review Item 725 but may be reviewed at three months if clinically indicated. Ongoing management and care is still provided through normal consultation items.

Team Care Arrangements

As with the GPMP, Team Care Arrangement (TCA) is available to any client with a chronic condition that has been in place for at least six months, or is likely to be in place for at least six months, or who has a terminal condition. The client must be living in the community or privately funded and living in an aged care facility. In addition to this, however, the client must have complex care needs that necessitate ongoing care by two other healthcare providers.

Steps involved in preparing a TCA include:

- identifying and confirming with the client which other treatment or service providers will be involved in their care and what information can be shared with them;
- collaborating with the participating providers to discuss potential treatment/services they will provide in order to achieve management goals for the client;
- documenting the goals, the collaborating providers, the treatment/services they have agreed to provide and client actions; and
- setting a review date.

The client's progress against the plan should be reviewed six monthly using the TCA Review Item 727 but may be reviewed at three months if clinically indicated. Ongoing management and care is still provided through normal consultation items.

Contribution to a multidisciplinary care plan

Two item numbers, Items 729 and 731, are for use by GPs asked to contribute to a care plan or to review a care plan prepared by an outside provider. Item 731 relates to a care plan for a resident of an aged care facility. If a GP contributes to this multidisciplinary plan and bills this item number, the resident is eligible to access allied health services under Medicare.

Case conferences

Case conferences (Item 734–779) involve the GP and at least two other health providers all of whom meet, in person or via a conference call, to discuss client management. The exact item numbers used depend on the length of the conference, whether or not the GP organised and participated in the conference or merely participated, and whether it is a discharge case conference or a community case conference or for a client in an aged care facility.

They are mentioned here for completeness. At this stage, the uptake on these item numbers is not high, possibly because they are time consuming and the remuneration is insufficient.

Allied health services under Medicare

For people with chronic conditions and complex care needs who have had a GPMP (Item 721) *and* a TCA (Item 723) done by their usual doctor, Medicare rebates are available for a maximum of five allied health visits per calendar year. There are currently fourteen allied health services covered. The relevant allied health providers must be registered with Medicare and have a provider number to enable them to participate in this service.

Once a GP has billed both the TCA and GPMP, the client is able to access this service by having a special EPC referral form for allied health services under Medicare filled out by the GP. A client may be referred to more than one allied health service but would need a referral form for each service; however, there is still a maximum of five visits available across all providers. Three dental services may be accessed under this system if the dentist has a Medicare provider number but there are conditions attached to this and a special referral form is required.

For clients in an aged care facility to access this allied health or dental service under Medicare, the GP would not do a GPMP and TCA but would need to participate in a care plan initiated by the aged care facility (Item 731).

Practice Incentive Program

In the area of chronic disease, the PIP pays out SIPs to practices on a quarterly basis when certain levels of care are provided for clients with diabetes and asthma. The SIP is intended to remunerate individual GPs for services and is in addition to the Medicare rebate payable for the consultation. Special item numbers are used that align with the level B, C and D consultation fees. These item numbers are the triggers for the SIP. The payment is independent of the length of the consultation.

MBS service incentive payments for PIP (as at 1 November 2006)

Condition	Item no	SIP	Outcomes payment
Asthma	Level B 2546 Level C 2552 Level D 2558 (Surgery consultation)	$100.00 (in addition to normal consultation fee)	No
Diabetes	Level B 2517 Level C 2521 Level D 2525 (Surgery consultation)	$40.00 (in addition to normal consultation fee)	Yes, $20/client ($5.00/quarter where over 20% of clients with diabetes have had annual cycle of care done)

Asthma

The Asthma Cycle of Care replaced the Asthma 3^+ Plan in November 2006. It consists of at least two asthma-related consultations within a twelve-month period for a client who has moderate to severe asthma. The second visit is a review visit and must be a planned visit.

The requirements of the Cycle of Care consist of a review of the client's asthma-related medication and devices, a documented individualised asthma action plan and self-management education. The review visit should assess the client's asthma control and ongoing management and the asthma action plan. This would involve a review of symptoms, spirometry (to assess lung function and response to treatment), medications, dosages and peak flow measurements (where appropriate).

Diabetes

To claim the SIP for diabetes, a diabetes register and a recall system must be in place. The relevant item numbers can be claimed when the annual cycle of care is completed. This annual cycle of care consists of a six-monthly review of weight, height, BMI and blood pressure, and a foot examination if considered necessary. It requires a yearly review of HbA_{1c}, microalbuminuria, total cholesterol, triglycerides and HDL cholesterol. Every two years (or earlier if indicated), an eye examination should be carried out. Other areas that should be reviewed include medications, physical activity, diet, smoking status and self-care education.

These are *minimum* requirements of care and elements should be carried out more frequently if clinically indicated. Group education sessions are now available through Medicare funding for all clients with type 2 diabetes.

Mental health

The PIP mental health incentive items ceased on 30 April 2007 after the introduction of the new GP Mental Health Care items, which were introduced in November 2006. These are the preparation of a GP Mental Health Care Plan (Item 2710, $150.00) and a review of a GP Mental Health Care Plan (Item 2712, $100.00). These items use the same three-step process—assess, plan and review—as do the GPMPs and TCAs. This plan will allow clients to have more access through new referral pathways to clinical psychologists, psychiatrists and other allied mental health professionals.

In addition, there is another item number (Item 2713, $66.00) which allows GPs to provide consultations for the continuing management of clients with mental disorders.

Domiciliary medication management review

The medication management review (Item 900, $134.10), while not strictly speaking an EPC item, should be used more frequently because of its value as a preventative health tool. The GP sends a referral to the client's local pharmacy which includes a copy of the client's medical history and recent blood chemistry. The pharmacy has a pharmacist meet with the client, usually in the client's own home, to review all medications. The pharmacist reviews the client's symptoms, compliance, blood results, drug device techniques, storage of drugs, and so on. The pharmacist responds to the GP in writing about the findings. The GP sees the client and gives him or her a copy of the medication plan (which would include any changes considered necessary) and sends a copy to the pharmacist.

The criteria for a medication review include, among other things, taking five or more regular medications, taking more than twelve doses per day, suspected non-compliance, significant changes to the medication regimen in last the three months, sub-therapeutic response to treatment, use of medications with a narrow therapeutic index, or recent hospitalisation. A client can have a medication review yearly but may have one done earlier if it is clinically indicated.

The equivalent of this item number for residents of an aged care facility is a Residential Medical Management Review (RMMR) (Item 903, $91.85).

Utilising these item numbers in general practice

When a client comes to the surgery, consider their cultural background firstly.

- If the client is of Aboriginal and Torres Strait Islander descent, then do the health assessment that correlates with their age (i.e. using Item 704, 706, 708 or 710).
- If the client is not ATSI and over 75 years old, do a health assessment (either an Item 700 or 702).
- If the client has an intellectual disability, use Item 718 or 719.

- If the client is between 45 and 49 years old, use Item 717.
- In the case of refugees or humanitarian entrants, an Item 714 or 716 is appropriate.

For all clients, other than residents of an aged care facility, ascertain whether or not they have a chronic or terminal condition. If so, and if the chronic condition has been in place for six months or will be in place for that long, consider doing a GPMP (Item 721). If in addition to this the client has complex care needs and requires the ongoing services of two other health providers, consider a TCA (Item 723). The client may be able to access the allied health services under Medicare, which would require a special referral form.

If the client's chronic condition is asthma or diabetes, decisions need to be made about whether to use or when to use PIP or CDMP, given that conditions apply. If the client has mental health issues as well as other chronic conditions, it may be relevant to use both CDMP and the Mental Health Care Plan (Item 2710). For clients with type 2 diabetes, there is now the opportunity to refer them for Medicare-funded group education sessions. This is independent upon there being a GPMP in place.

If the client resides in an aged care facility, a Comprehensive Medical Assessment (Item 712) is appropriate. Access to the allied health services is by a contribution to the aged care facility's care plan (Item 731). An RMMR (Item 903) would also be applicable.

For all clients other than those in an aged care facility, consider whether or not there is a need for a medication review (Item 900).

As of 1 July, 2007, a new item number (10997; $10.60) was introduced. This number can be utilised up to five times a calendar year by a practice nurse or registered Aboriginal health worker on behalf of the GP to provide monitoring and support to people with a chronic disease. The client must have a GPMP or TCA in place.

Further information

Further information is available from the Australian Government Department of Health and Ageing website (www.health.gov.au under 'Programs and Campaigns'). The 'Enhanced Primary Care Program' and 'Strengthening Medicare' sections contain a wealth of information, templates, case studies and check lists to assist practices to effectively provide enhanced primary care and chronic disease management.

practice tips

PRACTICE TIPS: USING THE EPC SYSTEM

	General practitioner or practice nurse
Assess	Check eligibility for a HA, GPMP or TCA.
	Use appropriate tools to ensure comprehensive assessment.
	Identify issues or problems.
	Identify risk factors.
	Use techniques to ensure the 'whole of person' is considered, not just the disease.
	Complete annual cycle of care requirements for diabetes and asthma clients.

Assist	Explain to the client how the plan or cycle of care works. Gain client's consent. Make an individual plan. Negotiate and set realistic goals. Ensure client's acceptance of plan. Give client a copy of assessment or plan. Gain permission to share plan with other providers as appropriate.
Arrange	Identify other health professionals to assist in multidisciplinary care. Refer to other health professionals and collaborate with them regarding client management. Negotiate a separate consultation to address other or ongoing issues. Organise a review date and place on recall system. Seek feedback from the other care providers.

Note: A practice nurse can assist with all of the above, but a GP must review and confirm all assessments and plans in order to comply with Medicare requirements.

key points

KEY POINTS FOR CLINICAL MANAGEMENT

- Maintain up to date registers for relevant clients, such as those clients who are ATSI or over 75 years old, or who have diabetes, asthma or mental health issues.
- Check that all clients over 75 years old are offered an opportunity for assessment.
- Encourage clients with asthma and diabetes to participate in an annual cycle of care.
- Implement a plan within the practice to target clients with chronic diseases with a view to developing GPMPs and TCAs, if needed.
- Ensure a GP does the final review of any plan or assessment undertaken.
- Maintain a recall system that adequately facilitates patient reviews.
- Develop good relations with allied health personnel in the catchment area to ensure timely feedback on clients.
- Overall, the aim of management is to improve quality of life.
- Encourage improvements in the areas of smoking, nutrition, alcohol and physical activity.

Index

B

C

D

E

F

G

H

N

O

P

Q

R

S

T

U

V

W